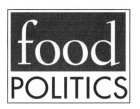

food
POLITICS

CALIFORNIA STUDIES IN FOOD AND CULTURE, 3
Darra Goldstein, Editor

MARION NESTLE

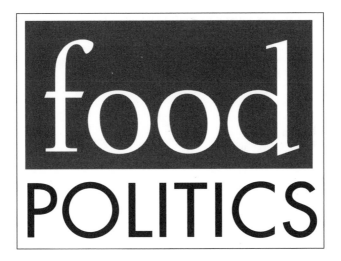

food
POLITICS

HOW THE FOOD INDUSTRY
INFLUENCES NUTRITION AND HEALTH

UNIVERSITY OF CALIFORNIA PRESS
Berkeley Los Angeles London

University of California Press
Berkeley and Los Angeles, California

University of California Press, Ltd.
London, England

© 2002 by the Regents of the University of California

Library of Congress Cataloging-in-Publication Data

Nestle, Marion.
    Food politics: how the food industry influences
nutrition and health / Marion Nestle.
       p. cm. —(California studies in food and
culture; 3)
    Includes bibliographical references and index.
    ISBN 0-520-22465-5 (cloth: alk. paper)
    1. Nutrition policy—United States. 2. Food—
Marketing—Moral and ethical aspects—United
States. 3. Food industry and trade—United States.
I. Title. II. Series.

TX360.U6.N47 F47 2002
363.8′5′0973—dc21   2001027678

Manufactured in the United States of America
10 09 08 07 06 05 04 03
10 9 8 7

CONTENTS

PREFACE

AS AN ACADEMIC NUTRITIONIST, I GRAPPLE ON A DAILY BASIS
with what I see as a central contradiction between nutrition theory and
practice. On the one hand, our advice about the health benefits of diets
based largely on food plants—fruits, vegetables, and grains—has not
changed in more than 50 years and is consistently supported by ongoing
research. On the other hand, people seem increasingly confused about
what they are supposed to eat to stay healthy. As a population, Americans are eating more animal-based foods—and more food in general—to
the point where half of us are overweight, even our children are obese,
and diseases related to diet are leading causes of death and disability. In
thinking about this contradiction, I have often wondered what role the
food industry might play in creating an environment so conducive to
overeating and poor nutritional practices and so confusing about basic
principles of diet and health.

I became interested in the role of the food industry in nutrition and
health because I have been a player—albeit a minor one—in some of the
events I describe in this book. I first experienced food companies in
action when I worked for the Department of Health and Human Services
as a nutrition policy advisor for two years in the late 1980s, and I continue to observe food industry actions as a member of federal committees
dealing with food and nutrition policy matters. In my current position
as chair of the Department of Nutrition and Food Studies at New York
University, I regularly receive public relations handouts from food
companies and trade associations. I talk to people who work for food,
beverage, and supplement companies at conferences, lectures, and press

conferences, and I often see them by appointment. I also speak with one or another newspaper, magazine, newsletter, or journal reporter nearly every day of my working life. Much of my understanding of the politics of nutrition comes from what I learn from such sources.

In thinking about such matters, I eventually came to the conclusion that food companies—just like companies that sell cigarettes, pharmaceuticals, or any other commodity—routinely place the needs of stockholders over considerations of public health. This conclusion may not surprise anyone who follows the political scene, but I had heard few discussions of its significance among my professional colleagues, despite its evident implications. Food companies will make and market any product that sells, regardless of its nutritional value or its effect on health. In this regard, food companies hardly differ from cigarette companies. They lobby Congress to eliminate regulations perceived as unfavorable; they press federal regulatory agencies not to enforce such regulations; and when they don't like regulatory decisions, they file lawsuits. Like cigarette companies, food companies co-opt food and nutrition experts by supporting professional organizations and research, and they expand sales by marketing directly to children, members of minority groups, and people in developing countries—whether or not the products are likely to improve people's diets.

For the most part, food company strategies are standard economic practices and are legal. Whether they are ethical or promote the health of the public is quite another matter. The ways in which food industry practices distort what Americans are told about nutrition—and compromise food choices—raise serious issues that are worth consideration by anyone concerned about nutrition and health.

This book discusses the issues raised by food industry marketing practices through a wide range of examples designed to interest—and be accessible to—a wide readership. I want everyone, whether trained in nutrition or not, to consider the issues discussed here, and I have written this book with the general reader very much in mind. I hope that food and nutrition professionals will read it, of course, but that others will do so as well: advocates for health, nutrition, and consumer issues; people concerned about public policy in food, nutrition, and health; federal officials working in these areas; staff of food companies, public relations firms, and magazines; students in agriculture, nutrition, and public policy courses; and anyone else who is at all curious about the ways in which food companies might influence how we think about nutrition and food choice. Although I have carefully researched this book and have documented my sources extensively, I have tried to make it accessible to nonspecialist readers by defining technical terms as they arise and by avoiding scientific jargon. For readers who might like a bit more technical information about nutrition before delving into the book, the Appendix introduces basic principles of nutrition and some of the issues that affect interpretation of nutrition research.

Because the book raises concerns about the food industry that are rarely discussed in academic or public circles, I have attempted to document the sources of my information more than might seem absolutely necessary. As this book reveals, much of what food companies do to create a favorable sales environment for their products—lobbying, marketing, engaging the services of nutrition experts—is conducted out of public view. For example, as an expert witness in cases involving food companies, I have seen documents attesting to lobbying interactions with Congress or with officials of federal agencies, but such documents are proprietary, subject to sworn confidentiality agreements, and unusable as sources of information. Given this situation, I have had to rely on personal experience and other "nonacademic" sources more than is usually the practice in studies of this kind.

Furthermore, I could not find *anyone* who would speak to me "on the record" for this book. When I told friends in government, food companies, and academia that I was writing a book about how the food industry affects nutrition and health, they offered to tell me anything I wanted to know, but not for attribution. I had to find other ways to document how food companies use the political system, marketing strategies, and nutrition experts to encourage people to buy more of their products— whether or not those products are likely to promote health.

I used books and professional journals, of course, but was especially reliant on government documents. I became an indefatigable reader of *Federal Register* notices, Congressional hearing reports, Acts of Congress, General Accounting Office reports, and agency advisory notices to industry. These materials used to be difficult to find, even with access to a law library as comprehensive and helpful as the one at my university. These days, such documents are readily available on the Internet, and I frequently cite Web addresses. I also used many "unofficial" sources: newspapers, magazines, newsletters, position papers, committee correspondence, speeches, package labels, press releases, advocacy materials, and materials collected from conference exhibits, supermarkets, and health food stores. To the extent permitted by space limitations, these sources are listed in the Notes at the end of the book.

The question of how much of myself to put in this book also proved knotty. Some colleagues who read chapters at early stages wanted more personal commentary; others found it intrusive. In the end, I felt I had to reveal my own participation and biases and to let the documentation speak for itself. Thus I must confess at the outset that in my current position, I find it impossible to avoid entanglements with food companies. Lobbying groups for the salt, sugar, vitamin, and omega 3–fatty acid industries routinely send me information and research articles about the nutritional benefits of these substances, as do trade associations for foods as diverse as wheat, soybeans, blueberries, peanuts, pistachios, and flax seed. Public relations and scientific staff of companies such as Procter & Gamble and Unilever visit my department regularly to consult about products under development. I give speeches at meetings overtly sponsored by food companies and at meetings organized by professional societies who receive funding from such companies. I read journals subsidized by food companies. I speak on panels with food company representatives. I have held grants from food companies. I have asked food company representatives for their newsletters, books, press materials, and teaching slides. I occasionally consult for food companies. Such interactions are the *norm* among academic nutritionists. Only questioning them is unusual. This book addresses that gap.

I also must confess that I am fully aware that not everyone is as able as I am to discuss these issues. I hold a tenured, "hard-money" full professorship, and New York University pays my entire salary. Furthermore, my research focuses on food and nutrition policy; unlike most other nutrition academics, I do not require expensive laboratories nor do I need to generate my own research funding. In this privileged position, I can afford to be independent of the food industry. Some years ago, concerned that accepting funding from food companies might compromise this independence, I attempted to develop a personal policy to deal with sponsorship matters. As I disclose in several places in this book, I go to meetings sponsored by food companies and accept travel funds and public relations materials, but I do not personally accept honoraria or any other payment. Instead, I ask companies to donate the funds to our department's scholarship fund. This policy, imperfect though it may be, works for me. In revealing it, I hope to stimulate debate about its merits and to encourage colleagues to consider creating their own versions.

In presenting this and the other issues discussed in this book, and in explaining how they developed and why opinions about them differ so greatly, I have tried to be accurate, balanced, and fair. My goal in writing the book is to encourage readers to view the food industry in a new light, to understand how food company actions dominate so much of what we are told about nutrition, to consider the issues raised here, and to make personal decisions about whether to address them and in what way.

As is always the case in such matters, I could not have acquired the information presented in this book—nor could I have written it—without help from many colleagues and friends. To begin with, Ann Snitow suggested how the book might be structured and insisted that I find an agent. Lydia Wills of Artists Agency assumed that responsibility and has been an inspiration throughout. Much of my early thinking about these issues was stimulated by conference invitations from the organizers of Oldways Preservation & Exchange Trust—Dun Gifford, Greg Drescher, Nancy Jenkins, and Sara Baer-Sinnott. Philip Lee and Sheldon Margen, who have done such things for me for many years, again wrote letters of support, as did Irv Rosenberg and Ann Marcus.

During the research phase, Michael Jacobson and his colleagues at the Center for Science in the Public Interest—Bonnie Liebman, Darren Mitchell, Bruce Silverglade, George Hacker, and David Schardt—opened their files and let me use what I wanted. Donna Marino of Unilever/Lipton's arranged with Teris Binder and Vicky Kranidiotis to permit me to spend a day at the company's enviable library. Annette Yonke thought I should be reading *Illinois Agrinews* and provided a subscription. Declan Conroy made it possible for me to subscribe to *Food Regulation Weekly* on terms continued by *Food Chemical News*. Lisa Bero, Matthew Cann, Arthur Levin, Leah Margulies, and Mark Ritchie provided papers, clippings, and historical documents. My NYU colleagues were especially generous: Fred Tripp provided an invaluable clipping service to the *Wall Street Journal*; Sharron Dalton, Ellen Fried, Kyle Shadix, and Lisa Young made sure I kept up on current events; Suzanne Rostler organized my files and found much more to put in them; and Monica Bhagwan and Stacey Freis provided enthusiastic and highly efficient research assistance.

Several friends and colleagues commented on sections of the manuscript at various stages: Barbara Abrams, LaRue Allen, Jeff Backstrand, Amy Bentley, Jennifer Berg, Abby Bloch, Larry Cohen, Joanne Csete, Dennis Dalton, Jon Deutsch, Jane Ellis, Loma Flowers, Alan Hausman, Janna Howley, Melinda Lee, Diane McFadden, Leslie Mikkelsen, Malden Nesheim, JoAnn Silverstein, and Sam Silverstein. I am especially grateful to Warren Belasco, Ellen Fried, Joan Gussow, Trish Lobenfeld, and Sheldon Margen for their stamina (heroism, really) in reviewing drafts of the entire manuscript, to Mitchell Davis who interrupted a vacation in Japan for emergency editorial assistance, to Kristie Lancaster for computer wizardry, and to Joanne Csete for testing the Index.

My NYU colleague Barbara Kirshenblatt-Gimblett introduced me to my editorial sponsor and now friend at the University of California Press, Stanley Holwitz. Among his many other good deeds, Stan helped recruit John Bergez to edit the manuscript; the book is better written and better constructed for both their efforts. The Dean of NYU's School of Education, Ann Marcus, granted me sabbatical leave in the spring and summer of 1999 to work on this book, and my colleagues in the Department of Nutrition and Food Studies let me delegate even more than the usual level of responsibility, then and subsequently. Alyce Conrad, Jessica Fischetti, and Kelli Ranieri provided daily support throughout the two years I worked on this project. I am blessed with colleagues—faculty, staff, and students—who make it a pleasure to go to work every day, and I thank them, as well as my beloved family, Rebecca Nestle and Michael Suenkel, Charles Nestle and Lidia Lustig, and the Moss cousins and their partners and children, for being in my life. Finally, I thank the many people who provided information or documents but preferred to remain anonymous. Preparation of this book was supported in part by research development grants from New York University and its Steinhardt School of Education.

INTRODUCTION
THE FOOD INDUSTRY AND "EAT MORE"

THIS BOOK IS ABOUT HOW THE FOOD INDUSTRY INFLUENCES what we eat and, therefore, our health. That diet affects health is beyond question. The food industry has given us a food supply so plentiful, so varied, so inexpensive, and so devoid of dependence on geography or season that all but the very poorest of Americans can obtain enough energy and nutrients to meet biological needs. Indeed, the U.S. food supply is so abundant that it contains enough to feed everyone in the country nearly twice over—even after exports are considered. The overly abundant food supply, combined with a society so affluent that most people can afford to buy more food than they need, sets the stage for competition. The food industry must compete fiercely for every dollar spent on food, and food companies expend extraordinary resources to develop and market products that will sell, regardless of their effect on nutritional status or waistlines. To satisfy stockholders, food companies must convince people to *eat more* of their products or to eat their products instead of those of competitors. They do so through advertising and public relations, of course, but also by working tirelessly to convince government officials, nutrition professionals, and the media that their products promote health—or at least do no harm. Much of this work is a virtually invisible part of contemporary culture that attracts only occasional notice.

This book exposes the ways in which food companies use political processes—entirely conventional and nearly always legal—to obtain government and professional support for the sale of their products. Its twofold purpose is to illuminate the extent to which the food industry determines what people eat and to generate much wider discussion of the food industry's marketing methods and use of the political system.

In my 25 years as a nutrition educator, I have found that food industry practices are discussed only rarely. The reasons for this omission are not difficult to understand. Most of us believe that we choose foods for reasons of personal taste, convenience, and cost; we deny that we can be manipulated by advertising or other marketing practices. Nutrition scientists and practitioners typically believe that food companies are genuinely interested in improving health. They think it makes sense to work with the industry to help people improve their diets, and most are outraged by suggestions that food industry sponsorship of research or programs might influence what they do or say. Most food company officials maintain that any food product can be included in a balanced, varied, and moderate diet; they say that their companies are helping to promote good health when they fund the activities of nutrition professionals. Most officials of federal agriculture and health agencies understand that their units are headed by political appointees whose concerns reflect those of the political party in power and whose actions must be acceptable to Congress. Members of Congress, in turn, must be sensitive to the concerns of corporations that help fund their campaigns.

In this political system, the actions of food companies are normal, legal, and thoroughly analogous to the workings of any other major industry—tobacco, for example—in influencing health experts, federal agencies, and Congress.[1] Promoting food raises more complicated issues than promoting tobacco, however, in that food is required for life and causes problems only when consumed inappropriately. As this book will demonstrate, the primary mission of food companies, like that of tobacco companies, is to sell products. Food companies are not health or social service agencies, and nutrition becomes a factor in corporate thinking only when it can help sell food. The ethical choices involved in such thinking are considered all too rarely.

Early in the twentieth century, when the principal causes of death and disability among Americans were infectious diseases related in part to inadequate intake of calories and nutrients, the goals of health officials, nutritionists, and the food industry were identical—to encourage people to eat more of all kinds of food. Throughout that century, improvements in the U.S. economy affected the way we eat in important ways: We obtained access to foods of greater variety, our diets improved, and nutrient deficiencies gradually declined. The principal nutritional problems among Americans shifted to those of *overnutrition*—eating too much food or too much of certain kinds of food. Overeating causes its own set of health problems; it deranges metabolism, makes people overweight, and increases the likelihood of "chronic" diseases—coronary heart disease, certain cancers, diabetes, hypertension, stroke, and others—that now are leading causes of illness and death in any overfed population.

People may believe that the effects of diet on chronic disease are less important than those of cigarette smoking, but each contributes to about one-fifth of annual deaths in the United States. Addressing cigarette smoking requires only a single change in behavior: Don't smoke. But because people must eat to survive, advice about dietary improvements is much more complicated: Eat this food instead of that food, or eat less. As this book explains, the "eat less" message is at the root of much of the controversy over nutrition advice. It directly conflicts with food industry demands that people eat more of their products. Thus food companies work hard to oppose and undermine "eat less" messages.

I first became aware of the food industry as an influence on government nutrition policies and on the opinions of nutrition experts when I moved to Washington, DC, in 1986 to work for the Public Health Service. My job was to manage the editorial production of the first—and as yet only—*Surgeon General's Report on Nutrition and Health*, which appeared as a 700-page book in the summer of 1988.[2] This report was an ambitious government effort to summarize the entire body of research linking dietary factors such as fat, saturated fat, cholesterol, salt, sugar, and alcohol to leading chronic diseases. My first day on the job, I was given the rules: No matter what the research indicated, the report could not recommend "eat less meat" as a way to reduce intake of saturated fat, nor could it suggest restrictions on intake of any other category of food. In the industry-friendly climate of the Reagan administration, the producers of foods that might be affected by such advice would complain to their beneficiaries in Congress, and the report would never be published.

This scenario was no paranoid fantasy; federal health officials had endured a decade of almost constant congressional interference with their dietary recommendations. As I discuss in Part I, agency officials had learned to avoid such interference by resorting to euphemisms, focusing recommendations on nutrients rather than on the foods that contain them, and giving a positive spin to any restrictive advice about food. Whereas "eat less beef" called the industry to arms, "eat less saturated fat" did not. "Eat less sugar" sent sugar producers right to Congress, but that industry could live with "choose a diet moderate in sugar." When released in 1988, the *Surgeon General's Report* recommended "choose lean meats" and suggested limitations on sugar intake only for people particularly vulnerable to dental cavities.

Subsequent disputes have only reinforced sensitivities to political expediency when formulating advice about diet and health. Political expediency explains in part why no subsequent *Surgeon General's Report* has appeared, even though Congress passed a law in 1990 requiring that one be issued biannually. After ten years of working to develop a *Surgeon General's Report on Dietary Fat and Health*—surely needed to help people understand the endless debates about the relative health consequences of eating saturated, monounsaturated, trans-saturated, and total fat—the government abandoned the project, ostensibly because the science base had become increasingly complex and equivocal. A more compelling reason must have been lack of interest in completing such a report in the election year of 2000. Authoritative recommendations about fat intake would have had to include some "eat less" advice if for no other reason than because fat is so concentrated in calories—it contains 9 calories per gram, compared to 4 each for protein or carbohydrate[3]—and obesity is a major health concern. Because saturated fat and trans-saturated fat raise risks for heart disease, and the principal sources of such fats in American diets are meat, dairy, cooking fats, and fried, fast, and processed foods, "eat less" advice would provoke the producers and sellers of these foods to complain to their friends in Congress.

Since 1988, in my role as chair of an academic department of nutrition, a member of federal advisory committees, a speaker at public and professional meetings, a frequent commentator on nutrition issues to the press, and (on occasion) a consultant to food companies, I have become increasingly convinced that many of the nutritional problems of Americans—not least of them obesity—can be traced to the food industry's imperative to encourage people to *eat more* in order to generate sales and increase income in a highly competitive marketplace. Ambiguous dietary advice is only one result of this imperative. As I explain in Part II, the industry also devotes enormous financial and other resources to lobbying Congress and federal agencies, forming partnerships and alliances with professional nutrition organizations, funding research on food and nutrition, publicizing the results of selected research studies favorable to industry, sponsoring professional journals and conferences, and making sure that influential groups—federal officials, researchers, doctors, nurses, school teachers, and the media—are aware of the benefits of their products.

Later sections of the book describe the ways in which such actions affect food issues of particular public interest and debate. Part III reviews the most egregious example of food company marketing practices: the deliberate use of young children as sales targets and the conversion of schools into vehicles for selling "junk" foods high in calories but low in nutritional value. Part IV explains how the supplement industry manipulated the political process to achieve a sales environment virtually free of government oversight of the content, safety, and advertising claims for its products. In Part V, I describe how the food industry markets "junk" foods as health foods by adding nutrients and calling them "functional" foods or "nutraceuticals." The concluding chapter summarizes the significance of the issues raised by these examples and offers some options for choosing a healthful diet in an overabundant food system. Finally, the Appendix introduces some terms and concepts used in the field of nutrition and discusses issues that help explain why nutrition research is so controversial and so often misunderstood.

Before plunging into these accounts, some context may prove useful. This introduction addresses the principal questions that bear on the matters discussed in this book: What are we supposed to eat to stay healthy? Does diet really matter? Is there a significant gap between what we are supposed to eat and what we do eat? The answers to these questions constitute a basis for examining the central concern of this book: Does the food industry have anything to do with poor dietary practices? As a background for addressing that question, this introduction provides some fundamental facts about today's food industry and its marketing philosophies and strategies, and also points to some common themes that appear throughout the book.

WHAT IS A "HEALTHY" DIET?

To promote health as effectively as possible, diets must achieve balance: They must provide *enough* energy (calories) and vitamins, minerals, and other essential nutrients to prevent deficiencies and support normal metabolism. At the same time, they must not include *excessive* amounts of these and other nutritional factors that might promote development of chronic diseases. Fortunately, the optimal range of intake of most dietary components is quite broad (see the Appendix). It is obvious that people throughout the world eat many different foods and follow many different dietary patterns, many of which promote excellent health and longevity. As with other behavioral factors that affect health, diet interacts with individual genetic variation as well as with cultural, economic, and geographical factors that affect infant survival and adult longevity. On a

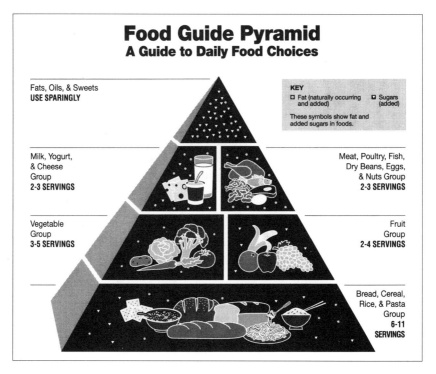

Food Guide Pyramid
A Guide to Daily Food Choices

Fats, Oils, & Sweets
USE SPARINGLY

KEY
☐ Fat (naturally occurring and added)   ◪ Sugars (added)

These symbols show fat and added sugars in foods.

Milk, Yogurt, & Cheese Group
2-3 SERVINGS

Meat, Poultry, Fish, Dry Beans, Eggs, & Nuts Group
2-3 SERVINGS

Vegetable Group
3-5 SERVINGS

Fruit Group
2-4 SERVINGS

Bread, Cereal, Rice, & Pasta Group
6-11 SERVINGS

FIGURE 1. The 1992 USDA *Food Guide Pyramid* recommends a hierarchical—and therefore controversial—dietary pattern based mainly on foods of plant origin, as discussed in Part I.

population basis, the balance between getting enough of the *right* kinds of nutrients and avoiding too much of the *wrong* kinds is best achieved by diets that include large proportions of energy from plant foods—fruits, vegetables, and grains.

The longest-lived populations in the world, such as some in Asia and the Mediterranean, traditionally eat diets that are largely plant-based. Such diets tend to be relatively low in calories but high in vitamins, minerals, fiber, and other components of plants (phytochemicals) that—acting together—protect against disease. Dietary patterns that best promote health derive most energy from plant foods, considerably less from foods of animal origin (meat, dairy, eggs), and even less from foods high in animal fats and sugars. The *Food Guide Pyramid* of the U.S. Department of Agriculture (USDA) is meant to depict a plant-based diet that promotes optimal health (see Figure 1). Chapter 2 describes the extent to which this *Pyramid* fails to illustrate an optimal dietary pattern, however, and explains the food industry's role in that failure.

DOES DIET MATTER?

In addition to consuming largely plant-based diets, people in long-lived populations are physically active and burn up any excess calories they obtain from food. An active lifestyle helps mitigate the harmful effects of overeating, but the evidence for the importance of diet in health also is overwhelming. Disease by chronic disease, scientists consistently have demonstrated the health benefits of diets rich in fruit and vegetables, limited in foods and fats of animal origin, and balanced in calories. Comprehensive reports in the late 1980s from the United States and Europe documented the evidence available at that time, and subsequent research has only strengthened those conclusions.[4]

Health experts suggest conservatively that the combination of poor diet, sedentary lifestyle, and excessive alcohol consumption contributes to about 400,000 of the 2,000,000 or so annual deaths in the United States—about the same number and proportion affected by cigarette smoking. Women who follow dietary recommendations display half the rates of coronary heart disease observed among women who eat poor diets, and those who also are active and do not smoke cigarettes have less than one-fifth the risk. The diet-related medical costs for just six health conditions—coronary heart disease, cancer, stroke, diabetes, hypertension, and obesity—exceeded $70 billion in 1995. Some authorities believe that just a 1% reduction in intake of saturated fat across the population would prevent more than 30,000 cases of coronary heart disease annually and save more than a billion dollars in health care costs. Such estimates indicate that even small dietary changes can produce large benefits when their effects are multiplied over an entire population.[5]

Conditions that can be prevented by eating better diets have roots in childhood. Rates of obesity are now so high among American children that many exhibit metabolic abnormalities formerly seen only in adults. The high blood sugar due to "adult-onset" (insulin-resistant type 2) diabetes, the high blood cholesterol, and the high blood pressure now observed in younger and younger children constitute a national scandal. Such conditions increase the risk of coronary heart disease, cancer, stroke, and diabetes later in life. From the late 1970s to the early 1990s, the prevalence of *overweight* nearly doubled—from 8% to 14% among children aged 6–11 and from 6% to 12% among adolescents. The proportion of overweight adults rose from 25% to 35% in those years. Just between 1991 and 1998, the rate of adult *obesity* increased from 12% to nearly 18%. Obesity contributes to increased health care costs, thereby becoming an issue for everyone, overweight or not.[6]

The cause of overweight is an excess of calories consumed over calories burned off in activity. People gain weight because they eat too many calories or are too inactive for the calories they eat. Genetics affects this balance, of course, because heredity predisposes some people to gain weight more easily than others, but genetic changes in a population occur too slowly to account for the sharp increase in weight gain over such a short time period. The precise relationship between the diet side and the activity side of the weight "equation" is uncertain and still under investigation, in part because we lack accurate methods for assessing the activity levels of populations. People seem to be spending more time at sedentary activities such as watching television and staring at computer screens, and the number of hours spent watching television is one of the best predictors of overweight, but surveys do not report enough of a decrease in activity levels to account for the current rising rates of obesity.[7] This gap leaves overeating as the most probable cause of excessive weight gain.

DO AMERICANS OVEREAT?

Overweight itself constitutes ample evidence that many Americans consume more calories than they burn off, but other sources of information also confirm the idea that people are eating too much food. The calories provided by the U.S. food supply increased from 3,300 per capita in 1970 to 3,800 in the late 1990s, an increase of 500 per day. These supply figures tend to overestimate amounts of food actually consumed because they do not account for wastage, but they do give some indication of trends (see the Appendix). Surveys that ask about actual dietary intake tend to underestimate caloric intake, because people find it difficult to remember dietary details, but easier to give answers that seem to please investigators. Even so, dietary intake surveys also indicate that people are eating more than they were in the 1970s. Then, people reported eating an average of about 1,800 calories per day. By 1996 they reported 2,000 calories per day. No matter how unrealistically low these figures may be and how imprecise the sources of data, all suggest a trend toward caloric intakes that exceed average levels of caloric expenditure.[8]

In addition to revealing how much people are eating, food supply and dietary intake surveys indicate changes in food habits over time. The increase in calories reflects an increase in consumption of *all* major food groups: more vegetables and more fruit (desirable), but also more meat and dairy foods, and more foods high in fat and sugar (less desirable). The most pronounced change is in beverage consumption. The supply of whole milk fell from 25.5 gallons per capita per year in 1970 to just 8.5 gallons in 1997. The supply of low-fat milk rose from 5.8 to 15.5 gallons during the same time, but that of soft drinks rose from 24.3 to 53 gallons. To reduce fat intake, people replaced whole milk with lower-fat varieties (same nutrients, fewer calories), but they undermined this beneficial change by increasing consumption of soft drinks (sugar calories, no nutrients). Despite the introduction of artificial sweeteners, the supply of calorie-laden sweeteners—sugars, corn sweeteners, and honey—has gone up. Because of the inconsistencies in data, the trend in fat intake is harder to discern. Fat in the food supply increased by 25% from 1970 to the late 1990s, but dietary intake surveys do not find people to be eating more of it. Although USDA nutritionists conclude that Americans are eating less fat, they also observe that people are eating more food outside the home, where foods are higher in fat and calories.[9]

In comparison to the *Pyramid*, American diets clearly are out of balance, as shown in Figure 2. Top-heavy as it is, this illustration *underestimates* the discrepancy between recommended and actual servings. For one thing, the USDA's serving estimates are based on self-reports of dietary intake, but people tend to underreport the intake of foods considered undesirable and to overestimate the consumption of "healthy" foods. For another, the USDA calculates numbers of servings by adding up the individual components of mixed dishes and assigning them to the appropriate *Pyramid* categories. This means that the flour in cookies is assigned to the grain category, the apples in pies to the fruit group, and the potatoes in chips to the vegetable group. This method may yield more precise information about nutrient intake, but it makes high-calorie, low-nutrient foods appear as better nutritional choices than they may be. The assignment of the tomatoes in ketchup to the vegetable group only reinforces the absurdity of the USDA's famous attempt during the Reagan administration to count ketchup as a vegetable in the federal school lunch program.[10]

The comparison hides other unwelcome observations. USDA nutritionists report that the average consumption of whole-grain foods is just one serving per day, well below recommended levels. And although the

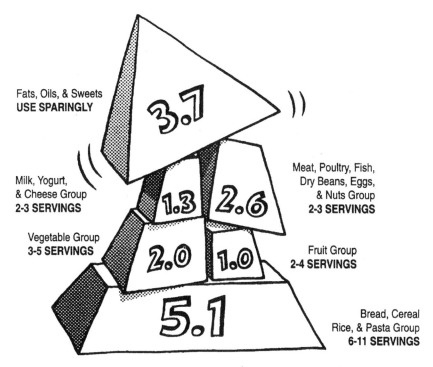

FIGURE 2. This "food consumption" pyramid compares the average number of servings consumed per day by the U.S. population in the mid-1990s to the servings recommended by the *Food Guide Pyramid*. (Courtesy National Cattlemen's Beef Association)

number of vegetable servings appears close to recommendations, *half* the servings come from just three foods: iceberg lettuce, potatoes (frozen, fresh, and those used for chips and fries), and canned tomatoes. When fried potatoes are excluded from the count, vegetable servings fall below three per day. Even though the consumption of reduced-fat dairy products has doubled since 1970, half the dairy servings still come from high-fat, high-calorie cheese and whole milk. Servings of added fats are at least one-third higher than they should be, and servings of caloric sweeteners are half again as high. From such observations, we can conclude that the increased calories in American diets come from eating more food in general, but especially more of foods high in fat (meat, dairy, fried foods, grain dishes with added fat), sugar (soft drinks, juice drinks, desserts), and salt (snack foods).[11] It can hardly be a coincidence that these are just the foods that are most profitable to the food industry and that it most vigorously promotes.

THE U.S. FOOD INDUSTRY

This book uses the term food industry to refer to companies that produce, process, manufacture, sell, and serve foods, beverages, and dietary supplements. In a larger sense, the term encompasses the entire collection of enterprises involved in the production and consumption of food and beverages: producers and processors of food crops and animals (agribusiness); companies that make and sell fertilizer, pesticides, seeds, and feed; those that provide machinery, labor, real estate, and financial services to farmers; and others that transport, store, distribute, export, process, and market foods after they leave the farm. It also includes the food service sector—food carts, vending machines, restaurants, bars, fast-food outlets, schools, hospitals, prisons, and workplaces—and associated suppliers of equipment and serving materials. This vast "food-and-fiber" system generates a trillion dollars or more in sales every year, accounts for 13% of the U.S. gross national product (GNP), and employs 17% of the country's labor force. Of the $800 billion or so a year that the public spends directly on food and drink, alcoholic beverages account for about $90 billion, and the rest is distributed among retail food enterprises (54%) and food service (46%).[12]

The U.S. food industry is the remarkably successful result of twentieth-century trends that led from small farms to giant corporations, from a society that cooked at home to one that buys nearly half its meals prepared and consumed elsewhere, and from a diet based on "whole" foods grown locally to one based largely on foods that have been processed in some way and transported long distances. These changes created a farm system that is much less labor-intensive and far more efficient and specialized. In 1900, 40% of the population lived on farms, but today no more than 2% do. Just since 1960, the number of farms has declined from about 3.2 million to 1.9 million, but their average size has increased by 40% and their productivity by 82%. Most farms today raise just a single commodity such as cattle, chickens, pigs, corn, wheat, or soybeans. Many are part of a system of "vertical" integration: ownership by one corporation of all stages of production and marketing. Chickens constitute an especially clear example. In the mid-1950s, chickens were raised in small flocks by many farmers; today, most are "factory-farmed" in massive numbers under contract to a few large companies.[13]

TABLE 1. Sales and advertising expenditures for the ten leading producers of packaged food products in the United States

Company and Examples	Food Sales [Total Sales], 1999 ($ Billions)	Advertising, U.S., 1998 ($ Millions)
Nestlé	34.9 [49.4]	534.4
Carnation foods		31.1
Lean Cuisine		16.4
Butterfinger candy		11.2
Unilever/Bestfoods*	32.4 [55.3]	
Unilever		1,015.0
Lipton's tea beverages		41.8
Wish-Bone salad dressing		15.2
Bestfoods		202.5
Thomas' English muffins		9.5
Skippy peanut butter		4.0
Philip Morris	27.8 [78.6]	2,049.3
Kraft Foods, Inc.		146.1
Jell-O desserts		65.6
Altoids mints		10.1
Pepsico	11.6 [18.7]	1,263.4
Pepsi and Diet Pepsi		145.2
Lay's potato chips		55.8
Tropicana fruit juices		23.3
Groupe Danone	9.8 [14.2]	*
H.J. Heinz	9.3	214.5
Nabisco	8.4	225.7
Kellogg	7.7	448.5
Cereals		278.7
Eggo frozen waffles		34.3
General Mills*	6.7	597.9
Cereals		296.7
Fruit-by-the-Foot snacks		10.3
Campbell Soup	6.2	336.8
Soups		108.0
Pepperidge Farm		37.2

PRINCIPAL SOURCES: Endicott RC. 44th annual 100 leading national advertisers. *Advertising Age* September 27, 1999:s1–s46. Hays CL. *New York Times* June 7, 2000:C1,C8. Thompson S. *Advertising Age* June 12, 2000:4.

*In 2000, Unilever purchased Bestfoods soon after acquiring Ben & Jerry's and Slim-Fast. General Mills bought the Pillsbury division of Diageo, making the combined company the fifth largest of U.S. foodmakers, with $12.2 billion in annual sales. Danone was not among the top 200 U.S. advertisers in 1998, because the company's principal markets are in Europe.

Economic pressures force food and beverage companies to expand to tremendous size. In 2000, seven U.S. companies—Philip Morris, ConAgra, Mars, IBP, Sara Lee, Heinz, and Tyson Foods—ranked among the ten largest food companies in the world. Nestlé (Switzerland) ranked first, Unilever (U.K./Netherlands) third, and Danone (France) sixth. Other U.S.

companies such as Coca-Cola, McDonald's, PepsiCo, Procter & Gamble, and Roche (vitamins) ranked among the top one hundred companies worldwide. In the United States alone, just three companies—Philip Morris (Kraft Foods, Miller Brewing), ConAgra, and RJR-Nabisco—accounted for nearly 20% of all food expenditures in 1997. Table 1 lists the ten leading producers of packaged food products in the United States in 2000, along with their annual sales and advertising budgets. The largest companies generated more than $30 billion each in annual sales, placing great pressure on smaller companies to merge. Such pressures also apply to supermarkets. Mergers among food and cigarette companies merit special interest. As described in Table 2, two of the four leading U.S. cigarette companies, R. J. Reynolds and Philip Morris, bought—and sometimes swapped—food and beverage companies in maneuvers designed to protect stockholders' investments against tobacco liability lawsuits.

The increasing consumption of food outside the home also has implications for the food industry—and for health. Table 3 lists the leading U.S. food service companies by category: fast foods, restaurant chains, contract corporations, and hotel operations. The highest-selling food service chains are sandwich houses and fast-food chains. First among them is McDonald's; its 12,804 U.S. outlets brought in $19.6 billion in 2000 sales, more than twice as much as its nearest competitor.

The greater efficiency, specialization, and size of agriculture and food product manufacture have led to one of the great unspoken secrets about the American food system: overabundance. As already noted, the U.S. food supply—plus imports less exports—provides a daily average of 3,800 calories per capita. This level is nearly twice the amount needed to meet the energy requirements of most women, one-third more than that needed by most men, and much higher than that needed by babies, young children, and the sedentary elderly. Even if, as the USDA estimates, 1,100 of those calories might be wasted (as spoiled fruit, for example, or as oil for frying potatoes), the excess calories are a major problem for the food industry: they force competition. Even people who overindulge can eat only so much food, and choosing one food means rejecting others. Overabundance alone is sufficient to explain why the annual growth rate of the American food industry is only a percentage point or two, and why it has poked along at that low level for many years. It also explains why food companies compete so strenuously for consumer food dollars, why they work so hard to create a sales-friendly regulatory and political climate, and why they are so defensive about the slightest suggestion that their products might raise health or safety risks.

TABLE 2. Cigarette companies' ownership of food and beverage companies: chronology

1969	Philip Morris, Inc. acquires 53% of Miller Brewing.
1970	Philip Morris buys the remaining 47% of Miller Brewing.
1978	Philip Morris acquires 97% of Seven-Up.
1985	R.J. Reynolds buys Nabisco Foods for $4.9 billion, creating RJR-Nabisco, a public company. Philip Morris buys General Foods for $5.6 billion.
1986	Philip Morris sells Seven-Up to PepsiCo.
1988	Philip Morris buys Kraft, Inc. for $13.6 billion. RJR-Nabisco announces plans to "go private"; offers to buy outstanding public shares for $17 billion.
1989	The investment firm Kohlberg Kravis Roberts leverages a buyout of RJR-Nabisco for $24.9 billion, leaving the private company with $20 billion in debt. Philip Morris combines Kraft and General Foods to form Kraft General Foods.
1990	Philip Morris acquires Jacobs Suchard, a Swiss coffee and confectionary company, for $4.1 billion.
1991	Kohlberg Kravis Roberts sells stocks in RJR-Nabisco to the public. The bestseller *Barbarians at the Gate* (New York: HarperCollins, 1991) describes the takeover events.
1993	Kraft General Foods (Philip Morris) buys Nabisco ready-to-eat cereals from RJR-Nabisco for $448 million.
1995	Kraft General Foods reorganizes into Kraft Foods, Inc. In an effort to shore up stock prices, RJR-Nabisco becomes a holding company for R. J. Reynolds (tobacco) and Nabisco Holdings (food); sells 19% of shares in Nabisco Holdings to the public.
1996	Philip Morris buys shares of Brazil's leading chocolate company, Industrias de Chocolate Lacta, S.A.; Kraft Foods acquires Taco Bell.
1999	RJR-Nabisco sells its international tobacco business; separates and renames its domestic tobacco (R. J. Reynolds Tobacco Holdings) and food businesses (Nabisco Group Holdings). This action leaves Nabisco Group Holdings with 81% of Nabisco as its sole asset (Nabisco Holdings has the remainder), only $1 billion in debt, but with uncertain liability for tobacco lawsuits. Philip Morris said to be interested in buying Nabisco; acquires Philadelphia cream cheese; reports revenues exceeding $78 billion.
2000	Philip Morris buys Nabisco Holdings for $14.9 billion, creating a company that earned combined revenues of $34.9 billion and profits of $5.5 billion in 1999. This purchase leaves R.J. Reynolds Tobacco Holdings with $1.5 billion in cash and the tobacco liability.

PRINCIPAL SOURCES: Philip Morris Companies, Inc. Online: http://www.kraftfoods.com/. Accessed February 24, 1999. Hays CL. *New York Times* March 10, 1999:A1,C8, and July 2, 2000:C7.

TABLE 3. Where Americans eat: the top two U.S. food service chain companies in 2000 sales, by category and number of units

Chain Category	2000 Sales, ($ Millions)	Number of Units, U.S.
Sandwich		
McDonald's	19,573	12,804
Burger King	8,695	8,064
Pizza		
Pizza Hut	5,000	7,927
Domino's	2,647	4,818
Chicken		
KFC (Kentucky Fried Chicken)	4,400	5,364
Chick-fil-A	1,082	1,958
Grill Buffet		
Golden Corral	968	452
Ryan's Family Steak House	745	324
Family		
Denny's	2,137	1,753
International House of Pancakes	1,199	925
Dinner-House		
Applebee's Neighborhood	2,625	1,251
Red Lobster	2,105	629
Contract		
Aramark Global	4,136	2,907
LSG/Sky Chefs	1,476	103
Hotel Food Service		
Marriott	1,045	248
Hilton	953	228

SOURCE: Liddle AJ. *Nation's Restaurant News* July 25, 2001:57–132.

MARKETING IMPERATIVES

To sell their products, companies appeal to the reasons why people choose to eat one food rather than another. These reasons are numerous, complex, and not always understood, mainly because we select diets within the context of the social, economic, and cultural environment in which we live. When food or money is scarce, people do not have the luxury of choice; for much of the world's population, the first consideration is getting *enough* food to meet biological needs for energy and nutrients. It is one of the great ironies of nutrition that the traditional plant-based diets consumed by the poor in many countries, some of which are among the world's finest cuisines, are ideally suited to meeting nutritional needs as long as caloric intake is adequate. Once people raised on such foods survive the hazards of infancy, their diets (and their active lifestyles) support an adulthood relatively free of chronic disease until late in life.[14]

Also ironic is that once people become better off, they are observed to enter a "nutrition transition" in which they abandon traditional plant-based diets and begin eating more meat, fat, and processed foods. The result is a sharp increase in obesity and related chronic diseases. In 2000 the number of overweight people in the world for the first time matched the number of undernourished people—1.1 billion each. Even in an industrialized country such as France, dietary changes can be seen to produce rapid increases in the prevalence of chronic disease. In the early 1960s, the French diet contained just 25% of calories from fat, but the proportion now approaches 40% as a result of increased intake of meat, dairy, and processed foods. Despite contentions that the French are protected from heart disease by their wine consumption (a phenomenon known as the French Paradox), they are getting fatter by the day and experiencing increased rates of diabetes and other health consequences of overeating and overweight. The nutrition transition reflects both taste preferences and economics. Food animals raised in feedlots eat grains, which makes meat more expensive to produce and converts it into a marker of prosperity. Once people have access to meat, they usually do not return to eating plant-based diets unless they are forced to do so by economic reversal or are convinced to do so for reasons of religion, culture, or health.[15]

Humans do not innately know how to select a nutritious diet; we survived in evolution because nutritious foods were readily available for us to hunt or gather. In an economy of overabundance, food companies can sell products only to people who *want* to buy them. Whether consumer demands drive food sales or the industry creates such demands is a matter of debate, but much industry effort goes into trying to figure out what the public "wants" and how to meet such "needs." Nearly all research on this issue yields the same conclusion. When food is plentiful and people can afford to buy it, basic biological needs become less compelling and the principal determinant of food choice is personal preference. In turn, personal preferences may be influenced by religion and other cultural factors, as well as by considerations of convenience, price, and nutritional value. To sell food in an economy of abundant food choices, companies must worry about those other determinants much more than about the nutritional value of their products—unless the nutrient content helps to entice buyers (see Parts IV and V).[16] Thus the food industry's marketing imperatives principally concern four factors: taste, cost, convenience, and (as we shall see) public confusion.

Taste: Make Foods Sweet, Fat, and Salty

Adults prefer foods that taste, look, and smell good, are familiar, and provide variety, but these preferences are influenced strongly by family and ethnic background, level of education, income, age, and gender. When asked, most of us say we choose foods because we like them, by which we mean the way we respond to their flavor, smell, sight, and texture. Most of us prefer sweet foods and those that are "energy-dense" (high in calories, fat, and sugar), and we like the taste of salt. The universality of such preferences suggests some physiologic basis for all of them, but the research is most convincing for sweetness. Ripe fruit is innately sweet and appealing, but many of us can and do learn to enjoy the complex and sometimes bitter taste of vegetables. Whether a taste for meat is innate or acquired can be debated, but many people like to eat steak, hamburgers, and fried chicken, along with desserts, soft drinks, and salty snacks. Such preferences drive the development of new food products as well as the menus in restaurants.

Cost: Add Value but Keep Prices Low

One result of overabundance is pressure to add value to foods through processing. The producers of raw foods receive only a fraction of the price that consumers pay at the supermarket. In 1998, for example, an average of 20% of retail cost—the "farm value" of the food—was returned to its producers. This percentage, which has been declining for years, is unequally distributed. Producers of eggs, beef, and chicken receive 50% to 60% of retail cost, whereas producers of vegetables receive as little as 5%. Once foods get to the supermarket, the proportion represented by the farm value declines further in proportion to the extent of processing. The farm value of frozen peas is 13%, of canned tomatoes 9%, of oatmeal 7%, and of corn syrup just 4%.[17]

As shown in Figure 3, the remaining 80% of the food dollar goes for labor, packaging, advertising, and other such value-enhancing activities. Conversion of potatoes (cheap) to potato chips (expensive) to those fried in artificial fats or coated in soybean flour or herbal supplements (even more expensive) is an example of how value is added to basic food commodities. Added value explains why the cost of the corn in Kellogg's

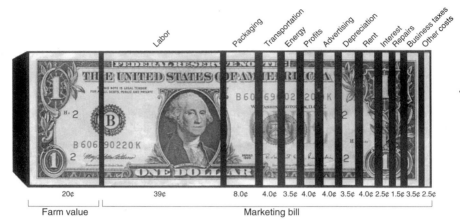

FIGURE 3. The distribution of the U.S. food dollar: 80% of food expenditures go to categories other than the "farm value" of the food itself. (Source: USDA *FoodReview* 2000;23(3):27–30)

Corn Flakes is less than 10% of the retail price. With this kind of pricing distribution, food companies are more likely to focus on developing added-value products than to promote consumption of fresh fruits and vegetables, particularly because opportunities for adding value to such foods are limited. Marketers can add value to fruits and vegetables by selling them frozen, canned, or precut, but even the most successful of such products—prepackaged and branded "baby" carrots, salad mixes, and precut fruit—raise consumer concerns about freshness and price.

Despite the focus on adding value, overabundance keeps food costs low compared to those anywhere else in the world, and this is due only in part to our high average income. The average American pays less than 10% of income for food. People in low-income countries like Tanzania pay more than 70% of income for food, and those in middle-income countries like the Philippines up to 55%, but even people in high-income countries like Japan pay as much as 20%. Americans, however, strongly resist price increases. In the United States, lower prices stimulate sales, especially the sale of higher-cost items; price is a more important factor in the consumer's choice of steak than of ground beef. Cost is so important a factor in food choice that economists are able to calculate the effect of a change in price on nutrient intake. They estimate that a decline in the price of meat, for example, causes the average intake of calcium and iron to rise but also increases the consumption of calories, fat, saturated fat, and cholesterol.[18]

A more important reason for low food prices is that the government subsidizes food production in ways that are rarely evident. The most visible subsidies are price supports for sugar and milk, but taxpayers also support production quotas, market quotas, import restrictions, deficiency payments, lower tax rates, low-cost land leases, land management, water rights, and marketing and promotion programs for major food commodities. The total cost of agricultural subsidies rose rapidly at the end of the twentieth century from about $18 billion in 1996 to $28 billion in 2000. As we shall see in Part II, the large agricultural corporations that most benefit from federal subsidies spare no effort to persuade Congress and the administration to continue and increase this largesse.[19]

Convenience: Make Eating Fast

Convenience is a principal factor driving the development of value-added products. The demographic causes of demands for convenience are well understood. In the last quarter of the twentieth century, the proportion of women with children who entered the work force greatly expanded, and many people began to work longer hours to make ends meet. In 1900, women accounted for 21% of the labor force, and married women for less than 6%, but by 1999, women—married or not—accounted for more than 60%. The structure of American families changed once there was no longer a housewife who stayed home and cooked. Working women were unable or unwilling to spend as much time grocery shopping, cooking, and cleaning up after meals.[20]

Societal changes easily explain why nearly half of all meals are consumed outside the home, a quarter of them as fast food, and the practice of snacking nearly doubled from the mid-1980s to the mid-1990s. They explain the food industry's development of prepackaged sandwiches, salads, entrees, and desserts, as well as such innovations as "power" bars, yogurt and pasta in tubes, prepackaged cereal in a bowl, salad bars, hot-food bars, take-out chicken, supermarket "home meal replacements," McDonald's shaker salads, chips prepackaged with dips, and foods designed to be eaten directly from the package. Whether these "hyper-convenient" products will outlast the competition remains to be seen, but survival is more likely to depend on taste and price than on nutrient content. Many of these products are high in calories, fat, sugar, or salt but are marketed as nutritious because they contain added vitamins (see Part V).

Nutritionists and traditionalists may lament such developments, because convenience overrides not only considerations of health but also the social and cultural meanings of meals and mealtimes. Many food products relegate cooking to a low-priority chore and encourage trends toward one-dish meals, fewer side dishes, fewer ingredients, larger portions to create leftovers, almost nothing cooked "from scratch," and home-delivered meals ordered by phone, fax, or Internet. Interpreting the meaning of these developments no doubt will occupy sociologists and anthropologists for decades. In the meantime, convenience adds value to foods and stimulates the food industry to create even more products that can be consumed quickly and with minimal preparation.

Confusion: Keep the Public Puzzled

Many people find it difficult to put nutrition advice into practice, not least because they view the advice as ephemeral—changing from one day to the next. This view is particularly unfortunate because, as I explain in Part I, advice to eat more fruits and vegetables and to avoid overweight as a means to promote health has remained constant for half a century. Confusion about nutrition is quite understandable, however. People obtain information about diet and health from the media—newspapers, magazines, television, radio and more recently the Internet. These outlets get much of their information from research publications, experts, and the public relations representatives of food and beverage companies. Media outlets require *news*, and reporters are partial to breakthroughs, simple take-home lessons, and controversies. A story about the benefits of single nutrients can be entertaining, but "eat your veggies" is old news. It is more interesting to read about a study "proving" that calcium does or does not prevent bone loss than a report that patiently explains the other factors—nutrients, foods, drinks, exercise—that might influence calcium balance in the body. Although foods contain hundreds of nutrients and other components that influence health, and although people eat diets that contain dozens of different foods, reporters rarely discuss study results in their broader dietary context.[21] News outlets are not alone in focusing on single nutrients or foods; researchers also do so. It is easier to study the effects of vitamin E on heart disease risk than it is to try to explain how current dietary *patterns* are associated with declining rates of coronary heart disease. Research on the effects of single nutrients is more likely to be funded, and the results are more likely to garner headlines, especially if they conflict with previous studies. In the meantime, basic dietary advice remains the same—constant, but dull.

Newspaper sales and research grants may benefit from confusion over dietary advice, but the greatest beneficiary of public confusion is the food industry. Part II explains how virtually every food and beverage product is represented by a trade association or public relations firm whose job it is to promote a positive image of that item among consumers, professionals, and the media. These groups—and their lobbyists—can take advantage of the results of single-nutrient research to claim that products containing the beneficial nutrient promote health and to demand the right to make that claim on package labels. If people are confused about nutrition, they will be more likely to accept such claims at face value. It is in the interest of food companies to have people believe that there is no such thing as a "good" food (except when it is theirs); that there is no such thing as a "bad" food (especially not theirs); that all foods (especially theirs) can be incorporated into healthful diets; and that balance, variety, and moderation are the keys to healthful diets—which means that no advice to restrict intake of their particular product is appropriate. The *Pyramid*, however, clearly indicates that some foods *are* better than others from the standpoint of health.

PROMOTING "EAT MORE"

In a competitive food marketplace, food companies must satisfy stockholders by encouraging more people to eat more of their products. They seek new audiences among children, among members of minority groups, or internationally. They expand sales to existing as well as new audiences through advertising but also by developing new products designed to respond to consumer "demands." In recent years, they have embraced a new strategy: increasing the sizes of food portions. Advertising, new products, and larger portions all contribute to a food environment that promotes eating more, not less.

Advertise, Advertise, Advertise

Advertising operates so far below the consciousness of everyone—the public, most nutritionists I know, and survey researchers—that it hardly ever gets mentioned as an influence on food choice. The subliminal nature of food and beverage advertising is a tribute to its ubiquity, as well as to the sophistication of the agencies that produce it. Extraordinary amounts of money and talent go into this effort. Food and food service companies spend more than $11 billion annually on direct media advertising in magazines, newspapers, radio, television, and billboards. Some examples of expenditures by specific companies are given in Table 1. In 1999 McDonald's spent $627.2 million, Burger King $403.6 million, Taco Bell $206.5 million, and Coke and Diet Coke $174.4 million on direct media advertising. Even small products have impressive advertising budgets, as illustrated by expenditures of $117 million for Wrigley's chewing gum and nearly $80 million for M&M candies.[22] For every dollar spent that "measured" way, the companies spend another two dollars on discount incentives—for example, coupons for consumers and "slotting fees" for retailers to ensure space on supermarket shelves. In total, food companies spent more than $33 billion annually at the turn of the century to advertise and promote their products to the public. Most of this astronomical sum is used to promote the most highly processed, elaborately packaged, and fast foods. Nearly 70% of food advertising is for convenience foods, candy and snacks, alcoholic beverages, soft drinks, and desserts, whereas just 2.2% is for fruits, vegetables, grains, or beans.[23] Figure 4 illustrates the disproportionate distribution of marketing expenditures relative to dietary recommendations. Although the costs of marketing may appear huge, they amount to just a small fraction of sales.

Advertising costs for any single, nationally distributed food product far exceed (often by 10 to 50 times) federal expenditures for promotion of the *Pyramid* or to encourage people to eat more fruit and vegetables. Of the more than $300 million that the USDA spends annually on nutrition education, most goes for research projects, the educational components of agricultural extension, and other activities that target relatively few people. Despite protestations by marketers that advertising is a minor element in food choice and that the ubiquity of advertising dilutes its impact, they continue to use it to sell products. Successful campaigns are carefully researched, targeted to specific groups, and repeated frequently. Advertising promotes the sales of specific food products and in proportion to the amount spent, as shown for commodities such as milk, cheese, grapefruit juice, and orange juice. Food sales increase with the intensity, repetition, and visibility of the advertising message.[24] Promotion of nutritional advantages (low-fat, no cholesterol, high-fiber, calcium-added) increases sales, as does the use of health claims (lowers cholesterol, prevents cancer). Cigarette company-owned food advertisers are particularly adept at using charity to sell food products, as shown in Figure 5. Advertising sells food to children, a phenomenon well understood by advertisers

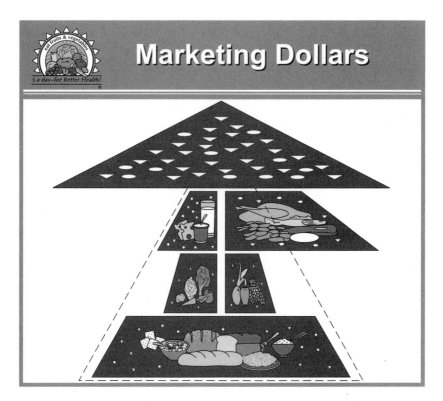

FIGURE 4. The Produce for Better Health Foundation, a government–industry partnership to promote consumption of fruits and vegetables, created this "food marketing" pyramid to illustrate the disproportionate expenditure of advertising dollars in comparison to dietary recommendations. (Courtesy Elizabeth Pivonka, ©Produce for Better Health Foundation, Wilmington, DE)

of tobacco and beer. As discussed in Part III, advertisers deliberately promote food brands among children and more active demands for advertised foods.

Introduce New Products

To food and beverage companies, added value and convenience are driving forces for new-product development. Whether the industry creates new products in response to consumer demand or generates demand by

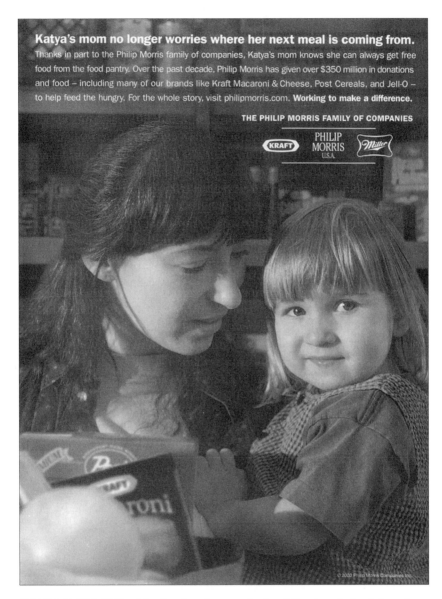

FIGURE 5. This Philip Morris advertisement for its philanthropic food donations appeared in *Walking*, a health and fitness magazine aimed at young women, in October 2000. No advertisements for cigarettes appear in the magazine. Philip Morris owns Kraft Foods and Miller Beer.

TABLE 4. Major categories of the 11,037 new food products introduced in 1998

Product Category	Number of New Products
Candy, gum, snacks	2,065
Condiments	1,994
Beverages	1,547
Bakery foods	1,178
Dairy foods	940
Processed meats	728
Entrees, pre-prepared	678
Fruits and vegetables	375
Soups	299
Desserts	117
Pet foods	105
Breakfast cereals	84
Baby foods	35

SOURCE: Gallo AE. *FoodReview* 1999;22(3):27–29.

creating the products is difficult to untangle; most likely, both interact. Regardless, new-product introductions have increased greatly since the mid-1980s when there were fewer than 6,000 annually. In the peak year of 1995, manufacturers introduced 16,900 food and beverage products, but the number has since declined. All told, 116,000 packaged foods and beverages have been introduced since 1990, and these joined a marketplace that now contains 320,000 items competing for supermarket shelf space large enough to hold just 50,000.[12] The glut of food products means that only the most highly promoted products will succeed; even these may encounter difficulties if they do not taste good, raise questions about health or safety, or cost too much.

In 1998, manufacturers introduced slightly more than 11,000 new products (Table 4). More than two-thirds of those products are condiments, candy and snacks, baked goods, soft drinks, and dairy products (cheese products and ice cream novelties)—foods largely allocated to the top of the *Pyramid*. Slightly more than one-fourth are "nutritionally enhanced" so that they can be marketed as low in fat, cholesterol, salt, or sugar or as higher in fiber, calcium, or vitamins. Some such products, among them no-fat cookies, vitamin-enriched cereals, and calcium-fortified juice drinks, contain so much sugar that they belong at the top of the *Pyramid*. Developing such foods has only one purpose: to attract sales.

Serve Larger Portions

"Eat more" marketing methods extend beyond billboards and television commercials; they also include substantial increases in the sizes of food packages and restaurant portions. When the *Pyramid* recommends 6 to 11 grain servings, these amounts seem impossibly large with reference to restaurant, fast, or take-out foods. The *Pyramid* serving numbers, however, refer to portion size *standards* defined by the USDA: A standard grain serving is one slice of white bread, one ounce of ready-to-eat cereals or muffins, or one-half cup of rice or pasta. Therefore, a single bakery muffin weighing 7 ounces, or one medium container of movie-theater popcorn (16 cups), easily meets or exceeds a day's grain allowances. Larger servings of course contain more calories. The largest movie-theater soft drink contains 800 calories if not too diluted with ice. Larger portions can contribute to weight gain unless people compensate with diet and exercise. From an industry standpoint, however, larger portions make good marketing sense. The cost of food is low relative to labor and other factors that add value. Large portions attract customers who flock to all-you-can-eat restaurants and order double-scoop ice cream cones because the relative prices discourage the choice of smaller portions. It does not require much mathematical skill to understand that the larger portions of McDonald's french fries are a better buy than the "small" when they are 40% cheaper per ounce.[25]

Taken together, advertising, convenience, larger portions, and (as we shall see) the added nutrients in foods otherwise high in fat, sugar, and salt all contribute to an environment that promotes "eat more." Because dietary advice affects sales, food companies also conduct systematic, pervasive, and unrelenting—but far less apparent—campaigns to convince government officials, health organizations, and nutrition professionals that their products are healthful or harmless, to undermine any suggestion to the contrary, and to ensure that federal *dietary guidelines* and food guides will help promote sales.

ISSUES AND THEMES

Overabundant food and its consequences occur in the context of increasing centralization and globalization of the food industry and of altered patterns of work, welfare, and government. The food system is only one aspect of society, but it is unusual in its universality: Everyone eats. Because food affects lives as well as livelihoods, the situations discussed in this book generate substantial attention from the industry and the government, as well as from advocates, nutrition and health professionals, the media, and the public at large. In this book's discussions of specific topics and incidents, several themes occur. Some of these themes touch on matters central to the functioning of democratic institutions and are worth noting as they emerge in the chapters that follow.

One such theme is the "paradox of plenty," the term used by historian Harvey Levenstein to refer to the social consequences of food overabundance, among them the sharp disparities in diet and health between rich and poor.[26] Wealthier people usually are healthier, and they choose better diets. They also tend to avoid smoking cigarettes, to drink alcohol in moderation if at all, and to be better educated and more physically active. Health habits tend to cluster in patterns, making it difficult to tease out the effects of diet from that of any other behavioral factor. Most paradoxical in the presence of food overabundance is that large numbers of people in the United States and elsewhere do not have enough to eat. The economic expansion of the twentieth century differentially favored people whose income was higher than average and provided much smaller gains for the poor. As noted earlier, when people in developing countries go through a "nutrition transition," they increase the intake of meat, fat, and processed foods, gain weight, and develop risk factors for diseases of overconsumption. In the United States, low-income groups seem to have about the same nutrient intake as people who are better off, but they choose diets higher in calories, fat, meat, and sugar, and they display higher rates of obesity and chronic diseases. The income gap between rich and poor can be explained by the functioning of economic and related educational systems. The gaps in diet and health are economically based, but they also derive in part from the social status attached to certain kinds of food—meat for the poor and health foods for the rich, for example. Food and beverage companies reinforce this gap when they seek new marketing opportunities among minority groups or in low-income neighborhoods. The alcoholic beverage industry is especially adept in marketing to "disenfranchised" groups.[27]

A second theme is the conflict between scientific and other kinds of belief systems. Although most scientists view scientific methods—testing hypotheses by controlled experiments—as inherently valid and truthful, we shall see that many people regard science as just one of a number of belief systems of equal validity and importance. Religious beliefs, concerns about animal rights, and views of the fundamental nature of society, for example, influence the way people think about food. So do vested interests. Like any other kind of science, nutrition science is more a matter of probabilities than of absolutes and is, therefore, subject to interpretation. Interpretation, in turn, depends on point of view. Government agencies invoke science as a basis for regulatory decisions. Food and supplement companies invoke science to oppose regulations and dietary advice that might adversely affect sales. Advocates invoke science to question the safety of products perceived as undesirable. In contrast, scientists and food producers, who might benefit from promoting research results, nutritional benefits, or safety, tend to view other-than-scientific points of view as inherently irrational. Debates about food issues that affect broad aspects of society often focus on scientific proof of safety whether or not safety constitutes the "real" issue, largely because alternative belief systems cannot be validated by scientific methods.[28]

The third theme constitutes this book's central thesis: diet is a political issue. Because dietary advice affects food sales, and because companies demand a favorable regulatory environment for their products, dietary practices raise political issues that cut right to the heart of democratic institutions. Nearly all of the situations discussed in this book involve struggles over who decides what people should eat and whether a given food is "healthy." As a result, they inevitably involve struggles over the way government balances corporate against public interests. Such struggles are fundamental to the functioning of the American political system. They are revealed whenever a company attacks its critics as "food police" or justifies self-interested actions as a defense of freedom of choice or exclusion of "Big Brother" government from personal decisions. They are expressed whenever food companies use financial relationships with members of Congress, political leaders, and nutrition and health experts to weaken the regulatory ability of federal agencies and whenever they go to court to block unfavorable regulatory decisions. Despite the overwhelmingly greater resources of food companies in defending their own interests we shall see that consumer advocates sometimes can be highly effective in convincing Congress, federal agencies, and the courts to take action in the public interest. On that optimistic note, let's begin by tracing the history of federal dietary advice to the public and the ways in which such advice has been influenced by the actions of the food industry.

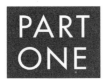

UNDERMINING DIETARY ADVICE

AS A NUTRITIONIST, I CANNOT GO ANYWHERE WITHOUT being asked why nutrition advice is so confusing. If it were not for public confusion, it would be difficult to explain to any rational person why dietary guidelines matter so much and why this book begins with an historical account of how the food industry affects them. As I will explain, dietary recommendations for prevention of chronic diseases have hardly varied for the past half-century, but the consistency of such advice is a well-kept secret. Americans may recognize the *Food Guide Pyramid* of the U.S. Department of Agriculture (USDA), but hardly anyone can recite federal dietary guidelines. Nutritionists know them and use them as a basis for counseling, but not everyone has access to a nutritionist. One reason for public confusion is that when it comes to nutrition education, no government agency has the funds to promote dietary recommendations in competition with food advertising. Instead, the major sources of nutrition advice for most people are the media and the public relations efforts of the food industry itself.

If nutrition guidelines have not seized public attention, it may be because they seem so obvious. Eat more fruit and vegetables? Nothing could be more self-evident. The banality of these guidelines belies their importance if not to the immediate health of the public then certainly to the health of the food industry. Dietary recommendations can be exploited to sell food products, but they also can turn the public away from entire categories of foods. The danger of such a catastrophe is sufficient to explain the ferocity of food industry arguments over the most minute, subtle, and seemingly inconsequential aspects of dietary advice. Thus the history of dietary guidance in the United States provides a fascinating introduction to food company attempts to compensate for the overabundance of food products—and to the ethical challenges that industry actions raise for government officials, nutrition experts, and company employees.

Nutrition advice might be less confusing and far less controversial if it were based solely on scientific knowledge, but research studies (as I explain in the Appendix) are subject to interpretation. Dietary guidelines necessarily are political compromises between what science tells us about nutrition and health and what is good for the food industry. As we shall see in Chapter 1, the government's current dietary guidelines are distinctly different from those issued a century ago. At that time, the goal of the USDA was to help people prevent nutrient deficiencies, and it did so by encouraging consumption of a wide variety of foods from the full range of American agricultural products—*eat more*. Today, federal agencies are far more concerned about preventing chronic diseases; they advise restrictions on intake of calories, fat, sugar, and salt—*eat less*. The "eat more" approach pleased everyone—agriculture officials, scientists, health professionals, and the food industry. Advice to eat less does not. Critics maintain that dietary restrictions are not justified by research, that only a small part of the population benefits from such advice, and that dietary guidelines represent too great an intrusion of government into habits that are none of its business. These arguments divert attention from the real issue, the perception that advice to eat less will reduce the profits of the food industry. In today's competitive and litigious food marketplace, any suggestion to eat less of a product is sure to elicit vigorous opposition and to galvanize lobbyists into action. Chapter 2 describes one such incident in detail: the USDA's 1991 withdrawal from publication of its *Food Guide Pyramid* in response to protests by meat and dairy producers. In Chapter 3, I analyze the subtleties of dietary advice to explain why each word of *dietary guidelines* is subject to such an intense level of dispute.

CHAPTER 1

FROM "EAT MORE" TO
"EAT LESS," 1900–1990

THE U.S. GOVERNMENT HAS BEEN TELLING PEOPLE WHAT TO
eat for more than a century, and the history of such advice reflects
changes in agriculture, food product development, and international
trade, as well as in science and medicine. In 1900, for example, the leading causes of death were infectious diseases such as tuberculosis and
diphtheria made worse by the nutrient deficiencies and overall malnutrition that were especially prevalent among the poor. Life expectancy at
birth for both men and women barely exceeded 47 years. To overcome
nutritional deficiencies and related disorders, government nutritionists
urged people to eat more of a greater variety of foods. Throughout the
twentieth century, an expanding economy led to improvements in housing, sanitation, and nutrition. Diseases resulting from nutritional deficiencies declined, and by 2000 life expectancy had increased to an average of 77 years. Today, the leading causes of death are chronic diseases
associated with excessive (or unbalanced) intake of food and nutrients.
Table 5 compares the ten leading causes of death in the United States in
1900 and 2000. Despite the great advances in public health during the
twentieth century, the leading conditions related to diet—coronary heart
disease, cancers at certain sites, diabetes, stroke, and liver cirrhosis, for
example—could be reduced in prevalence or delayed until later in life if
people ate less of dietary components that increase disease risk. Advice to
eat less, however, runs counter to the interests of food producers.

The conflict between more recent ideas about diets that promote
health and the interests of the food industry accounts for much of the
public confusion about nutrition. As this chapter will explain, dietary

TABLE 5. The ten leading causes of death in 1900 and 2000

1900	% Total[a]	2000	% Total[b]
Tuberculosis	11.3	Diseases of heart[c]	31.4
Pneumonia	10.2	Cancer	23.3
Diarrheal diseases	8.1	Stroke	6.9
Heart disease[c]	8.0	Lung disease	4.7
Liver disease	5.2	Accidents	4.1
Injuries	5.1	Pneumonia and influenza	3.7
Stroke	4.5	Diabetes mellitus	2.7
Cancer	3.7	Suicide	1.3
Bronchitis	2.6	Kidney diseases	1.0
Diphtheria	2.3	Liver disease and cirrhosis	1.0

Data from Hinman AR. *Public Health Reports* 1990;105:374–380. National Center for Health Statistics. *Health, United States*, 1999. Hyattsville, MD, 1999. Online: **http://www.cdc.gov/nchs/**. Accessed May 3, 2000.

[a] These percentages are based on data from just ten states and the District of Columbia, accounting for 23% of the population; data for the entire country did not become available until 1933.

[b] In 1997, 2,314,245 people died from all causes in the United States.

[c] Atherosclerosis of the coronary arteries—what we now call coronary heart disease—was not recognized as a clinical entity in 1900. Consequently, "heart disease" does not necessarily refer to the same condition for 1900 and 1999, and the 1900 figures may underestimate the extent of coronary heart disease in the population.

advice issued by the government never has been based purely on considerations of public health. The agencies that issue dietary advice inevitably have other constituencies as well as the public, most notably the agricultural and food industries. When the interests of these industries conflict with current thinking about nutrition, as in the examples described here, the result is controversy, confusion, and the invocation of science to support one or another point of view.

"EAT MORE":
PREVENTING DIETARY DEFICIENCIES, 1890s TO 1960s

The federal role in promoting food consumption developed as a result of colonial history. As far as one can tell, the diet of the earliest American settlers depended on foods obtained through farming, hunting and gathering, and—to a limited extent—internal and external trade. As trade increased, and as the country became more industrialized and urbanized, methods of food preservation, storage, and distribution improved. What people actually were eating before the twentieth century, however, is known only from anecdotal accounts or small surveys. The U.S. Department of Agriculture (USDA) began collecting information about the supply of basic food commodities in 1909, about household food consumption practices in 1936-37, and about the food intake of individuals only in 1965.[1] Earlier dietary practices can only be inferred, and cannot easily be correlated with health status except indirectly through changes in disease rates or life expectancy.

Nevertheless, from the time of its creation in 1862, the USDA was expected to perform two functions. One was to ensure a sufficient and reliable food supply. The other was to "diffuse among the people of the United States useful information on subjects connected with agriculture in the most general and comprehensive sense of that word."[2] This last was interpreted as a mandate to issue dietary advice. In early years, the two functions seemed perfectly compatible. Both promoted a greater and more varied food supply. By the early 1890s, the USDA began to sponsor studies on the relationship between agriculture and human nutrition, and it appointed W. O. Atwater as the first director of research activities. Atwater published tables that listed the content of calories, protein, carbohydrate, fat, and "mineral matters" in common American foods. He also estimated the amounts of food needed to meet the nutrient requirements of people performing different levels of work. His analysis of the eating habits of New England laborers and professionals, for example, confirmed "the general impression of hygienists that our diet is one-sided and that we eat too much . . . fat, starch, and sugar. This is due partly to our large consumption of sugar and partly to our use of such large quantities of fat meats. . . . How much harm is done to health by our one-sided and excessive diet no one can say. Physicians tell us that it is very great."[3]

Atwater believed that American men required more calories and protein than recommended by European physiologists of that era because people in this country worked harder. He suggested that men doing moderate work required about 3,500 calories daily, with a distribution that calculates to about 15% of calories from protein, 33% from fat, and 52% from carbohydrate. This intake level exceeds current recommendations by about 1,000 daily calories, but Atwater was ahead of his time; the proportions of protein, fat, and carbohydrate are quite similar to those currently advised.

Atwater's advice said nothing about vitamins. Although classic vitamin-deficiency diseases such as scurvy, beriberi, and pellagra were understood to be associated with diet in some way, their specific causes were unknown and no vitamin had as yet been isolated. Early in the twentieth century, as scientists began to identify the structure and function of one vitamin after another, the USDA immediately translated these scientific advances into advice for consumers. By 1915 or so, the agency had produced at least 30 pamphlets to inform "housekeepers" about the nutritive value of foods, the role of specific foods in the diet, and foods appropriate for young children at home or at school.

Food Groups

In 1917, the USDA issued its first set of overall dietary recommendations as a 14-page pamphlet, titled *How to Select Foods*. This document is remarkable for establishing precedents to which the agency still firmly adheres. It established the food-group format by organizing the food sources of nutrients then known to be needed for health into five categories: fruits and vegetables; meats and other protein-rich foods (including milk for children); cereals and other starchy foods; sweets; and fatty foods. It also established principles that continue to govern USDA policy on dietary advice. The pamphlet did not "recommend any special foods or combinations of foods. It tells very simply what the body needs to obtain from its food for building its tissues, keeping it in good working order, and providing it with fuel or energy for its muscular work. It shows in a general way how the different food materials meet these needs and groups them according to their uses in the body."[4] As we shall see, this approach permits all foods to be recommended as part of healthful diets and precludes suggestions to restrict foods in one or another group.

At the time, the USDA ignored Atwater's advice to limit intake of fat and sugar, and its publications emphasized the newly discovered "micronutrients," the vitamins and minerals that are essential for life but are needed only in small amounts. Food manufacturers and agricultural producers readily supported this emphasis because they grasped its marketing potential. They knew that the market for their products was limited. Food *already* was overabundant in the United States and *already* supplied more than enough calories for the population. Food producers could exploit the discoveries of vitamins and minerals to promote their products as vital for health and longevity. Because all food animals and plants contain vitamins and minerals, *all* could be promoted on this basis. A 1923 USDA publication emphasized this point: "The number of different food materials available in most parts of the United States is very great and is constantly increasing as a result of improved methods of agriculture. . . . There is no one of all these many foods that cannot be introduced into the diet in such a way as to contribute to its wholesomeness or its attractiveness."[5]

During the 1920s, the USDA used five food groups—still including fat and sugar—as the basis of its dietary advice to families, mothers of young children, and teenagers. By the 1930s, the agency had identified certain "protective" foods as especially rich sources of vitamins and minerals. It issued many pamphlets emphasizing the need to prevent deficiencies of essential nutrients by eating more servings from groups of such foods. The number of these groups varied, however, in part because of concerns about the effect of the high cost of "protective" foods on consumer purchases. A Depression-era food guide, for example, explained that food selection has far-reaching implications for agriculture and that producers want "to know how much of different foods may well appear in the diets of different consumer groups, and to what extent consumption may rise or fall as the economic situation changes."[6] That particular guide increased the number of food groups to 12 and, for the first time, included milk as a separate category.

In 1940, the U.S. National Academy of Sciences established a committee to advise the government about nutrition problems that might affect national defense; this committee became the Food and Nutrition Board in 1941. One of its first tasks was to establish standards for daily nutrient intake for the armed forces and for the general population.[7] The committee suggested Recommended Dietary Allowances (RDAs) for energy and eight nutrients at a conference in May 1941. Beginning in 1943, and continuing to the present day, such committees produced revisions of the RDAs at intervals of five to ten years. The USDA responded to the development of RDAs by making sure that its food guides described a dietary pattern that met those standards.

During World War II, the rationing of meat, sugar, butter, and canned goods inspired various federal agencies to develop food guides based on pragmatic considerations of food availability as well as theoretical considerations of nutrient standards. The result was a bewildering array of food groupings issued by various agencies. In 1942, federal pamphlets instructed Americans to "do your part in the national nutrition program" by eating foods from eight groups every day; four of these groups were milk, meat, eggs, and butter—all sources of fat and cholesterol as well as of essential vitamins and minerals.[8] The following year, the USDA issued the *National Wartime Nutrition Guide*: "U.S. needs us strong: eat the Basic 7 every day."[9] This guide combined meat, eggs, fish, and beans into one group, kept milk as a separate category, and retained fats and sugars as separate groups. The changing number of food groups revealed a lack of coordination not only among federal agencies but also within the same agency. In 1943, for example, the USDA published the *Basic 7* but also told wartime homemakers how to plan low- and moderate-cost meals based on foods from 11 groups.

Immediately following the end of World War II, USDA publications continued these inconsistencies. In 1946, the agency issued a peacetime version: "This is the Basic 7 guide for well-balanced meals. In time of emergency, you need to eat less of the scarce foods, more of the plentiful. Food is needed to feed the hungry—don't waste it."[10] Two months later, it issued *Food for Growth: Food for Freedom*, targeted to children in the fourth through sixth grades. This publication was the first to recommend selections from just four food groups—milk; vegetables and fruits; eggs, meat, poultry, or fish (sometimes dried beans or peas); and a fourth category that included bread, cereal, cookies, and cakes.[11] These guides actively promoted consumption of fats and sweets, even to children. Together, they continued to promote "eat more."

Eating more received further support in the early 1950s when USDA nutritionists compared the results of a survey of nationwide food consumption practices to the most recent RDAs, realized that the diets of many Americans were below standard for several nutrients, and decided to construct a new food guide to help "the average person choose his food more wisely."[12] They simplified the four groups: milk (retaining its position as a separate category); meats (including beans and peas as alternatives); vegetables and fruits; and breads and cereals. To ensure that the guide would describe a diet that met RDA standards they also—for the first time—specified the number and size of servings within each group.

In an effort to achieve consensus on these innovations, the USDA invited leading nutrition authorities in government, research, the food industry, and agricultural commodity groups to review preliminary drafts because it "felt that food industry groups would have a vital interest in any food guide sponsored by the government." Indeed they did. Dairy producers were pleased with the treatment given to milk and milk products—the guide placed the milk group first. Meat industry groups were said to be "unhappy about the serving size indicated for meat. . . . They pointed out that this size is smaller than average."[12] The proposed serving sizes included two daily portions of 2–3 ounces of cooked meat, then (as now) less than what people usually eat at any one time.

Despite the complaints, the USDA incorporated these serving sizes first into a handbook for nutrition professionals and later into a guide for the general public known popularly as the *Basic Four*. This last is illustrated in Figure 6. Remarkably, the USDA used versions of the *Basic*

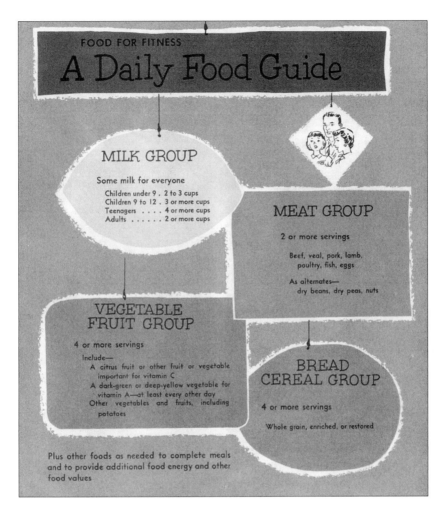

FIGURE 6. The 1958 *"Basic Four"* food guide established minimum levels of daily servings to prevent nutritional deficiencies. Milk and meat producers appreciated its "eat more" implication. This guide became obsolete in the late 1970s when the focus of dietary advice shifted from prevention of nutrient deficiencies to prevention of chronic diseases.

Four for the next 22 years, although it continued to base family meal and cost plans on 11 food groups. Except for the concern about portion size (an early warning of battles yet to come) food producer groups supported the USDA's efforts to promote consumption of more—and more varied—foods.

More "Eat More": Preventing Hunger

In the late 1960s, support for promoting "eat more" came from an entirely new direction. In 1967, a report of an investigation of hunger and malnutrition among low-income groups in the United States became the subject of a CBS television documentary, *Hunger in America*. At the time, the idea that people were going hungry in the land of plenty seemed so shocking that the program elicited widespread demands for expansion of federal food assistance programs. As a later report explained, "The failure of federal efforts to feed the poor cannot be divorced from our nation's agricultural policy, the congressional committees that dictate that policy, and the Department of Agriculture that implements it; for hunger and malnutrition in a country of abundance must be seen as consequences of a political and economic system that spends billions to remove food from the market, to limit production, to retire land from production, to guarantee and sustain profits for large producers of basic crops."[13]

In July 1968, the Senate responded to the public outcry by appointing George McGovern (Dem-SD) to chair a Select Committee on Nutrition and Human Needs that would lead "the war against hunger among the nation's young, old and poor."[14] For the next nine years, McGovern's committee created laws to expand food assistance for families, children, and the elderly through programs such as Food Stamps that still constitute the basis of the nation's "safety net" for the poor. Both the public and Congress strongly encouraged these "eat more" activities, giving the McGovern committee license to meddle in other areas of nutrition and health.

THE SHIFT TO "EAT LESS": PREVENTING CHRONIC DISEASE, 1969–1990

The ironic result of the McGovern committee's subsequent meddling was a sharp transition in federal dietary advice from "eat more" to "eat less" and from dietary advice as a relatively uncontroversial government activity to one that brought on outraged protest. By telling the public about dietary risks for chronic disease, the committee alarmed producers of foods that might be targeted as "bad." As one of its first actions, for example, the committee helped organize the 1969 White House Conference on Food, Nutrition, and Health. Participants not only discussed

TABLE 6. Ancel and Margaret Keys' 1959 dietary guidelines for prevention of coronary heart disease

1. Do not get fat, if you are fat, reduce.
2. Restrict saturated fats, the fats in beef, pork, lamb, sausages, margarine, solid shortenings, fats in dairy products.
3. Prefer vegetable oils to solid fats, but keep total fats under 30% of your diet calories.
4. Favor fresh vegetables, fruits, and non-fat milk products.
5. Avoid heavy use of salt and refined sugar.
6. Good diets do not depend on drugs and fancy preparations.
7. Get plenty of exercise and outdoor recreation.
8. Be sensible about cigarettes, alcohol, excitement, business strain.
9. See your doctor regularly, and do not worry.

Keys A, Keys M. *Eat Well and Stay Well.* New York: Doubleday, 1959.

nutritional deficiencies in the United States, but also the "health problems of adults in an affluent society—the degenerative diseases of middle age" caused by "overconsumption of calories with food choices that are not necessarily the wisest on the basis of available nutritional information."[15] Among hundreds of conference recommendations were suggestions to eat less of the "unwise" food choices—those containing too many calories and too much fat, cholesterol, salt, sugar, and alcohol.

The "affluent-society" panel at the conference—and the staff of the McGovern committee—were well aware of the emerging research that linked the high levels of these factors in American diets to risks for chronic disease. Much of this research had been accomplished by cardiologists appalled by the apparent "epidemic" of coronary heart disease among Americans that followed World War II. They could not help but be impressed by the contrasting absence of this disease among populations consuming largely plant-based diets. In 1959, the physician-researcher Ancel Keys and his wife published a "healthy-heart" cookbook suggesting the now-classic dietary principles summarized in Table 6. The American Heart Association had sponsored research on dietary fat and atherosclerosis in the mid-1950s; in the 1960s, it advised people to reduce calories from fat, and it recommended dietary changes and public policies to reduce risk factors for coronary heart disease in the early 1970s. These changes were to reduce intake of fat (to 35% of calories or less), saturated fat (to 10%), and cholesterol (to 300 milligrams per day) and by implication to eat less of foods containing those substances.

On that basis, the McGovern committee urged the National Institutes of Health (NIH) to support research on the ways in which dietary changes might prevent coronary heart and other chronic diseases. Committee staff members considered it odd that so little attention had been paid to the role of diet in health. They viewed classic problems of undernutrition as "a problem for a small but significant part of the population." As they explained, "malnutrition had two faces and . . . overconsumption was a major health concern for at least 30 million Americans."[16] To focus national attention on the *overconsumption* aspect of malnutrition, the committee held hearings on how diet affected obesity, diabetes, and heart disease in 1973 and issued a staff report on diet and chronic disease in 1974. In 1976, the committee initiated a new series of hearings with the riveting title "Diet Related to Killer Diseases." At the very first of these hearings, more than 30 witnesses described how eating too much of the wrong kinds of food would increase risks for cancer, cardiovascular disease, and obesity.[17] "Eat less" recommendations had become inevitable.

Dietary Goals: Issued, Opposed, Revised, 1977

On the basis of such testimony, the committee staff wrote the soon-to-be-infamous report, *Dietary Goals for the United States,* and released it at a press conference in January 1977. The report stated six goals, of which the first was to *increase* carbohydrate consumption to 55–60% of caloric intake. The remaining five, however, clearly meant *eat less;* reduce fat (to 30% of calories), saturated fat (to 10%), cholesterol (to 300 milligrams per day), sugar (to 15% of calories), and salt (to 3 grams per day). To meet the goals, Americans would need to eat more fruit, vegetables, whole grains, poultry, and fish. However, they also would have to *reduce* their intake of meat, eggs, and foods high in fat, butterfat, sugar, and salt, and to substitute nonfat milk for whole milk. These last recommendations generated nothing less than an uproar.

Cattle ranchers, egg producers, sugar producers, and the dairy industry registered strong protest at the very idea that Congress might be telling the public that their products were bad for health. The cattle industry, especially in McGovern's home state of South Dakota, demanded the report's immediate withdrawal. Meat and egg producers called for—and got—additional hearings to express their views. The hearing transcripts make fascinating reading that clearly reveals the interests at stake. For example,

Senator Robert Dole (Rep-KS), then a minority member of the committee, offered the president of the National Cattlemen's Association, Mr. Wray Finney, a compromise on the wording of the most disputed recommendation, "decrease consumption of meat" (here referred to as No. 2):

> SENATOR DOLE: I wonder if you could amend No. 2 and say "increase consumption of lean meat"? Would that taste better to you?
>
> MR. FINNEY: Decrease is a bad word, Senator.[18]

Members of the committee who represented states with large meat producer constituencies insisted that the report be revised. Senator McGovern himself was quoted as saying that "he did not want to disrupt the economic situation of the meat industry and engage in a battle with that industry that we could not win."[19]

In all fairness, food producers had plenty of company in their objections to the *Dietary Goals*. Some scientists were unhappy with the report, citing unproven science and the need for further expert review. One went so far as to call it "a nutritional debacle."[20] The American Medical Association (AMA) argued that treating individual patients (by its physician members of course) was preferable to the government's giving dietary advice that applied to everyone. The AMA also noted that "the recommendations carry with them the underlying potential for . . . discouraging the agricultural production of certain food products which may not in the view of the government be supportive of the *dietary goals*."[21]

Although opposition to the *Dietary Goals* often was expressed as skepticism about the quality of the underlying science, it derived more directly from the profound economic implications of the advice. For example, meat (beef, lamb, pork), poultry, fish, dairy foods, and eggs provided 50% of the fat, 62% of the saturated fat, and 94% of the cholesterol in the food supply in 1970.[22] To advise the public to consume less fat, saturated fat, and cholesterol was to advocate eating less of these foods, as well as of processed foods high in fats and oils. By 1977 this message was well understood by nutrition scientists, dietitians, and consumer activists and had already been reflected in declining sales of whole milk and eggs. When these trends continued—and beef sales also began to decline—food producer groups made more serious attempts to discredit, weaken, and eliminate dietary advice to eat less of their products.

Under intense pressure, the McGovern committee capitulated and issued a revised edition of the *Dietary Goals* late in 1977. The second edition strengthened advice about obesity and alcohol but made three changes designed expressly to placate food producers. The new recommendations

· Increased the salt allowance from 3 to 5 grams per day.
· Added the statement "some consideration should be given to easing the cholesterol goal for pre-menopausal women, young children and the elderly in order to obtain the nutritional benefits of eggs in the diet."
· Replaced the statement "reduce consumption of meat" with the less offensive "choose meats, poultry, and fish which will reduce saturated fat intake."[23]

The aftermath constituted its own drama. Nick Mottern, the committee staff member who had drafted the original report, objected to the compromises and was asked to resign. When Senator McGovern said that McDonald's and other such foods were "on the whole . . . a nutritious addition to a balanced diet," it seemed that "still another industry has thrown its weight around."[24] Regardless, publication of the *Dietary Goals* was the committee's last accomplishment. In February 1977, shortly after the appearance of the first edition, the Senate voted to "merge" McGovern's committee into a subcommittee of the Committee on Agriculture, Nutrition, and Forestry by the end of that year. The furor over the *Dietary Goals* did nothing to help Senator McGovern's political career. He was defeated when he ran for reelection in 1980.

Mobilizing Support for "Eat Less" Advice, 1978–1979

Despite the compromises, the *Dietary Goals* proved to be a turning point; the report set a standard for all subsequent dietary recommendations and changed the course of nutrition education in the United States. For example, the American Society for Clinical Nutrition (an organization of professors and physicians who conduct research on human nutrition) convened a committee in 1978 to respond to the "biased arguments" of scientists who had opposed the *Dietary Goals* and to conduct a major review of the existing research. The committee would "avoid the advocacy role and . . . constitute a consensus that would be of help to public officials in formulating national policy."[25] To the surprise of many, the committee concluded that research demonstrated impressive increases in disease risks from consuming too much fat, cholesterol, salt, sugar, and alcohol, and that the risks could be reduced by eating less of these factors and, therefore, their food sources.

The American Heart Association provided additional professional support for the *Dietary Goals* in 1978 when its scientists reiterated their long-standing advice to eat less fat, saturated fat, and cholesterol. In 1979 the National Cancer Institute (NCI) issued recommendations consistent with the *Dietary Goals* in its first statement on the role of diet in cancer risk. By the late 1970s, scientists were in substantial (if not perfect) agreement that similar dietary changes could help prevent the two most important causes of death in the United States—coronary heart disease and cancer.[26]

Healthy People In 1979 the Department of Health, Education, and Welfare (DHEW) issued *Healthy People*, a report from the surgeon general, intended to "encourage a second public health revolution in the history of the United States. And let us make no mistake about the significance of this document. It represents an emerging consensus among scientists and the health community that the Nation's health strategy must be dramatically recast to emphasize the prevention of disease."[27]

This report kicked off the Public Health Service's subsequent—and still ongoing—development of ten-year plans to improve the health of the nation. In a small section on nutrition, *Healthy People* advised eating more complex carbohydrates, more fish, and more poultry but less of the usual culprits (calories, saturated fat, cholesterol, salt, and sugar) and also *less red meat*. Noting that half the diet consists of processed foods, it also suggested that the nutritional qualities of those foods needed attention. Because advice to eat less meat and be wary of processed foods might be expected to attract unwelcome attention, officials released the report without a press conference as one of the last official acts of Joseph Califano, who had been fired from his position as DHEW Secretary by President Carter the month before. Even so, the report elicited a "storm of protest" from the meat industry. The president of the National Live Stock and Meat Board summarized industry views by noting that the report started with the words "the health of the American people has never been better, and we think it should have ended right there."[28]

Healthy People became the last federal publication to explicitly advise "eat less red meat." When later questioned about that statement, Surgeon General Julius Richmond speculated that subsequent editions of the report might instead advise people to switch to *lean* meat.[29] Table 7 charts the progress of this creatively euphemistic approach to advice about meat, from the *Basic Four* to reports issued at the end of the twentieth century.

TABLE 7. Evolution of federal recommendations to reduce dietary fat through changes in meat consumption

Year	*Report,* Agency	Meat Recommendation	Amount (oz/day)
1958	*Basic Four*, USDA	2 servings	4–6
1977	*Dietary Goals*, U.S. Senate	Decrease consumption of meat	*
1977	*Dietary Goals*, 2nd ed., U.S. Senate	Choose meats . . . which will reduce saturated fat intake	*
1979	*Healthy People*, DHEW	[Consume] relatively . . . less red meat	*
1979	*Food*, USDA	2 servings Cut down on fatty meats	4–6
1980	*Dietary Guidelines,* USDA and DHHS	Choose lean meats	*
1985	Dietary Guidelines, 2nd ed., USDA and DHHS	Choose lean meats	*
1988	*Surgeon General's Report*, DHHS	Choose lean meats	*
1990	*Dietary Guidelines*, 3rd ed., USDA and DHHS	Have 2 or 3 servings	6
1992	*Food Guide Pyramid*, USDA	Choose lean meat (2–3 servings)	5-7
1995	*Dietary Guidelines*, 4th ed., USDA and DHHS	Choose 2 to 3 servings of lean . . . meats Limit intake of high-fat processed meats Limit intake of organ meats	4–9
2000	*Dietary Guidelines*, 5th ed., USDA and DHHS	Choose 2 to 3 servings of . . . lean meats Limit . . . intake of high-fat processed meats Limit . . . intake of liver and other organ meats Limit use of animal fats	4–9

*Indicates that the report did not specify number of servings, ounces, or ounces per serving.

The USDA's Food Books   USDA nutritionists, meanwhile could not believe that people might actually follow diets that seemed "so disruptive to usual food patterns," and they wrote a series of publications to help people meet the *Dietary Goals*.[30] Their first attempt, *Food: The Hassle-Free*

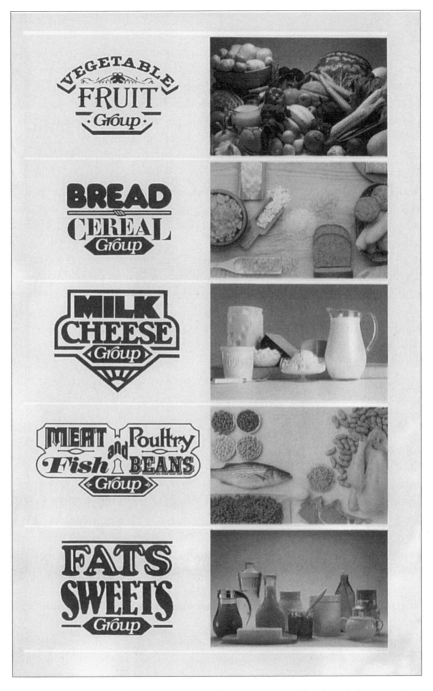

FIGURE 7. Food producers objected to this 1979 USDA food guide because it displayed the dairy and meat groups *below* the fruit, vegetable, and grain groups and close to the "eat less" category of fats, sweets, and alcohol.

Guide to a Better Diet, appeared cautiously neutral on matters of diet
and health: "Many scientists say the American diet is contributing to
some of the chronic diseases that hit people in later life. . . . Other scientists believe just as strongly that the evidence doesn't support such conclusions. So the choice is yours."[31] This guide, however, displayed the
vegetable/fruit and bread/cereal groups above the dairy and meat groups,
and it added a fifth group of foods at the bottom—fats/sweets/alcohol—
that keep bad "nutritional company" (see Figure 7). To reduce fat intake,
it suggested, "cut down on fatty meats." This time, the meat, dairy, and
egg industries complained not only about the eat less advice, but also
about what they perceived as the unfavorable placement of their food
groups below the plant food groups.

According to Carol Tucker Foreman, then Assistant USDA Secretary
for Food and Consumer Services, *Food* was the USDA's most requested
publication in 1979.[32] After the 1980 election, however, she and other
proponents of such advice lost their politically appointed positions, and
food producers found a more favorable reception for their complaints.
The new regime at the USDA did not reprint the guide and suspended work
on subsequent publications in the series. Instead, the USDA gave the completed page boards to the American Dietetic Association, which issued the
guide as two separate booklets in 1982.[33] *Food* was the last USDA publication to suggest *any* restriction on meat intake for the next 16 years.

Seeking Compromise: Dietary Guidelines for Americans, *1980*

In an attempt to give the public advice that would not cause a political
backlash, the USDA and the agency that succeeded DHEW, the Department of Health and Human Services (DHHS)—"with the fanfare of Moses
unveiling the tablets," —jointly released the *Dietary Guidelines for Americans* in February 1980.[34] Its seemingly innocuous recommendations
were to "Eat a variety of foods; Maintain ideal weight; Avoid too much
fat, saturated fat, and cholesterol; Eat foods with adequate starch and
fiber; Avoid too much sugar; Avoid too much sodium; If you drink alcohol, do so in moderation."[35]

Because they had replaced the unacceptable *eat less* phrases with the
vague *avoid too much*, agency officials expected few objections from
food producers. As USDA Secretary Bob Bergland said during the press
conference, "They feared we might issue edicts like eat no meat, or
eggs, and drink less whole milk. They have been waiting for the other
shoe to fall. There is no shoe."[34] Indeed, the Food Marketing Institute

(FMI), a trade organization representing supermarket chains, promised to distribute the *Guidelines* to its members because they are "simple, reasonable and offer great freedom of choice." Even the American Meat Institute (AMI) found the *Guidelines* helpful as they called for "a continuing and central role for meat."[29]

Other segments of the food industry, however, read between the lines and realized that the *Guidelines* merely repeated the *Dietary Goals* in less direct terms. Although they might have seemed bland and uncontroversial, they too elicited an "unbelievable outcry of charges and countercharges, editorials in prestigious newspapers, and congressional hearings."[36] One reporter readily explained the outcry: "The political *raison d'etre* for the Department of Agriculture is to make it easier for farmers to make money. And that purpose is not well served by permitting the people in Bethesda, Md., to run loose on such politically sensitive matters as red meat, butter, and eggs."[34]

In May, the National Academy of Sciences' Food and Nutrition Board issued a counter-report stating that healthy people should not have to restrict intake of fat or cholesterol. Critics charged that the report's dissent from the new Dietary Guidelines came from scientists with demonstrable ties to the meat, dairy, and egg industries.[37] Embarrassed by the disclosure, the Academy reorganized the Board. In 1982 its new members—with fewer ties to industry—issued a report on diet and cancer that supported the *Guidelines* and advised limits on intake of meats high in fat and salt, particularly cured meats such as bacon, hot dogs, and sausages, to reduce carcinogens. Meat producers, incensed, held the report responsible for a subsequent fall in livestock prices, and pork producers induced seven members of Congress to demand an investigation.[38] Protests were joined by some scientists concerned that the evidence relating diet to cancer was less than compelling: "The credibility of nutritional science is not enhanced by lowering the standards for critical assessment of evidence."[39]

Heading toward Consensus, 1981–1990

One of the more ironic aspects of this history is that federal agencies were able to forge a broad—and unexpected—consensus on dietary advice during the conservative era of the Reagan administration. When Ronald Reagan was elected president in November 1980, the *Dietary Guidelines* seemed doomed. Congress, ostensibly to ensure that all government agencies would speak with "one voice" on the subject of diet and health, immediately directed federal agencies to work with the Food and Nutrition Board to revise them. The new USDA Secretary, John Block, was an Illinois hog farmer; during his confirmation hearings, he had remarked that he was "not so sure government should get into telling people what they should or shouldn't eat."[40] Two high-level USDA positions had been filled by a former executive director of the American Meat Institute and a lobbyist for the National Cattlemen's Association (a tradition cherished to this day). In addition, one of Secretary Block's first acts had been to eliminate the USDA's Human Nutrition Center, a unit that promoted the interests of consumers rather than producers. Further, when the USDA and DHHS first appointed the new committee to revise the *Dietary Guidelines*, consumer groups charged that five of the six USDA nominees had close connections to food companies with vested interests in the advice. One prospective DHHS appointee threatened to resign, stating that he had "no intention of being part of a process that guts the guidelines."[41]

To the surprise of critics, however, the revised *Guidelines* appeared in 1985 with trivial changes in just three words: "maintain ideal weight" became "maintain desirable weight," and "alcohol" became "alcoholic beverages."[42] USDA Secretary Block, joined by the National Cattlemen's Association, endorsed the new *Guidelines*, explaining that "all of us have changed in our thinking."[43] This reversal came about as a result of a growing agreement that the preponderance of scientific evidence really did support *Dietary Goals* and *Guidelines*. One group after another issued dietary recommendations for prevention of one disease or another, all of the advice strikingly similar. The strongest support continued to come from heart disease groups such as the American Heart Association, which issued policy statements on diet and heart disease risk throughout the 1980s; its recommendations were endorsed by many other groups such as the American Medical Association and an NIH consensus panel. In the mid-1980s, the National Heart, Lung, and Blood Institute (NHLBI) announced a national campaign to lower blood cholesterol across the entire population, beginning with advice to reduce intake of fat and saturated fat. Although some physicians argued that people did not need to restrict their diets until doctors told them to, the NHLBI judged scientific support for a population-wide campaign sufficiently strong to justify its implementation. Groups concerned about cancer, diabetes, and high blood pressure also issued guidelines. Because the similarities of the various sets of recommendations far exceeded their differences, the *Dietary Guidelines* appeared to constitute a universal and commonly accepted approach to reducing risks for a broad range of chronic diseases.

The idea that the *Dietary Guidelines* represented a broad consensus received substantial support when four authoritative research reviews appeared one right after the other in the late 1980s. Oddly, the first was a report on meat from the National Academy of Sciences' Board on Agriculture. It had been sponsored by trade associations such as the American Meat Institute, the National Cattlemen's Association, and the National Pork Producers Council, whose members were becoming alarmed about the potential effect of fat guidelines on meat consumption. Indeed, the report confirmed the need to reduce fat intake and challenged the industry to start raising leaner meat. It was followed just months later by the massive *Surgeon General's Report on Nutrition and Health* and by the even lengthier *Diet and Health* report from the Food and Nutrition Board in 1989. An analogous summary from the World Health Organization's 32-country European region also had been issued in 1988.[44] All four reports identified the need to restrict fat, particularly saturated fat, as a public health priority. Because none elicited much critical comment, it appeared that scientists at last had agreed on dietary principles and that the food industry was resigned to dealing with the consensus rather than fighting it. We shall soon see that neither of these assumptions proved correct.

Consensus at the Expense of Clarity: Dietary Guidelines, 1990

Despite the apparent scientific agreement, USDA political appointees argued that emerging research established a need to reexamine the *Dietary Guidelines*. Claiming that the USDA was the "lead agency" for dietary advice to the public, they pressed for and obtained appointment of yet another new committee to reconsider the issue. This one consisted of nutrition scientists and physicians with few apparent ties to the food industry, although groups representing food producers, trade associations, or organizations allied with industry submitted written suggestions, as had become customary during committee reviews.

The revision process revealed that a consensus of sorts had been achieved—but at the price of clarity. To address concerns that some foods might be perceived as "bad," the committee noted that *any* food that supplies calories or nutrients should be recognized as useful in a nutritious diet. Furthermore, the committee altered the wording of some guidelines to make them more positive and less restrictive. For the phrase "avoid too much," it substituted "choose a diet low in." For "choose lean meat," it substituted "have two or three servings of meat." The committee did suggest upper limits of 30% of calories from fat and 10% from saturated fat—precisely those recommended by the 1977 *Dietary Goals*—but lest that advice appear too restrictive, it emphasized that the goals for fat "apply to the diet over several days, not to a single meal or food. Some foods that contain fat, saturated fat, and cholesterol, such as meats, milk, cheese, and eggs, also contain high-quality protein and are our best sources of certain vitamins and minerals."[45] This edition of the *Guidelines* elicited no public complaints from food producers, reinforcing the apparent consensus.

Thus many scientists in government and in the private sector had become convinced by 1990 that the preponderance of evidence supported recommendations for dietary restrictions. Increasing public interest in nutrition during the 1980s also had affected receptivity to such advice. Consumer demands for information, purchase of foods perceived as "healthy," and rejection of foods perceived as "unhealthy," created a public base of support for federal pronouncements on the role of diet in health. As a result—and perhaps most important—the food industry came to recognize the potential uses of dietary goals and guidelines for marketing purposes. Companies stopped complaining about dietary precepts and instead began *using* them, noting that guidelines "will encourage companies to develop products for nutrition conscious consumers" and that consumer demand would prompt "food companies to call attention to healthful properties of existing products and introduce a wide array of high fiber, low sodium, low fat and low cholesterol products."[46]

The food industry also pressured federal agencies to develop labeling regulations that would permit them to use health claims on food products. By 1989, some of us who had worked on the *Surgeon General's Report on Nutrition and Health* concluded that "the fundamental consistency of dietary recommendations for health promotion and disease prevention, though long obscured by controversy, is now generally accepted."[47] We believed that with consensus achieved and the controversy resolved, we could now focus attention on ways to put the guidelines into practice. Such optimism turned out to be naive as the next chapter reveals.

CHAPTER 2

POLITICS VERSUS SCIENCE

OPPOSING THE FOOD PYRAMID, 1991–1992

LATE IN APRIL 1991, I RECEIVED A PHONE CALL FROM MALCOLM Gladwell, then a reporter at the *Washington Post*, asking for an opinion on the latest furor over dietary advice. The recently appointed Secretary of the U.S. Department of Agriculture (USDA), former Congressman Edward R. Madigan, had just blocked the printing of the Department's latest food guide—the *Eating Right Pyramid*—because it was "confusing to children." That guide is illustrated in Figure 8. Unlike the *Basic Four*, which presented the food groups in squares of roughly equal size (see Figure 6), the *Pyramid* is explicitly hierarchical; it illustrates a dietary pattern in which most daily food servings are to be derived from the grain, vegetable, and fruit groups, with fewer servings from the milk and meat groups, and even fewer from foods high in fat and sugar.[1]

Secretary Madigan's explanation seemed so patently absurd that it immediately suggested an alternative interpretation: pressure from the meat industry. My reaction was a surprised "Oh no, not this again." As I explained to Mr. Gladwell, the food industry had often been involved in dietary guidance, and the USDA "is in the position of being responsible to the agriculture business. That is their job. Nutrition isn't their job."[2] These comments appeared in the *Washington Post* on April 27. In the following week, copies of the *Eating Right Pyramid* and internal USDA letters and memoranda related to its development, approval, production, and withdrawal suddenly appeared in my "in" box. These items invariably arrived either in plain, unmarked envelopes with no return addresses or as anonymous transmissions from Washington, DC, hotel fax machines. When reporters called, I passed these materials

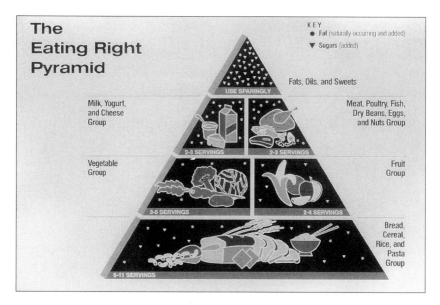

FIGURE 8. The USDA blocked publication of the 1991 *Eating Right Pyramid* under pressure from meat and dairy groups objecting to the position of their products in its hierarchy. This suppressed guide differs from the *Food Guide Pyramid* (Figure 1) mainly in its title and in the placement of the numbers of servings.

along. Much of what I know of this episode is based on such documents, the use that reporters made of them in press accounts, unofficial USDA memoranda, and telephone conversations with people who insisted on anonymity.

The USDA could not possibly have been acting in the interest of schoolchildren; that age group never had been the designated audience for federal food guides. Instead, the USDA was responding to meat and dairy producers complaining that the placement of their food groups in the narrower, "eat less" sectors of the *Pyramid* caused their products to be "stigmatized."[3] The ensuing controversy differed from previous incidents in one critical respect—the intensity of public scrutiny. Reporters seized on this story right from the start and never let go of it. For a year, the *Pyramid* remained front-page news. Then, after spending nearly a million dollars on further research, the USDA released a revised version— The *Food Guide Pyramid*—differing from the original in only minor details (see Figure 1). Those details, however, sufficiently appeased meat and dairy producers who withdrew their overt objections.[4]

Although the withdrawal of the *Pyramid* can be viewed as just another example of government's caving in to industry pressure, it merits especially close attention as an indicator of two issues of much broader public importance: the conflict of interest created by the USDA's dual mandates to protect agriculture and to advise the public about diet and health, and the undue influence of lobbyists in this area, as well as in other areas of federal policy decisions.

BUILDING THE PYRAMID:
RESEARCHING AN "EAT LESS" FOOD GUIDE

This saga begins in the mid-1970s, in the wake of the controversy over the 1977 *Dietary Goals*. Congress was under pressure to support health promotion as a means to reduce the costs of health care. Some officials—but certainly not others—in each of two federal agencies, the USDA and the Department of Health, Education, and Welfare (DHEW), were competing for control of nutrition education and research. Although it might seem logical that oversight of nutrition belongs in a health agency rather than one devoted to agriculture, USDA officials appointed by President Jimmy Carter, a Democrat, wanted control over this policy area. The conflict was resolved in favor of the USDA when the ailing Senator Hubert Humphrey (Dem-MN) said that "HEW has avoided the area of prevention like the plague, and it's about time that USDA moves in. It's going to take this aspect of the nutrition program whether it wants to or not."[5] In the 1977 Farm Bill (Public Law 95-113), Congress granted the USDA responsibility for a wide range of nutrition activities shared with DHEW—including dietary advice to the public. With this mandate, USDA staff nutritionists pressed forward with plans for a new food guide to help the public prevent nutrient deficiencies and also meet the *Dietary Goal* percentage targets for prevention of chronic diseases.

In 1988, in an effort to force the two agencies to issue consistent dietary advice and speak with "one voice," the House Appropriations Committee reaffirmed USDA's "lead-agency" responsibility for dietary guidance.[6] "Consistency" in this case meant advice favorable to agriculture. The committee's explicit intent was to prevent the successor agency to DHEW, the Department of Health and Human Services (DHHS), from issuing independent dietary advice that might adversely affect agricultural interests. DHHS objected strongly to the wording of the House report on the grounds that agencies under its jurisdiction—the Food and Drug Administration (FDA), the Centers for Disease Control (CDC), and the National Institutes of Health (NIH)—were more appropriately responsible for education and research on diet and health. DHHS also noted that it shared responsibility with USDA for ongoing editions of *Dietary Guidelines*. Congress ignored these objections and continued to grant USDA lead-agency responsibility for dietary advice to the public. But because dietary advice increasingly meant "eat less," USDA's dual mandates to protect agricultural producers and to advise the public about diet created increasing levels of conflict.

With this background, we can now return to the origins of the *Pyramid*. As we have seen, the 1980 *Dietary Guidelines* were designed to alleviate the food industry's concerns about the *Dietary Goals* and yet advise the public about ways to reduce dietary risks for chronic disease. The specific precepts of the *Guidelines* referred mainly to nutrients—fat, salt, and sugar—not to foods that contain them. Although the *Guidelines* govern the content of all government nutrition programs and educational materials, they are not generally known or understood by the public, and nutritionists in USDA's Human Nutrition Information Service (HNIS) thought it would be helpful to develop a new guide that translated advice about nutrients into more readily understandable advice about food choices. They particularly wanted to establish a research basis for the guide and to conduct a study—scientific, fully documented, and open to peer review—to determine the optimal numbers and sizes of servings from each food group.[7]

During the next three years, HNIS staff developed and documented the research basis for a food guide. They established nutritional goals, defined food groups, assigned serving sizes, and determined the number of servings that would prevent nutrient deficiencies and yet be low in fat, saturated, fat, and cholesterol. The basic elements of the new guide were well established by 1984 when HNIS used them in a Food Wheel for a course run by the American Red Cross. This wheel was divided into sectors proportional to the number of daily servings recommended for each group: 6–11 grains, 2–4 fruits, 3–5 vegetables, and 2–3 servings each from the meat and dairy groups. Fats, sweets, and alcohol were placed in a narrow sector labeled "moderation." This design seemed especially cluttered and difficult to interpret, and food industry officials requested changes in the text to downplay any "eat less" suggestions.[8] Thus the HNIS staff wanted to try something different, preferably something with an "appealing" illustration that would help people remember the most important messages: *variety* (multiple food groups), *proportionality* (appropriate numbers of servings), and *moderation* (restrictions on fat and sugar). Unlike previous USDA food guides, the *Pyramid* had a conceptual basis and, as we shall see, a research basis.

During the mid-1980s, HNIS staff thoroughly reviewed the food grouping system and the numbers and sizes of servings and used them without incident in several publications, most prominently a set of brochures to help people implement the *1985 Dietary Guidelines*.[9] The comprehensive reports on diet and health published in the late 1980s provided all the research support necessary to confirm the need for the new food guide. In 1988, HNIS contracted with the Washington office of Porter–Novelli, a public relations and consumer research firm, to develop a graphical illustration that would convey the concepts of variety, proportionality, and moderation to adults with at least a high school education and average income. Porter–Novelli conducted focus groups to evaluate design options and found that people understood the concepts best when the food groups were displayed in an equilateral triangle ("pyramid") in horizontal bands. Focus group participants easily caught on to the proportionality concept: "One thing the pyramid idea gives you, as opposed to the '*Basic Four*,' is trying to remember how many of each—you look at it, and you know you are supposed to eat more of the bread and cereal and less of the dairy."[10]

During 1988 and 1989, HNIS staff worked on the text of the *Eating Right Pyramid*. The 1990 *Dietary Guidelines* brochure incorporated the *Pyramid* serving numbers, thereby granting them status as official components of federal nutrition policy. In 1990 and 1991, HNIS sent drafts of the *Pyramid* booklet to 36 leading nutrition experts for review, presented the design at 20 professional conferences, and discussed the guide with more than 20 newspaper, magazine, radio, and television reporters. Because the lead time for textbook publishing is long, they met with at least 30 publishers to arrange substitution of the *Pyramid* for older guides in forthcoming texts. In short the *Pyramid* was no secret. HNIS staff presentations at professional meetings were fully open, and anyone who attended knew that the guide was in progress. Furthermore, HNIS had submitted the manuscript of the *Pyramid* brochure to the entire USDA bureaucracy through its exhaustive review and "clearance" procedures. A committee representing ten USDA units as well as DHHS had thoroughly vetted the *Pyramid*; the brochure had successfully passed six levels of USDA policy review and three divisional reviews.[11] The *Pyramid* was public information. It was fully cleared for publication at every political level within USDA. In February 1991, 11 years after beginning work on the project, HNIS staff sent the page boards to the printer, where the

Pyramid was assigned a March publication date. Although color adjustments delayed the printing, HNIS staff expected the *Pyramid* to be issued in a press run of a million copies by late April 1991.

TOPPLING THE PYRAMID:
A DAY-BY-DAY STREAK OF BAD LUCK

The color adjustment turned out to be just the first setback in a run of spectacularly bad luck that culminated in the *Pyramid*'s withdrawal. The next setback, which occurred in March, was the appointment of Edward R. Madigan as the new Secretary of Agriculture. An 18-year Congressman (Rep-IL), and the ranking Republican on the House Agriculture Committee, Mr. Madigan had been encouraged to seek the position by commodity and farm groups. Whatever his personal views on dietary advice, he was new to the job and more accustomed to the do-as-you-please culture of Congress than to that of a federal agency with a permanent professional staff. Then, early in April, the bad luck continued one day after the next.

Wednesday, April 10

In her weekly "Eating Well" column, Marian Burros of the *New York Times* reported that a health-advocacy group based in Washington, DC, The Physicians Committee for Responsible Medicine (PCRM), had asked the USDA to replace the *Basic Four* with new food groups that were entirely *vegetarian*—fruits, grains, vegetables, and legumes—and included meat and dairy products only as minor options.[12] In case anyone might miss the "eat less meat" message, an accompanying cartoon displayed vegetables aggressively driving a tractor over meat with a sidebar headlined "Move over meat: four new food groups." Outraged protests followed. John Block, who had been USDA secretary during the Reagan administration but at that point was head of a pork industry trade association, called the proposed guidelines "the height of irresponsibility."[12] Other critics charged that the PCRM's "potentially dangerous" dietary advice disguised an underlying animal-rights agenda.[13] This story elevated the advice to eat less meat to front-page news.

Thursday, April 11

Joe Crea, then a food reporter for the *Orange County Register* in Southern California, often wrote stories based on interviews with Betty

Peterkin, a veteran USDA staff nutritionist. She told him about the *Pyramid*. Crea wrote an article comparing the *Pyramid*'s recommendations to those of the Physicians Committee. His story appeared with an illustration comparing the two guides and a quote from a representative of the American Dietetic Association "lamenting" that the PCRM recommendations had appeared first, because the *Pyramid* was "a far more balanced and sensible approach."[14] As was standard practice, this story went out over news wire services.

Saturday, April 13

Washington Post reporter Malcolm Gladwell noticed the *Orange County Register* story on the wire services and thought it worth pursuing; his editor advised him to expand it with interviews. His April 13 account featured the remarks of Dr. Joan Gussow, a professor of nutrition education at Columbia University. Praising the *Pyramid*, she said, "[T]here is no question that the basic food groups . . . gave the impression that the most important things were meats and dairy products. This is a real mark of progress." Mr. Gladwell also quoted William Castelli, the director of the Framingham Heart Study, saying that he thought it was great that USDA "is going to suggest that we pig out on cereals and legumes and use the other foods as a complement. The societies that do that now live healthier lives."[15] The story appeared with an illustration of the *Pyramid* on the front page. In yet another improbable coincidence, the National Cattlemen's Association (a lobbying group for beef producers) happened to be holding its annual meeting in Washington, DC, that very weekend. Its members could hardly miss the *Washington Post* story or its significance.

Monday, April 15

The final stroke of bad luck was this: the Cattlemen's meeting agenda included a scheduled visit with Secretary Madigan two days after the story appeared. According to one account, the secretary had "also learned of the *Pyramid* for the first time in Saturday's paper. 'I bet a lot of you were surprised,' he said to the ranchers when he walked into their April 15 meeting. . . . 'I'm the Secretary of Agriculture, and I was surprised too.'"[16] The cattlemen complained that the *Pyramid* would cause people to eat less meat and that meat should not be displayed so close to the fats and sugars. They joined the National Milk Producers Federation in demanding that USDA withdraw the *Pyramid*.[17] During the next ten days, other trade associations also protested. The head of the American Meat Institute, for example, was said to have written a letter to Secretary Madigan explaining that although he had "neither seen the *Pyramid* nor been consulted about it," he thought that to clear up confusion USDA should reject its adoption.[18]

Saturday, April 27

The *Washington Post* story containing my quote appeared two weeks later. It contained Secretary Madigan's statement about withdrawing the guide so it could be tested on schoolchildren and low-income adults. It also quoted a USDA spokeswoman who confirmed that the *Pyramid* had been "killed" but denied that industry complaints were the reason; instead, she said that it might confuse children. The article, however, led off with the phrase "Yielding to pressure from the meat and dairy industries," and it quoted a lobbyist for the National Milk Producers Federation claiming that "her group's concerns were one of the reasons the proposal was pulled."[2] It and the article in the *New York Times* used comments from interviews to highlight USDA's conflicts of interest related to dietary advice and the department's consistent history of responding to the interests of agricultural producers at the expense of public health.

DEFENDING THE PYRAMID: MOBILIZING SUPPORT

In the aftermath of the *Pyramid*'s withdrawal, the USDA received hundreds of protest letters from organizations such as the American Cancer Society, the Society for Nutrition Education, the Center for Science in the Public Interest, and the United Fresh Fruit and Vegetable Association. The American Medical Association passed a resolution calling on President Bush to transfer responsibility for dietary guidance from USDA to DHHS. In early May, the House Committee on Government Operations demanded that USDA provide all of its records on the *Pyramid* as a basis for holding hearings (these never were held). At hearings of the House Agricultural Subcommittee, however, George Brown (Dem-CA) argued that USDA's actions regarding the *Pyramid* and other matters made it clear that "it is time to assess the pros and cons of moving nutrition research, education and monitoring responsibilities to another department."[19]

During the next weeks and months, the national press wrote one story after another about the *Pyramid*'s demise and its larger significance for the USDA's—and the government's—favoritism to corporate interests. The press reports were remarkable on other grounds, as well: They cited anonymous USDA staff as sources of the information, included illustrations of the suppressed *Pyramid* design, and voiced strong skepticism about Mr. Madigan's explanations. The *New York Times*, for example, ran a story under the headline "Are cattlemen now guarding the henhouse?"[18] and *Time* published one titled "While the Food and Drug Administration reforms labels, the Agriculture Department drags its feet, thanks to its cozy relations with the meat industry."[20] Because the USDA had claimed that the *Pyramid* would confuse children, *USA Today* did an experiment; it challenged children to draw their own symbols for a healthful diet. More than 400 schoolchildren took up the challenge; their designs indicated that although many children understood the *Pyramid*, others did not. The winning design was a Diet Dinosaur.[21] As might be expected, political cartoonists also had a field day with these events. Figure 9 gives a particularly pointed example. Overall, the press attention produced one outstanding benefit: It educated the public. As a reporter expressed it, "Had it not been for the ham-handed manner in which the *Pyramid* was withdrawn . . . it might have glided into relative obscurity. Now everyone who follows nutrition politics knows about it."[22]

At this point, I should disclose that my role as a conduit for USDA documents led to frequent discussions with reporters; as a result, I was quoted in many of these accounts or participated in them in other ways. The *Newsweek* story, for example, featured an original color illustration of the *Pyramid* attributed to an "unofficial USDA draft." *Newsweek* asked me for a color graphic, and I became its source, indirectly. I had only a black-and-white photocopy, but—shades of Watergate—I was able to find a "deep throat" who agreed to drop off color slides in my name at the concierge desk of the Four Seasons hotel in Washington, DC. Someone from *Newsweek* collected them and later sent them to me.

The well-publicized controversy took a toll at USDA. The department's politically appointed officials moved quickly to exclude HNIS staff from decision making about the *Pyramid* and from talking to the press. This situation came to light when a high-ranking USDA science official, Dr. Gerald Combs, coincidentally retired from the agency and became free to say what he pleased. He confirmed that "USDA's professional staff of nutrition educators has been silenced. The staff that produced the *Food Guide Pyramid* was never allowed to speak to the Secretary; presentations . . . were canceled; and letters and phone calls to the Cooperative Extension Service instructed them not to use the *Pyramid*."[17]

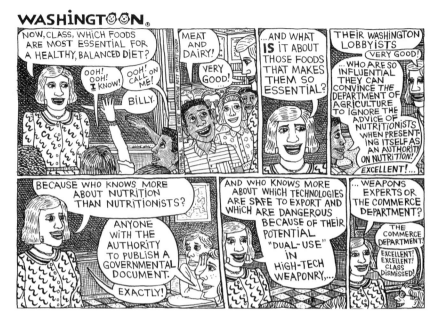

FIGURE 9. Mark Alan Stamaty's 1991 "Washingtoon" ridiculed the USDA for caving in to pressures from meat and dairy lobbyists in designing the *Pyramid*. It appeared in the *Washington Post* and the *Village Voice*. (Courtesy © 1991 Mark Alan Stamaty. Reprinted with permission.)

HNIS staff were understandably upset by these events, and many talked of quitting or taking early retirement. The *Pyramid*'s withdrawal had reinforced their impression that they were the Department's poor step-children . . . not taken very seriously . . . suddenly persona non grata—out of the loop."[16] Concerned that the scientific credibility of their work was at risk, they spoke with reporters under conditions of anonymity: "It's very clear this is the effect of pressure from the cattlemen . . . no one is going to believe us . . . [but this] is tainting everything the department is doing."[18] Such statements kept the press actively engaged in the story.

In defending his decision against persistent press criticism, Secretary Madigan held to his original statement. To the *New York Times,* he wrote, "The *Pyramid* symbol . . . found its way into the public domain prematurely. I didn't release it because the *Pyramid* was and is under review. . . . But we should not release any symbol until it has tested well with our target audiences, children and the undereducated."[23] He responded to the statement in *Time* about USDA's "cozy relations" with the meat industry in another letter: "For the record, I did not cancel the printing of the new eating right pyramid symbol because of pressure from the cattle and dairy industries. . . . Sixty percent of this department's 1992 budget is devoted to nutritional programs, but no beneficiary of any of these programs was included in the focus groups that chose the *Pyramid* symbol."[24] Later, he added: "Replacing the popular 'food wheel' that has graced the classrooms of America since the 1950s, produced "an avalance of news stories [saying that USDA] had caved in to opposition from the meat and dairy industries. That's simply not true."[25]

These explanations were misleading at best and revealed that Mr. Madigan was not consulting his own agency's staff. The release of the *Pyramid* was not premature; the proposed graphic design and text had been thoroughly tested and cleared. USDA's food guides—including the *Pyramid*—targeted adults of average income and education and were not aimed specifically at recipients of USDA food assistance programs. The Food Wheel had never been used in classrooms or, for that matter, by anyone outside the Red Cross. Such misunderstandings only reinforced reporters' skepticism.

RENEGOTIATING THE RESEARCH

Given Secretary Madigan's explanation, the USDA now was obliged to conduct the "missing" research. In July 1991, the agency announced that it had awarded a six-month, $400,000 contract to Bell Associates, a Boston consulting firm, to test the value of the *Pyramid* against other graphic designs in communicating dietary advice to adults and children receiving food assistance. To "keep USDA honest," DHHS also contributed to the research funding (reportedly $200,000) and became involved in its oversight.[26] Eventually, the agencies paid Bell Associates at least $855,000 for this work, an amount substantially in excess of the $160,000 reportedly paid to Porter–Novelli (and that sum itself was rumored to have been considerably less).

Bell's initial focus-group research produced ambiguous results that appeared to confirm that the *Pyramid* design was at least as effective as any other at conveying the concepts of variety, proportionality, and moderation. At that point, USDA asked for more testing. Bell conducted the additional research in two phases, qualitative and quantitative. During the qualitative phase of the research, Bell reviewed design options such as wheels and the children's submissions to *USA Today*, and developed several alternative graphics such as pyramids, bowls, pie charts, and

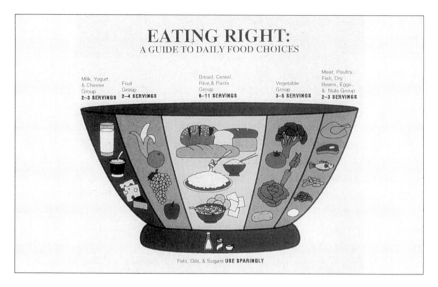

FIGURE 10. Meat and dairy producers preferred a bowl design over a pyramid because they thought the bowl shape suggested greater equivalence among food groups.

shopping carts. It tested these designs with groups of school children, low-income adults, science and home economics teachers, representatives of food commodity groups, and nutrition professionals and advocates. Bell also interviewed children and adults who received Food Stamps. The results: Industry representatives preferred pie chart and bowl designs that did not "stack" the food groups into evident hierarchies, but nutrition professionals preferred pyramids because they more clearly conveyed the intended messages. At this point, the field narrowed to two design options: pyramids and bowls. The bowl alternative is shown in Figure 10.

In the quantitative phase, Bell addressed the newly intended audience by collecting responses to messages conveyed by pyramid and bowl shapes from more than 3,000 children and low-income adults. The results, sent to USDA and DHHS in a draft report in January 1992, indicated that the effects of the two designs were virtually indistinguishable. On the basis of some remarkably slight scoring differences, however, Bell concluded that children, minorities, and low-income adults preferred bowl designs, not because they understood the intended messages any better, but because they associated bowls with food.[27]

At that point, USDA officials were faced with a particularly difficult dilemma. With no significant research suggesting that either design was more effective, they had to choose between two courses of action, both unattractive. They could select a pyramid design and run the risk of embarrassment over the delay, additional costs, and continued opposition from food producers, or they could choose the bowl design for what would evidently be political rather than scientific reasons. This dilemma was revealed to the nutrition community early in January 1992.[28]

To resolve it, USDA and DHHS appointed an advisory committee to respond to the Bell draft report. The committee recommended that Bell analyze the data again, this time using a scoring system weighted to emphasize the concepts of proportionality and moderation. This scoring system suggested that both pyramid and bowl designs effectively conveyed the need for variety in food intake (with composite message scores of 85 and 87, respectively, on a scale of 1 to 100) but that pyramids did somewhat better with proportionality (43 versus 37) and moderation (33 versus 27). The low scores, however, meant that *neither* design was particularly effective. The scores also differed from those presented in an earlier draft of the Bell Report (dated March 13), and this discrepancy suggested that the analysis was under constant revision until the very last moment. In late March, Marian Burros of the *New York Times* publicly revealed these problems in a story illustrated with drawings of the two competing designs constructed by a *New York Times* staff artist. Her exposé was the result of brilliant reporting; Ms. Burros never had seen the bowl design but deduced its details from conversations with her sources.[26] Her article increased the pressure on USDA to get the *Pyramid* out to the public as quickly as possible.

RELEASING THE "NEW" PYRAMID

On April 28, 1992—a year and a day and $855,000 after the announcement of its withdrawal—Secretary Madigan proclaimed the release of the USDA's *Food Guide Pyramid*. Without apology, he explained, "[W]e spent $855,000 on comprehensive tests to answer concerns raised by commodity groups, nutritionists and health care professionals. . . . The results clearly indicated that the *Food Guide Pyramid* was the most effective symbol."[29]

The new version differed from the one shown in Figure 8 in at least 33 ways, most of them utterly trivial. Two, however, were not. The term "Eating Right" had been changed to "Food Guide" in response to complaints from Kraft Foods (owned by Philip Morris) that the title infringed on its copyrighted line of prepared meals, and to complaints from ConAgra that the *Pyramid* might give Kraft a marketing advantage.[30] The most important change also was designed to appease food producers. The numbers of recommended servings had been moved outside the design and set in boldface type to suggest that the diet should include *at least* 2–3 servings of meat and dairy foods each day. This change implied an increase in servings from the *Basic Four*. Ironically, given who had registered the most complaints, the *Pyramid* had increased the upper range of the meat allowance. It specified that the two servings should be "the equivalent of 5 to 7 ounces of cooked lean meat" rather than the 4–6 ounces suggested in the *Basic Four* guide.

Such "improvements" might explain Secretary Madigan's pronouncement that the *Pyramid* would no longer mislead people into "believing that some foods were good while others were bad, or that some foods were more important than others,"[29] a statement that in itself was misleading because the intent of the *Pyramid* all along had been to illustrate hierarchies of food groups. Reportedly, Secretary Madigan preferred bowl designs and was unhappy with the decision to release the *Pyramid*, but he denied being under any pressure. Instead, he said that two assistant secretaries (presumably, one each from USDA and DHHS) "came to me with their conclusions and the reasons why the *Pyramid* was superior and I accepted that."[31]

How the agencies decided to select the *Pyramid* can only be surmised. Internal memoranda indicate that USDA staff and the advisory committee argued that pyramids were superior to bowl designs in conveying proportionality and moderation and that Bell's conclusions had to reflect the research findings. One hypothesis was that DHHS, having contributed to the costs of the research, insisted on the outcome favored by the investigations. According to one HNIS nutritionist, "The political people were forced into this decision by the internal staffers, the Department of Health and Human Services, and the professional community. . . . The political people wanted to drop it and said it would be a one-day story, but it just didn't die. The research would never have been done if it hadn't been for the pressure. . . . When the results came out it was so clear-cut that they could not manipulate it.[31] One official of DHHS, however, discounted any suggestion of conflict. He was said to have admitted that there had been some disagreement between the two agencies but maintained that the *Pyramid* research project had involved "a high degree of collegiality both at the professional staff level and the political level."[30]

Despite these assurances, one source of contention between the agencies soon emerged publicly. In August 1992, USDA released yet another version of the *Pyramid*, this time with the agency's name removed from the title. Now called *The Food Guide Pyramid* (rather than *USDA's Food Guide Pyramid*), the booklet acknowledges the support of DHHS for aiding development of this "research-based food guidance system."[32]

SURVIVAL OF THE *PYRAMID:* IMPLICATIONS

During the years when USDA nutritionists were developing the *Pyramid*, they tried hard to ensure that its principal features—the food groups and serving numbers and sizes—were substantiated by research, reviewed by experts, understood by consumers, discussed at professional meetings, and approved for publication by USDA. Because they had done more than expected to conceptualize, research, and review the guide, they had no reason to believe that it would be controversial. If anything, their work was *too* successful. The *Pyramid* design made it all too evident that food choices should be hierarchical and that some food groups are preferable to others. Nevertheless, the guide might have been released with only modest public interest had not the National Cattlemen's Association been meeting in Washington during that fateful weekend in April 1991.

The ultimate rescue of the blocked guide occurred because nutritionists in government and the private sector worked behind the scenes to strengthen the research and bring the dispute to the attention of the press. Reporters used the incident to highlight the conflicts of interest at USDA and to criticize the role of lobbyists in influencing federal policy. The period following the *Pyramid*'s withdrawal coincided with a recession, as well as with a changing political climate. The Republican administration's *laissez-faire* attitude toward business was becoming less popular. This shift, which culminated in the election of a Democratic president, Bill Clinton, in 1992, reduced public tolerance of a government that favored business interests over those of the public—at least for that moment.

For the USDA—and for health professionals—the *Pyramid* controversy had been resolved satisfactorily. In this instance, science conquered politics; the slightly more effective design survived. The delay and persistent press reports brought the *Pyramid* extraordinary publicity that may well have been worth its extra cost. The design was used immediately in schools and on package labels, and it soon become the most widely distributed and best-recognized nutrition education device ever produced in this country. The *Pyramid* now is an icon. It appears not only in nutrition education materials, posters, and textbooks but also in food advertisements, cookbooks, and board games—and even on Christmas ornaments. Within three years of its release, nearly half of American adults said they had heard of it, and the proportion has since increased to an astonishing 67%.[33] The *Pyramid* has spawned numerous offshoots illustrating the dietary pattern of one or another cultural or ethnic group, and there are Mediterranean, Asian, Vegetarian, Kosher, Soul Food, and other pyramids to suit almost any dietary preference. *Pyramid* serving numbers constitute a standard for evaluation of dietary intake patterns, of the quality of foods advertised on children's television programs, and of the categories of foods most frequently advertised. By any criterion of recognition or dissemination, the *Pyramid* has been highly influential.

Whether it has improved dietary intake is quite another matter. In 1992, the *Wall Street Journal* predicted that the *Pyramid* would "accelerate shifts in consumption patterns away from products high in animal fat, such as red meat and cheese, while spurring further development of low-fat products."[34] This prediction has proved only partially correct—consumption of premium ice cream and American cheese, for example, has increased. Thus the effectiveness of the *Pyramid* as an educational tool to encourage consumption of more healthful diets is debatable, as the following chapter explains.

CHAPTER 3

"DECONSTRUCTING"
DIETARY ADVICE

AS NOTED EARLIER, DESPITE THE CONSTANTLY RECURRING themes of dietary advice for health promotion—eat more plant foods and less of animal and processed foods—many people feel confused about what they should be eating. Because public discussion of nutrition issues tends to focus on single nutrients and on the distinctions between one set of guidelines and another, the fundamental similarity of five decades of dietary advice becomes hopelessly obscured. The contradiction between the constancy of the advice and the public's confusion can be explained in part by deliberate or unconscious efforts to undermine "eat less" precepts. Pressures from food companies have led government officials and nutrition professionals to produce dietary guidelines that disguise "eat less" messages with euphemisms. Their true meaning can be detected only through careful reading, interpretation, and analysis—"deconstruction"—as this chapter demonstrates. But first, let's take a look at how the *Pyramid* has fared since its release in 1992 and at the events surrounding the preparation and issuing of the *Dietary Guidelines* in 1995.

CRITICIZING THE *PYRAMID*

When the USDA released the *Food Guide Pyramid* in 1992, some nutrition and industry groups lauded the guide as an improvement over the *Basic Four*, but others challenged its most basic premises—its conceptual framework, scientific validity, and effectiveness as a teaching tool. The *Pyramid* was supposed to help dispel public misunderstanding of nutrition advice, resolve conflicting interpretations of research studies, and clear up confusion even among experts about the applicability of broad public health recommendations to the dietary practices of individuals. Yet critics even have challenged the value of such basic advice as avoiding overweight and eating more fruits and vegetables. Alliances of nutrition societies, federal agencies, and food industry groups have added to the confusion by adopting as a fundamental premise of their partnership that no specific foods or food groups should be categorized as good or bad— thereby contradicting the *Pyramid*'s explicit food-group hierarchies.

Table 8 lists issues raised by critics of the *Pyramid*, by category. Many seem trivial (such as the geometric matter), silly (the botanic issue), or flawed (some of the biochemical concerns). The ideological criticism attacks one of the design's founding tenets, "proportionality"—the idea that diets should include more servings from plant food groups than from other groups. The gastronomic, pedagogic, and conceptual categories, however, raise more difficult issues. Critics complain that the *Pyramid* does not adequately assign foods to groups, define serving sizes, or distinguish "good" from "bad" kinds of fat, nor does it explain that some serving numbers are meant to be upper limits (meat, dairy, and the fat/sweets groups), whereas others are meant to be lower limits (grains, fruits, and vegetables). Advice about fat raises particularly complex issues. A leading nutrition researcher argues, for example, that appropriate dietary advice should explain critical differences in the health effects of various types of fat, but the *Pyramid* fails to indicate that monounsaturated fats (such as those in olives, nuts, and avocados) promote health, whereas saturated and *trans*-saturated fats do not.[1]

It is difficult to imagine how any single graphical design might address all of these concerns. As some analysts explain, "The issues surrounding dietary guidance are complex" but the *Pyramid* would work better if it clarified and promoted its key themes of variety, moderation, and proportionality.[2] Other groups have attempted to correct some of the *Pyramid*'s perceived flaws by creating versions of their own: Mediterranean, Vegetarian, and a variety of Asian *Pyramids* generally place even greater emphasis on adherance to plant-based, as opposed to meat-based, diets. Such alternatives solve some of the problems of the USDA *Pyramid*, but not all. The great strengths of the USDA *Pyramid* are its conceptualization, its basis in research, the overwhelming support it has received from studies linking largely plant-based diets to health, its representation of a much more healthful diet than that typically consumed, and its ready adaptability to almost any personal, ethnic, or cultural dietary preference. Most of all, the *Pyramid* is distinguished by its hierarchical

TABLE 8. Principal problem categories and criticisms of the USDA's 1992 *Food Guide Pyramid*

Problem Category	The Pyramid Does Not, But Should:
Geometric	Represent a pyramid (it is a triangle).
Botanic	Classify fruits and vegetables appropriately (tomatoes and peppers are fruits).
Biochemical	Recognize the biochemical equivalency of sugars and starches in the body. Ensure adequate intake of essential fatty acids. Distinguish the health impact of total fat from the effects of saturated, monounsaturated, polyunsaturated, and *trans*-saturated fatty acids.
Ideological	Emphasize that all food groups are equivalent and that there are no good or bad foods (this was its point).
Gastronomic	Emphasize whole, minimally processed—as opposed to refined—grains. Separate beans (a vegetable) from meats. Equate fresh beans (now in the vegetable group) with dried beans (in the meat group). Distinguish high-fat from low-fat meat and dairy foods. Emphasize nontropical oils as opposed to tropical oils and animal fats. Distinguish high-fat from low-fat cooking methods.
Pedagogic	Guide educators and the public in placing commonly consumed foods in appropriate groups. Explain serving sizes adequately or consistently. Convey the complexities of information about nutrition and health.
Conceptual	Distinguish serving recommendations that should be considered upper limits (meat and high-fat dairy foods) from those that should be considered lower limits (grain, fruit, and vegetable groups). Meet the concerns and needs of vegetarians. Reflect the replacement of Recommended Dietary Allowances (RDAs) by the new Dietary Reference Intakes (DRIs). Reflect the emphasis of more recent dietary guidelines on physical activity, plant-based diets, food safety, and appropriate use of salt and alcohol.

depiction of the benefits of a plant-based diet, and it is no accident that this aspect is also its most controversial.

Controversy over such matters is not confined to the United States. The Canadian health agency, for example, attempted to avoid any suggestion of hierarchy by displaying food groups as colors of a rainbow.

Even so, food producers complained that the guide appeared to favor vegetarian diets, to reinforce the "myth that meat is not good for you," and to give the impression that meat, dairy, and eggs are bad foods. In response, officials increased the number of servings in the guide and made other conciliatory changes.[3] Industry-friendly food guides avoid controversy by omitting "eat less" recommendations. The Food and Agriculture Organization (FAO) of the United Nations, for example, explains that its recommendations deliberately address the total diet rather than single nutrients or foods, because "various dietary patterns can be consistent with good health."[4] Its four guidelines are unlikely to cause trouble: "Enjoy a variety of foods. Eat to meet your needs. Protect the quality and safety of your food. Keep active, and stay fit." Despite rapidly rising rates of obesity and related diseases in FAO's constituent countries, its guide contains no hint that people might be healthier if they ate less of some foods than of others. When it comes to dietary advice, the science that favors consumption of some foods more than others is difficult to disentangle from the commercial implications of such advice.

THE MAKING OF THE 1995 DIETARY GUIDELINES

One reason why nutrition advice appears to change so frequently is that Congress *requires* USDA and the Department of Health and Human Services (DHHS) to revisit the *Dietary Guidelines* at frequent intervals. Title III of the National Nutrition Monitoring and Related Research Act of 1990 specifies that

> At least every five years the Secretaries shall publish a report entitled "*Dietary Guidelines for Americans.*" Each such report shall contain nutritional and dietary information and guidelines for the general public, and shall be promoted by each Federal agency in carrying out any Federal food, nutrition, or health program. . . . [These] shall be based on the preponderance of the scientific and medical knowledge which is current at the time the report is prepared.[5]

To implement this requirement, the agencies appoint a joint committee to decide whether revision is necessary. Because no committee would ever deny the need for revisions (otherwise, why bother to serve on it?), its members then carry out congressional intent by reviewing research, writing guidelines, drafting text to accompany them, and submitting a report explaining the changes from the previous version. The agencies determine the final design and text.

I was a member of the 1995 Advisory Committee, the first appointed as a result of the congressional mandate, and I can attest to the fact that once a committee is appointed, it will want to tinker. Indeed, *Dietary Guidelines* is best understood as a *committee* report—the result of the interplay of give-and-take, bullying, boredom, and (eventually) compromise among a group of people who entered the process with differing opinions and agendas. Whether the members change their opinions as a result of the ensuing meetings, hearings, comments, or research review is questionable, if only because the time is short and the amount of required reading staggering. By the end of my committee tenure, the accumulated documents formed a stack five feet high.

The most contentious issue during preparation of the 1995 report concerned hierarchies. A majority of committee members voted to divide the existing guidelines into two tiers. The lower tier was to include the guidelines for sugar, salt, and alcohol, which some members viewed as less well supported by science. This suggestion received enthusiastic endorsement from the relevant industries. I was in the minority on this issue, mainly because I believe that the separate dietary guidelines are meant to be followed as a whole—all at the same time—and that each one defines a particular aspect of a healthful diet. I also was concerned that establishing two levels of recommendations would suggest that the second-tier guidelines were less important. To resolve such concerns, the agencies asked a group of experts to comment on how the public might perceive a two-tier format. Practically everyone who was invited to reply to this question said that people would assume that first-tier guidelines were more important and that a two-tier system would influence the ways in which educators, the media, and the industry conveyed nutrition messages:

> There is no doubt in my mind that such a change would result in public perceptions—and possibly behaviors—that in fact the "second tier" issues are of less importance than the " first tier" guidelines, and possibly that they are in fact inconsequential. . . . A third effect, one that is especially troubling to me, might be that certain segments of the food industry would seize the opportunity to promote products with low nutrient density related to the "second tier" guidelines.[6]

To most experts in communicating nutrition advice, a second tier would imply little need to limit intake of sugar, salt, and alcohol. On that basis, our committee dropped the two-tier idea, but as I shall explain, the committee in charge of the 2000 edition adopted that idea with a vengeance.

Aside from the usual hearing testimony and written comments, lobbying of committee members by meat and dairy groups was not particularly evident during preparation of the 1995 *Guidelines*. Our advice about meat retained the usual "choose two to three servings of lean . . . meats." Our text suggested the benefits of eating moderately from the meat-and-beans group and avoiding sources of saturated fat in the diet. For the first time, we recommended meals with rice, pasta, potatoes, or bread at the center of the plate and included a section on vegetarian diets. In view of the demonstrable health benefits of such diets, our statement—a hard-fought compromise—seemed unnecessarily cautious ("Meat, fish, and poultry are major contributors of iron, zinc, and B vitamins in most American diets, and vegetarians should pay special attention to these nutrients").[7]

Although the *Dietary Guidelines* document is a statement of federal policy and is supposed to govern the design of the *Pyramid*, the popularity of the *Pyramid* changed this relationship and caused the two guides to be linked more closely. The 1995 *Guidelines* included an illustration of the *Pyramid* and the directive "Use foods from the base of the *Food Guide Pyramid* as the foundation of your meals." For meat, the *Guidelines* used the *Pyramid*'s serving numbers and sizes (2–3 servings of 2–3 ounces) but failed to mention the upper limit of 5–7 ounces. The effect of this omission was to extend the recommended range of intake to 9 ounces per day (Table 7), which perhaps explains the lack of objections from meat producers. Instead, as discussed below, the 1995 *Guidelines* sparked controversy about—of all things—the alcohol guideline. Because the *Pyramid* is supposed to translate federal nutrition policy into food choices, revision was required to ensure its consistency with the 1995 *Dietary Guidelines*. USDA did that in 1996, indicating that the agency would continue to revise the *Pyramid* in response to later editions of the *Dietary Guidelines* produced in subsequent years.

DECONSTRUCTING *DIETARY GUIDELINES* 2000

In 1998 the agencies appointed the advisory committee for the congressionally mandated fifth edition of the *Dietary Guidelines* to be published in 2000. At its first meeting, the committee revealed that it would be doing more than the usual level of tinkering. According to one account, the committee chair explained that "the role of nutrition in health is changing, and the guidelines are going to have to reflect that," and a member said that the current guidelines "represent the end of an era in

TABLE 9. Industry affiliations of members of the *Dietary Guidelines* 2000 Advisory Committee[a]

> *Dairy industry groups*
> > Dannon Company (yogurt)
> > National Dairy Council
> > National Dairy Promotion and Research Board
> > Mead Johnson Nutritionals (milk-based infant formulas)
> > Nestlé (milk-based formulas, condensed milk, and ice cream)
> > Slim-Fast (milk-based diet products)
>
> *Egg industry groups*
> > The American Egg Board
>
> *Meat industry groups*
> > The American Meat Institute
> > National Livestock and Beef Board

[a]Affiliations include service as visiting lecturer, scientific advisory board member, trustee, grant recipient, grant review committee member, symposium organizer, or author. (Physicians Committee for Responsible Medicine. Washington, DC, December 13, 1999)

regard to how people think about nutrition."[8] In short order, it also became clear that pressures on the process would come from unusual sources and that debate would be even more contentious than usual. For example, the congressional Black Caucus complained that the *Guidelines* "demonstrate a consistent racial bias" in recommending dairy products as part of a balanced diet, because most nonwhite people are unable to digest the lactose in milk after the age of five or so.[9] This was not the first time that such charges had been leveled, but it was by far the most highly publicized. In a campaign organized by the Physicians Committee for Responsible Medicine (PCRM), the Washington, DC-based group that had issued the vegetarian food guide discussed in the previous chapter, the Black Caucus demanded that dairy products be listed as optional rather than as superior sources of calcium.[10]

Late in 1998, PCRM filed a federal lawsuit based on this and one other charge: 6 of the 11 members of the *Guidelines* committee had significant ties to the meat, dairy, or egg industries. PCRM charged that these members—all university-based academics—had received research grants from, lectured to, consulted for, published with, or served on boards of the organizations with commercial interests in specific guidelines and what was said about them. Table 9 lists such organizations. Eventually, the court denied PCRM's request for a preliminary injunction but agreed that the methods for appointing committee members deserved further scrutiny.

Although previous advisory committees also were obliged by federal law to hold open meetings, the workings of this one were especially public because transcripts and documents could be posted immediately on USDA's Internet Web site. Thus reporters and anyone else from industry or advocacy groups could follow the development of the committee's thinking. A journalist reporting on an August 1999 working draft noted that three of the first four proposed guidelines had nothing to do with food choices but instead focused on uncontroversial issues of food safety, exercise, and weight maintenance.[11] A later draft released for public comment revealed that the committee had reintroduced tiers—this time three of them—and made other changes that minimized "eat less" messages.[12]

President Clinton announced the 2000 *Guidelines* in his weekly radio address on May 27, and they were released at a National Nutrition Summit meeting held in Washington, DC, two days later. Table 10 summarizes the 2000 *Dietary Guidelines*. Although the summit was largely devoted to discussions of obesity prevention, neither of the agency secretaries suggested that the guidelines might help people eat less. Instead, USDA Secretary Dan Glickman said,

> These guidelines reflect the latest in scientific knowledge on nutrition and health. They recommend that all Americans use the *Food Guide Pyramid* to make informed food choices, choosing a *balanced* diet that includes a *variety* of grains, fruits and vegetables every day. They also encourage all Americans to *moderate* how much saturated fat, cholesterol, total fat, sugars, salt and alcohol are in their diets [emphasis added].[13]

DHHS Secretary Donna Shalala made similar remarks:

> We always made sure that our policy decisions on nutrition were driven by medical science—not political science. . . . These new guidelines continue to emphasize balance, moderation, and variety in food choices. . . . They also offer more practical advice and scientific information than ever before to help American consumers make the smartest possible decisions when it comes to what we eat.[14]

The National Cattlemen's Beef Association issued a press statement: "Beef fits in the *Dietary Guidelines for Americans*, which call for balance, variety and moderation of all foods."[15]

As noted earlier, dietary guidelines are meant to be followed as a whole to achieve a *Pyramid*-like dietary pattern—one that contains more servings from the plant food groups—fruit, vegetables, and grains—but fewer from the meat, dairy, and fat/sugar groups. The "Aim, Build, Choose" approach, however, introduces a *new* hierarchy: fitness first,

TABLE 10. Federal recommendations for diet and disease prevention: *Nutrition and Your Health: Dietary Guidelines for Americans*, 5th edition, 2000

Aim for fitness.
  Aim for a healthy weight.
  Be physically active each day.
Build a healthy base.
  Let the *Pyramid* guide your food choices.
  Choose a variety of grains daily, especially whole grains.
  Choose a variety of fruits and vegetables daily.
  Keep foods safe to eat.
Choose sensibly.
  Choose a diet that is low in saturated fat and cholesterol and moderate in
    total fat.
  Choose beverages and foods to moderate your intake of sugars.
  Choose and prepare foods with less salt.
  If you drink alcoholic beverages, do so in moderation.

next a mixture of dietary and other issues that include the "eat more" precepts, and last the "eat less" advice. As might be expected, food industry groups appreciated this change: "The ABC approach will complement our industry's objective. The messages continue to build on a solid foundation whereby diet is viewed in the context of all the foods we eat and the lifestyle we follow."[16] The committee's report gave no indication that the members considered the significance of the new hierarchy. The report merely states that the intent of the three-tier system was "to help the user to organize the guidelines in a memorable, meaningful way" and that the prominent placement of the weight and physical activity guidelines was "essential for clarity."[12] With this introduction, we can begin examining the meaning of each of the guidelines, word by deconstructed word.

Aim for Fitness

That the first two guidelines deal with body weight makes sense; obesity is an extraordinarily important public health problem. The verb *aim* is weak, however, and conveys a lack of expectation that people can change their weight. The "Aim" guidelines could not be less controversial, but they are remarkable for the prominence they give to activity rather than diet. People become overweight when they take in more calories than needed for daily activities. Although some people can lose weight through exercise alone, most must attend to both sides of the equation—

calories eaten as well as calories expended—and must *eat less*. The accompanying text hardly says so. Instead, it talks about "sensible eating" and raises issues about risk factors, genetics, and eating disorders. Weight-loss advice is to "do so gradually." Only in a small box on "sensible" portion sizes do we find the single "eat less" suggestion—a good one: "Be especially careful to limit portion size of foods high in calories, such as cookies, cakes, other sweets, French fries, and fats."

Build a Healthy Base

The "Build" section also is uncontroversial. "Let the *Pyramid* guide . . ." is a gentle approach demanding no active change on anyone's part. The next two guidelines mean "eat more"; they call for positive action and confirm the benefits of plant-based diets. Variety also conveys an "eat more" message: choose different kinds of foods from among a large selection. It is no accident that the two "eat more" guidelines are the only ones that refer to *foods*—grains, vegetables, and fruits. The "eat less" guidelines, in contrast, talk about nutrients or food chemicals (fat, cholesterol, sugar, salt, alcohol)—not their food sources. The food-safety guideline also is uncontroversial (*of course* people should prepare safe food) but shifts attention away from the need for dietary change. The committee explains this guideline "as a step in unifying and strengthening the focus of the *Dietary Guidelines* on actionable measures that can be taken by consumers and public officials to keep Americans healthy." Such advice, reasonable as it is, reinforces the idea that consumers—rather than food producers or processors—bear the primary responsibility for protection against food-borne illness.

Choose Sensibly

In this third tier set of guidelines, the words *low, moderate,* and *less* suggest "eat less." *Moderate* means different things to different people, as one investigator has shown,[17] but USDA research reveals that most people understand moderation to mean "small amounts." Other terms used in food guides and guidelines also require deconstruction, as shown in Table 11. The committee downplayed the "eat less" guidelines by placing them in the bottom tier, but also by stating them as self-canceling phrases: *choose* is an "eat more" word attached to an "eat less" guideline. Note that the "eat less" guidelines invariably address nutrients, not food. They refer to fat, saturated fat, and cholesterol, but not to the most

TABLE 11. "Deconstruction" of terms used in food guides and dietary guidelines

Term	Translation
2–3 servings of meat/day	Eat less red meat.
2–3 servings of dairy/day	Eat less of high-fat dairy products.
Grains, vegetables, fruits	Eat a largely plant-based diet.
Low in saturated fat and cholesterol	Eat less red meat and less of fried foods, high-fat dairy foods, and processed foods.
Variety	Eat foods low in fat, saturated fat, cholesterol, sugar, and salt.
Choose	Eat less.
Moderate	Eat less.

important food sources of fats—meat, dairy, eggs, and fried and processed foods. They refer to salt and sugar, not to pretzels or soft drinks, and they say alcoholic beverages, not beer, wine, or hard liquor. Trade associations guard vigilantly against suggestions to eat less of their particular foods, but they can live with more abstract advice to limit intake of one or another nutrient.

UNDERMINING "EAT LESS" GUIDELINES

As noted earlier, the history of food industry pressures on "eat less" guidelines began with the 1977 *Dietary Goals,* although even then scientists had for many years debated the effects of diets high in meat, dairy, and eggs on heart disease risk. Each separate guideline has its own lengthy history of lobbying pressures, but in the interest of brevity, I will review industry pressures on only the fat, sugar, salt, and alcohol guidelines. Because of my personal involvement in the 1995 alcohol guideline, I will examine that one in greater detail.

Choose a Diet Low in Saturated Fat and Cholesterol and Moderate in Total Fat

Fat is fattening; it contains more than twice the caloric value of equal amounts of protein or carbohydrate. For this reason, studies cannot easily distinguish the effects of fat on disease risk from those of calories, or the effects of diets high in total fat and those relatively high in one or another fatty acid (the building blocks of fats). All food fats are mixtures of saturated, monounsaturated, and polyunsaturated fatty acids, but they vary in the relative amounts of each type. Decades ago, researchers discovered that high levels of cholesterol in blood predispose individuals to coronary heart disease and that saturated fat (most prominent in meat and dairy products) raises blood cholesterol levels more than monounsaturated fats (typical of olive oil). They also observed that polyunsaturated fats (most prominent in vegetable seed oils) reduces blood cholesterol levels. More recently, *trans*-saturated fats (found in margarine, hydrogenated vegetable oils, and, to a lesser extent, meat and dairy foods) also have been shown to raise blood cholesterol levels.

Because high-fat diets also tend to be high in calories and saturated fat, "total fat" became a convenient shorthand term for more complicated advice about calories, fatty acids, and food sources. Today, we know more about the effects of specific fatty acids on blood cholesterol levels and on the risk of heart disease. Some scientists interpret this knowledge to mean that advice to reduce total fat is unnecessary and simplistic and that the fat guideline should instead advise limits on saturated and *trans*-saturated fats.[1] The 2000 *Guidelines* use saturated fat as a euphemism for the meat and dairy foods that provide more than half of its amount in current American diets.[18] Because reducing intake of total fat means limiting the principal food sources of saturated fats—meat, dairy, and foods fried in animal fats—doing so is still good advice.

Meat In Table 7, we saw how objections from meat producers shifted 1977 recommendations about meat from "decrease consumption" to the euphemistic "choose meats . . . which will reduce saturated fat intake." Since then, the guideline has evolved to the even more euphemistic "choose lean meat." Advice to consume two daily servings of 4–6 ounces shifted to the encouraging "have 2 or 3 servings" and later to the positively directive "choose 2–3 servings," now amounting to 4–9 ounces. What is most remarkable about the increasingly positive tone of this guideline, and about its increase in the number and size of recommended servings, is that the change occurred during a period of increasing scientific consensus that saturated fat is the primary offender in raising risks of heart disease. The meat industry can live with euphemistic advice to consume diets "low in saturated fat." It is only when that term gets translated into food sources—"animal fat" or "eat less meat"—that industry groups are galvanized into action, and nutrition scientists and educators become uncomfortable and advise "moderation."

Dairy   As a means to reduce saturated fat, the 2000 guideline advises, "Choose fat-free or low-fat dairy products." Thus it merely suggests substitution of low-fat for high-fat options and says nothing about eating less. Dairy foods are sources of calcium, but they are also high in fat, saturated fat, and lactose, a sugar that cannot always be digested by most people in the world over the age of five years.[19] The "Let the *Pyramid* guide . . ." section suggests that people *require* 2–3 servings of dairy foods daily, preferably fat-free or low-fat, and it also lists high-fat cheeses as recommended sources of calcium. How dairy foods came to be considered *essential* despite their high content of fat, saturated fat, and lactose is a topic of considerable historical interest. As it turns out, nutritionists have collaborated with dairy lobbies to promote the nutritional value of dairy products since the early years of the twentieth century. Recently, however, some scientists have raised doubts about whether dairy foods confer special health benefits. In addition to concerns about lactose intolerance, some question the conventional wisdom that dairy foods protect against osteoporosis or, for that matter, accomplish *any* public health goals.[20] Others suggest that the hormones, growth factors, and allergenic proteins in dairy foods end up doing more harm than good.[21] The scientific issues related to the use of dairy products—or to that of any other single nutrient or food—are unlikely to be resolved easily or soon, but they focus attention on the role of the dairy industry as a primary source of information about these foods.

During the days of nutrient deficiencies, nutritionists considered milk an especially protective food, and many continue to embrace that view. Certainly, much of the credit for the public's favorable views must go to the National Dairy Council, which adopted the *Basic Four* for its own purposes and made its version of the guide widely available in schools. The Dairy Council made one critical design change, however; it stacked the food groups vertically and placed the milk group at the top. Subsequent versions continue to give greatest prominence to the milk group, to recommend 2–4 servings per day, and to make no distinction between full-fat and low-fat products. Indeed, the current version does not even refer to the fat content of dairy products.[22] The Dairy Council's interpretation of the *Pyramid* also evades the fat issue and, as shown in Figure 11, raises the number of suggested servings from the milk group to 3–4 per day.

The education and research activities of the Dairy Council and the promotional activities of the National Fluid Milk Processor Promotion

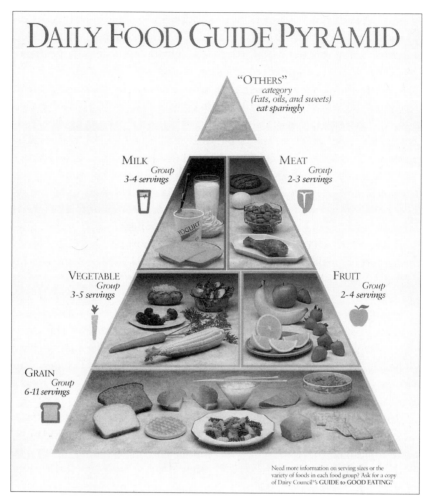

DAILY FOOD GUIDE PYRAMID

"OTHERS"
category
(Fats, oils, and sweets)
eat sparingly

MILK
Group
3-4 servings

MEAT
Group
2-3 servings

VEGETABLE
Group
3-5 servings

FRUIT
Group
2-4 servings

GRAIN
Group
6-11 servings

Need more information on serving sizes or the
variety of foods in each food group? Ask for a copy
of Dairy Council's GUIDE to GOOD EATING.

FIGURE 11. The Dairy Council's version of the *Pyramid* makes no visual distinction between high-fat and low-fat dairy products and increases the recommended number of dairy servings to 3–4 per day. (Courtesy National Dairy Council, Rosemont, IL, 1999)

Board are funded through a generous "check-off" (generic marketing) program run by USDA. Through this board, the industry invests heavily in advertising campaigns aimed at reversing a 30-year decline in milk consumption. In 1999 the Council's $130 million "milk mustache" celebrity campaign was credited with increasing milk sales by 0.7%, an achievement considered a triumph even though 40% of the increase came

from sales of flavored—mostly chocolate—milk.[23] Dairy funds also paid
for full-page advertisements in the *New York Times* announcing low calcium intake as a "major health emergency. The best way to get calcium is
through your diet . . . Three glasses of milk a day."[24] Although many scientists support this approach, others do not. Thus the appearance by
DHHS Secretary Donna Shalala in a milk mustache advertisement surprised many observers (see Figure 12). Although the advertisement
emphasized the calcium needs of teenagers, it was placed in the *New
York Times* and other venues more likely to appeal to adults. And
although Secretary Shalala was not paid for her participation, the advertisement could easily be construed as federal endorsement of the milk
industry's agenda at the very time DHHS and USDA were appointing the
advisory committee for the 2000 *Dietary Guidelines.*[25]

"Check-off" boards are not supposed to lobby. Presumably as part of
its *educational* mission, the Dairy Council filed objections to several proposed features of the draft guidelines. The Council argued for setting a
higher standard for definitions of "high fat," opposed the inclusion of soy
beverages in the dairy food group, objected to the suggestion that lactose-
intolerant people could choose sources of calcium other than dairy foods,
and called for special guidelines for children with more liberal allowances
for dietary fat—all in the name of health benefits. In one instance, the
complaints worked; the agencies deleted soy beverages from the list of
dairy servings in the final guidelines, which may help explain why the
Dairy Council ultimately commended them: "New findings make 2–3
daily servings of dairy 'a powerful action step.'"[26]

Choose Beverages and Foods to Moderate Your Intake of Sugars

Sugar was one of the more contentious guidelines in the 2000 edition,
largely because of industry arguments that research on sugar and disease
did not support a recommendation to "eat less." The progression of this
guideline is especially revealing [emphasis added]:

- Committee report, September 1999: *go easy* on beverages and foods
  high in *added* sugars.
- Committee report, February 2000: choose beverages and foods that
  limit your intake of sugars.
- Agency override, May 2000: choose beverages and foods to *moderate*
  your intake of sugars.

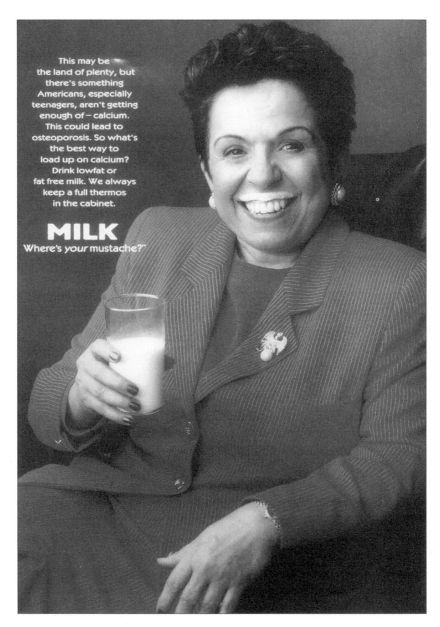

FIGURE 12. The National Fluid Milk Processor Promotion Board featured Donna Shalala, then Secretary of Health and Human Services, in this milk marketing advertisement (the pin was given to her by President Clinton). The advertisement appeared in the *New York Times Magazine*, February 1, 1998.

Go easy means "eat less," and *added* distinguishes processed foods from fruits and vegetables that naturally contain sugar. The committee report explains that added sugars displace nutrient-containing foods in the diet and that a "focus on total sugars is not supported by the literature and causes confusion among consumers." Although the text of the final version states that soft drinks, candy, cakes, cookies, fruit drinks, and dairy desserts are the major sources of added sugars, the guideline itself obscures that point, as does the positive "choose" as opposed to the restrictive "go easy." The report offers no explanation for the softening of this recommendation, leading readers to surmise that the committee must have agreed with the Grocery Manufacturers of America that the "minimum burden of scientific proof has not been met" for more restrictive advice.[16]

Investigative reports revealed fierce industry lobbying to retain the 1995 wording, "Choose a diet moderate in sugars." Sugar trade associations viewed *limit* as a potential disaster for their $26 billion industry, and their lobbyists induced 30 senators, half from sugar-growing states, to question whether the USDA had the right to "change the sugar guidelines based on existing science."[27] The trade associations also objected to singling out individual foods and beverages as major food sources of sugars. Instead, according to another account, the Grocery Manufacturers wanted "recommendations related to meals and snacks . . . [which] would avoid creation of good food vs. 'bad' food scenarios and would be more in line with the practical advice of health professionals, who urge consumers to look at their food intakes over time instead of on a 'single food or beverage basis.'"[16]

Choose and Prepare Foods with Less Salt

The survival of the salt guideline is somewhat surprising, given that debates over its role in health are nothing short of ferocious. Everyone agrees that salt has something to do with blood pressure.[28] The arguments revolve around how much and for whom. The 2000 committee noted "an unusually high level of controversy" about whether advising the entire population to restrict salt is warranted or whether this advice should be applied only to people diagnosed with high blood pressure or at risk for it. Like pretty much every committee that has considered the issue, this one viewed the preponderance of the evidence as favoring a population-based approach—meaning a recommendation that *everyone* cut down on salt intake—on the grounds that prevention always is preferable to treatment and that not everyone has access to medical diagnosis. Indeed, the committee strengthened the guideline by substituting *less* for the previous edition's *moderate*, but it retained the self-canceling *choose*. Although the text identifies processed foods as the major sources of salt in American diets, it does not advise "eating less" of such foods. Instead, it suggests reading package labels to compare the salt content of packaged dinners, cereals, cheeses, soups, and sauces (all high in salt). It says "go easy" only with respect to condiments—soy sauce, ketchup, pickles, and olives—without mentioning potato chips or other high-salt processed foods, many of which also are high in calories and fat.

Salt is absolutely essential to the processed food industry. It binds water and increases the weight of foods at very low cost. It makes processed foods palatable, and it makes people thirsty. Salt promotes "eat more." Therefore, the food industry wants to convince scientists and policy makers that the following propositions hold true: (1) salt raises blood pressure in only a small fraction of the population, (2) even modest reductions in salt intake could be dangerous to health, and (3) experts so strongly disagree about the effects of salt that no restrictive advice is warranted. Some scientists also support these propositions. The salt foods industry is represented by the Salt Institute, a lobbying group particularly adept at fostering doubt that salt has anything to do with high blood pressure. The Salt Institute distributes to nutrition scientists a newsletter, now delivered via electronic mail, that tracks research and policies relevant to salt intake. These accounts invariably publicize studies that seem to show no adverse effects but minimize research that might contradict that agenda. Despite the wide reach of the Salt Institute's public relations efforts and the controversy it has fostered, its tactics have gone largely unexamined in the United States. They have, however, received pointed attention from British scientists.[29]

If You Drink Alcoholic Beverages, Do So in Moderation

Alcohol raises difficult public policy issues. Some people do not drink at all, whereas others drink to abuse. Only a small proportion of the population drinks moderately by the definition given in the *Dietary Guidelines*: an upper limit of one drink a day for women and two for men (a drink is 12 ounces of regular beer, 5 ounces of wine, or 1.5 ounces of 80-proof distilled spirits, which provide 150, 100, and 100 calories, respectively). Because the *average* intake of alcohol in a population predicts the proportion of people who abuse alcohol, a principal objective of public health policy is to keep overall intake as low as possible.

Advice to "drink less" makes excellent sense for preventing the accidents, violence, and social problems that arise from alcohol abuse. What especially complicates advice about alcohol consumption, however, is the inconvenient finding that moderate drinking provides health *benefits*— alcohol protects against coronary heart disease. Thus the alcohol guideline must balance potential benefits against the known risks of alcohol abuse. As though this balance were not hard enough to achieve, the alcoholic beverage industry wants to use health benefits for heart disease prevention as a marketing tool to counteract the required warning statements about the adverse effects of alcohol, particularly those related to birth defects, driving ability, and overall health.

Using Health Claims on Wine Labels   In the late 1980s, in an effort to counteract declining sales and protests against drunk driving, the wine industry began to press for bottle labels extolling the benefits of wine consumption. The Mondavi company, for example, placed the following "wine and civilization" label on its 1988 Fumé Blanc: "Wine has been with us since the beginning of civilization. It is the temperate, civilized, sacred, romantic mealtime beverage recommended in the Bible. Wine has been praised for centuries by statesmen, philosophers, poets, and scholars. Wine in moderation is an integral part of our culture, heritage, and the gracious way of life."[30]

In March 1991, in response to complaints from the Center for Science in the Public Interest (a Washington, DC-based advocacy group), the Bureau of Alcohol, Tobacco and Firearms (BATF), an arm of the Treasury Department, informed California vintners that federal rules did not permit them to refer to wines as *sacred*. By 1990, BATF had received many inquiries about health claims on wine labels but explained that its rules also precluded statements suggesting that "wine has curative or therapeutic effects if such statement is untrue in any particular or tends to create a misleading impression."[31] The term *misleading*, according to BATF, applied to statements that were not properly qualified, gave only one side of the issue, and were unbalanced as to risks and benefits. BATF especially wanted to avoid any suggestion to nondrinkers that they should start drinking to improve their health. Once Mondavi deleted the word *sacred* and the phrase *recommended in the Bible*, BATF allowed the label to be used.

By this time, the wine industry had become happily aware of the French and Mediterranean "paradoxes." In the late 1980s, French researchers observed that the fat content of the French diet was as high as that of Americans but that heart disease rates among the French were much lower. They attributed this anomaly to the large amounts of alcohol consumed in France, mostly in the form of wine, and especially red wine.[32] In November 1991, this work was featured on the popular CBS television show *60 Minutes,* a program that is considered especially credible. The results were spectacular: sales of red wine increased nearly 45%, and shortages of red grapes caused prices in California to rise sharply. One amazed analyst called the program "the 20 minutes that changed the industry." BATF, however, threatened to close wineries or stores that quoted from the broadcast in promotional materials.[33]

Despite the inability of most research studies to distinguish among the health effects of beer, wine, and spirits, the wine industry continued to promote "moderate drinking" as synonymous with drinking wine. In October 1992, in a move viewed as "highly surprising and highly desirable for the wine industry," BATF agreed; it permitted Beringer Vineyards to hang a tag from its wine bottles with a quotation from the *60 Minutes* broadcast: "Alcohol, in particular red wine, reduces the risk of heart disease." When numerous medical, consumer, religious, education, and antialcoholism groups, along with other federal agencies involved in nutrition research, advertising, and labeling filed vigorous protests, Beringer withdrew the tags, if a bit ungraciously: "Beringer continues to feel that California wineries should be able to disseminate to the public balanced information about the potential benefits of moderate wine drinking. In no way does the winery wish to encourage inappropriate or irresponsible alcohol consumption. Beringer believes that all communication on the subject should present a balanced perspective and should stress the concept of moderation." [34]

During the next few years, the wine industry and its supporters continued to publicize the French paradox and research studies demonstrating connections between wine and reduced mortality from heart disease and other causes. For example, Dr. Curt Ellison said, during another *60 Minutes* broadcast, "It seems quite clear that we should not do anything that would decrease moderate drinkers in the population. I think that would be bad for the public health."[35]

Writing the 1995 Alcohol Guideline   I must confess immediately to being a member of the three-person subcommittee that drafted the 1995 alcohol guideline and its accompanying text. This guideline elicited so little comment from members of the larger committee that it was the first to be adopted. At the time, I was unaware of the dispute about the wine labels, and other committee members also did not mention it. Although the alcohol industry had lobbied the committee through the usual channels of written comments and public testimony, so did many other food industries likely to be affected by the new guidelines. Of the 152 written comments on the alcohol guideline, 88 called for a more positive statement about moderate wine and health; most of the letters were identically worded and evidently the result of an organized campaign. I doubt whether any of us paid special attention to them. We knew that two decades of studies supported the benefits of moderate drinking, and we did not think we could ignore this research. Furthermore, we ourselves drank wine in moderation. If we drank at all, it was likely to be a glass or two of wine (and good wine at that) with dinner. We could see little harm in permitting an upper limit of two drinks a day for men but just one for women (because women metabolize alcohol less rapidly, demonstrate a higher risk of breast cancer with even small amounts of alcohol, and if pregnant, can induce alcohol toxicity in the fetus).

Knowing the risks of exceeding these amounts, we were taken aback when a spokeswoman for Women for WineSense, an industry group, called for elimination of restrictions against moderate drinking during pregnancy on the grounds of weak evidence and the "unnecessary anxiety" it might cause.[36] Given that the lowest level of alcohol that might damage a fetus was uncertain, we thought anxiety a small price to pay for prudence. Because of the social consequences of alcohol abuse, and because other behavioral changes such as smoking cessation, weight loss, and eating less saturated fat could help prevent heart disease, we saw no reason to suggest that nondrinkers start drinking.

In short, we believed that we were following mainstream scientific thought and had achieved a balance between the troublesome societal risks of alcohol abuse and the health benefits of moderate drinking. We thought we were writing the text of that guideline on the basis of science and did not even consider marketing or moralistic issues. Although we kept the guideline identical to the previous edition's "If you drink alcoholic beverages, do so in moderation," we deliberately made the tone of the accompanying text less prohibitionist. We deleted the 1990 statement "Drinking has no health benefit . . . consumption is not recommended" and substituted "Alcoholic beverages have been used to enhance the enjoyment of meals by many societies throughout human history." We were flabbergasted when the *New York Times* headlined its story about the 1995 *Dietary Guidelines*, "In an about-face, U.S. says that alcohol has health benefits" and gave as its quote of the day a statement from Dr. Philip Lee, then Assistant Secretary of DHHS: "Wine with meals in moderation is beneficial. There was a significant bias in the past against drinking. To move from antialcohol to health benefits is a big change."[37]

Promoting Wine with Dietary Guidelines   The industry, of course, could not have been more delighted with this turn of events. Alcohol accounted for more than $50 billion in sales in 1994, but the amount consumed per person—particularly the amount of hard liquor—had been declining steadily since the early 1980s. Critics soon charged that the alcohol industry had been behind the text changes in the guidelines. The Marin Institute, a California organization devoted to prevention of alcohol and other drug problems, interviewed committee members and wrote an investigative report that focused on two text items: the "enjoyment" statement and a sentence on "physiologic drug" effects that USDA and DHHS had deleted from our proposed text. According to the Marin Institute reporter, the agencies had done so in response to lobbying by the Wine Institute, a California-based trade association.[38]

The Marin Institute had good reason to make this claim. In addition to documenting meetings between the Wine Institute and federal officials, the reporter was familiar with the long history of aggressive lobbying tactics by the alcohol industry. The Wine Institute, for example, was well known for its strategies to promote wine as a health food: manipulation of research findings, exaggeration of health benefits, and failure to mention health risks—all in the name of public education.[39] Indeed, the Wine Institute had immediately placed the "enjoyment" statement on the masthead of its wine-and-culture newsletter series. It "worked tirelessly" to persuade Congress to earmark funding for studies of moderate drinking, and to convince the public to consider wine not as a "gateway drug" but rather as a "legitimate component of the nation's lifestyle."[40] The Wine Institute pressed BATF to approve another label, this one saying, "To learn the health effects of moderate wine consumption, send for the federal government's *Dietary Guidelines for Americans*." This idea elicited strong objections from DHHS and the Federal Trade Commission. In response, the president of the Wine Institute, John De Luca, explained that the

> Wine Institute's proposed label statement is not part of a marketing program. It is an essential education component of our public policy mission to counter

the political campaigns pushing for higher taxes on our products, trade limitations, advertising restrictions and infringements on constitutional rights. This
label is voluntary, and simply refers consumers to the updated section on alcoholic beverages in the *Dietary Guidelines for Americans* for information on
the "health effects" (not health benefits) of moderate wine consumption.[41]

In March 1998, Senator Strom Thurmond (Rep-SC) wrote to DHHS Secretary Donna Shalala protesting the "enjoyment" statement, which, he
said, "reads as if it were written as an advertisement for the alcohol
industry . . . after reading these guidelines, I had the impression that the
Federal government is encouraging moderate consumption of alcohol."[42]

Despite the senator's concerns, BATF was said to be favoring approval
of two label statements on wine bottles, the one referring buyers to the
Dietary Guidelines and the other saying, "The proud people who made
this wine encourage you to consult your family doctor about the health
effects of wine consumption."[43] When a survey found wine drinkers to
deny that such statements would encourage them to drink more, the
Treasury Department approved them, saying that "under existing law,
[B]ATF can only deny labeling statements if they are false or misleading";
these were neither, because all they did was to direct consumers to
sources of information.[44] The Wine Institute heralded this decision as an
"historic breakthrough . . . a defining new chapter in the evolution of federal policy towards wine in America."[45] Observers viewed this decision
as opening the door to the use of labels to make similar claims for *all*
alcoholic beverages—and as a clear win for the industry: "lobbyists 1,
public interest 0."[46]

The Treasury Department then drafted legislation to strengthen warnings about the health hazards of alcohol, especially to pregnant women
and young people, an action decried by the industry as "not needed, not
warranted, and a bureaucratic effort to expand [BATF's] base."[47] Senator Thurmond introduced a bill that would prohibit health messages on
wine labels, transfer authority over alcohol labeling from the Treasury
Department to DHHS, and raise taxes on wines: "Generally, I do not
favor increased taxes . . . but in this era of shrinking budgets, the only
way in which we will be able to finance adequate, impartial and trust-
worthy research into alcohol-induced diseases such as hypertension,
breast cancer, and birth defects is to generate a new revenue flow that will
be used specifically for investigating such killers."[48]

The Senator's proposals, designed to add 59 cents to the cost of each
bottle of wine and to raise $8 billion annually for research, were not
expected to get very far, given that the Wine Institute is "well-financed

and has the ear of many on Capitol Hill."[49] For example, a 53-member, bipartisan congressional Wine Caucus led by a California representative from the Napa Valley, held tasting receptions, dinners, and meetings with noted vintners and wine industry leaders.[50] In March 1999, Senator Thurmond asked the inspectors general of DHHS and USDA to investigate whether the Wine Institute had conspired with senior government officials to manipulate the 1995 *Dietary Guidelines* to promote the use of alcohol. The senator said that he was not "interested in outlawing alcoholic beverages or legislating morality" but that he wanted to know whether "public policy has been compromised by a lobbying organization to the detriment of the nation's public health."[51] As part of this investigation, DHHS sent me a questionnaire about my participation in drafting the 1995 alcohol guideline. Did I have expertise in the area of alcohol and health? [yes] Did I participate in writing the guideline? [yes] Had I corresponded or talked with wine industry representatives, known of undue influence, or had business affiliations with the wine industry during the time the guidelines were in preparation? [no] The questionnaire did *not* ask: Were you aware of the history of alcohol policy in the United States and the ways in which the industry has promoted the benefits of its products while downplaying their risks? [not nearly enough]

Backtracking: The 2000 Alcohol Guideline   The 2000 *Dietary Guidelines* committee learned from this example. It kept the wording of the 1990 and 1995 guidelines but revised the text to place "more emphasis on adverse effects of excess intake"—in fact, much more. It began, "Alcoholic beverages are harmful when consumed in excess. Excess alcohol impairs judgment and can lead to dependency and a great many other serious health problems." The remainder of the paragraph lists such problems in detail. As the committee explained in its report,

> [T]he proposed text now begins with a paragraph that addresses adverse effects of excess alcohol intakes and mentions no beneficial effects. . . . The committee suggests that the sentence in the previous guideline "Alcoholic beverages have been used to enhance the enjoyment of meals by many societies throughout human history" be omitted from the current text. Although that statement is factually correct, a similar statement could be made for many other foods and nutrients, for example, salt or sugar.[12]

The only surviving mention of benefit is this carefully worded statement: "Drinking in moderation may lower risk for coronary heart disease, mainly among men over age 45 and women over age 55." The final text included a statement added by USDA and DHHS: "However, there are other factors that reduce the risk of heart disease, including a healthy diet, physical activity, avoidance of smoking, and maintenance of healthy weight."

Thus, at one stroke, this committee made sure that the *Dietary Guidelines* could no longer be used to promote wine, let alone beer or hard liquor, and ended the need for Senator Thurmond's investigation and legislative proposals. In this case, the Wine Institute's heavy-handed efforts to use the guidelines as an "education" tool had succeeded, but with the wrong audience. The efforts had "educated" the committee and the sponsoring agencies, none of which was likely to make the same mistake again.

Reconstructing Dietary Advice

Surveys indicate that people are interested in nutrition and health but are confused by conflicting information, suffer from "nutritional schizophrenia," and cannot figure out how to achieve "nutritional utopia."[52] Surely, ambiguous guidelines must contribute to the confusion. This chapter explained how food industries insist that guidelines be expressed positively and focus on nutrients rather than foods. Instead, food companies prefer thoroughly permissive principles that encourage consumption of all foods regardless of nutritional value: "balance, variety, and moderation are the keys to healthful diets; there is no such thing as a good or a bad food; all foods can be part of healthful diets; it's the total diet that counts."

Consciously or unconsciously, such principles have been internalized, adopted, and promoted by nutrition researchers and practitioners and, therefore, by the government agencies for which they consult. The result has been consistent pressure to make dietary advice more positive despite the lack of compelling evidence that this approach is more effective in helping people eat more healthfully. Food industry pressures on Congress and federal agencies, ties between nutritionists and the food industry, and the inability of just about everyone to separate science from personal beliefs and opinions (whether recognized or not) affect dietary advice. Although dietary guidelines are not wholly responsible for consumer confusion and frustration, they contribute to it and do little to help people understand how to choose better diets.

In retrospect, it seems clear that those of us working on the 1995 *Dietary Guidelines* should have been more aware of the marketing consequences of our statements and of their potential to mislead the public. In our defense, the benefits of wine were "in the air"—on television, in books and magazines, and at professional meetings. The role of the industry in deliberately creating that environment took place below our level of consciousness. As the next chapters demonstrate, the subliminal nature of food industry lobbying efforts is itself a deliberate strategy for promoting and protecting product sales.

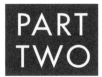

PART TWO

WORKING THE SYSTEM

FOOD COMPANIES USE EVERY MEANS AT THEIR DISPOSAL—
legal, regulatory, and societal—to create and protect an environment
that is conducive to selling their products in a competitive marketplace. To begin with, they lobby. They lobby Congress for favorable
laws, government agencies for favorable regulations, and the White
House for favorable trade agreements. But lobbying is only the most
obvious of their methods. Far less visible are the arrangements made
with food and nutrition experts to obtain approving judgments about
the nutritional quality or health benefits of food products, and the personal connections made with legislators or agency officials who might
be in a position to promote favorable regulations. The chapters in Part
II explain how this system works.

I first encountered lobbying in action during the two years that I
worked for the Public Health Service as managing editor of the 1988
Surgeon General's Report on Nutrition and Health. This report was to
be the first comprehensive review of research linking dietary factors to
the risk of chronic disease. When I arrived in Washington, DC, in the
fall of 1986, the report had been in production for two years and was
widely understood to be leading to policy recommendations for "eat
less" dietary changes. Representatives of every food or food category
that might be affected by the report's recommendations paid a visit to
the office. Although I was largely protected from these interactions, I
did meet at various times with delegations of sugar, salt, and meat producers who were understandably curious about what the report might
say. These groups were explicit about their concerns, and they made

sure that we were completely aware of research supporting their products' health benefits.

These visits met the definition of lobbying: activities designed to influence *government*—Congress, federal agencies, and the White House. Chapter 4 explains the historical context in which lobbying takes place and the ways in which food lobbying continues that tradition. Chapter 5 describes a different form of lobbying—the deliberate fostering of connections between food companies and nutrition professionals through the companies' sponsorship of research and educational activities, and other forms of partnership. Food companies also go to great pains to befriend federal officials, develop legislation in their own self-interest, and use public relations to create a positive image for their activities, as described in Chapter 6. When all else fails, food companies engage in "hardball" tactics and file lawsuits to intimidate critics. These activities, discomfiting as they may be, are entirely legal. Occasionally, however, companies get caught in patently illegal actions such as bribery or price fixing. Chapter 7 describes situations that place food companies on one or the other side of the legal line, as either plaintiffs or defendants. Together, these chapters illustrate how lobbying and related activities raise questions about the undue influence of food companies not only on the health of the public but also on democratic political processes and institutions.

CHAPTER 4

INFLUENCING GOVERNMENT

FOOD LOBBIES AND LOBBYISTS

TO UNDERSTAND HOW FOOD COMPANIES ARE ABLE TO EXERT disproportionate influence on government nutrition policy, we must begin with a discussion of lobbying and its integral position in American political processes. Lobbying is any *legal* attempt by individuals or groups to influence government policy or action, a definition that explicitly excludes bribery. Historically, lobbying always has involved three elements: (1) promoting the views of special-interest groups, (2) attempting to influence government laws, rules, or policies that might affect those groups, and (3) communicating with government officials or their representatives about laws, rules, or policies of interest.[1] Food lobbyists, therefore, are people who ask government officials to make rules or laws that will benefit their clients' companies, whether or not they benefit anyone else.

At their best, lobbyists provide federal officials with well-researched technical advice about proposed legislation, regulation, and public education. The value of this expertise has been the ostensible reason for congressional reluctance to limit lobbying activities. Offering expertise, however, is only one strategy. More important are personal contacts established through meetings and social occasions. Other lobbying methods include arranging campaign contributions, staging media events, organizing public demonstrations, harassing critics, and encouraging lawsuits. Such efforts have been—and are—so successful that lobbyists have sometimes been considered to constitute their own branch of government.

Lobbyists, however, are hired, not elected. They differ from advocates and independent experts in that they are paid to represent private—not public—interests, and many of their activities are hidden from public view. Thus lobbying raises questions about undue influence and misuse of power. Our political system must balance the rights of individuals and groups against the rights of society as a whole, and it requires elected officials to listen to groups demanding self-interested actions. What concerns us here is the differential ability of food companies to obtain laws and rules that act in their favor at the expense of public health.

SETTING THE STAGE FOR FOOD LOBBYING: THE HISTORICAL CONTEXT

That food lobbies are permitted to do what they do derives directly from the long tradition of acceptance of lobbying as an integral part of the American political system. That lobbying would create tensions in that system was known from the outset. In 1787 James Madison wrote of the "dangerous vice" of *factions*—his term for lobbying groups. He viewed factions as an inevitable result of basic human nature, as well as of the unequal distribution of property. He believed that the "mischiefs" caused by special-interest groups would be controlled inevitably as a natural outcome of majority rule: "There are two methods of curing the mischiefs of faction: the one, by removing its causes; the other, by controlling its effects . . . [a faction] may clog the administration, it may convulse the society; but it will be unable to execute and mask its violence under the forms of the Constitution."[2]

As Madison predicted, public exposures of excessive and dishonest lobbying were followed by investigations and demands for its regulation. For the next 150 years, various states and Congress made sporadic but unsuccessful attempts to control lobbying—so much so that beginning in 1911, nearly every session of Congress involved some attempt to address lobbying abuses. When Congress finally did act on the matter, it made lobbying *legal*. It required only that persons paid to lobby register and disclose their sources of funds. Furthermore, Congress did not specify enforcement procedures, which may be one reason why the law resulted in only a single conviction—and that in 1959. Lobbying regulations were universally viewed as unenforceable and, therefore, ineffective.

Legislation passed in 1995 closed some, but by no means all, of the loopholes.[3] That law defines lobbyists as people who spend at least 20% of their time on such activities, have contact with government officials or staff, and are paid more than $5,000 in a six-month period for this work.

Because all three of these criteria had to be met, people whose activities met just one or two did not need to register.[4] At about the same time, amendments to federal election laws limited the value of gifts and meals that legislators could accept from lobbyists. The House rule barred lobbyists from buying meals for members and aides except at stand-up receptions attended by 25 people (the "toothpick" rule), although small gift items were still permissible. The Senate's rules were somewhat less restrictive. Senators and aides, for example, could not accept paid travel to *recreational* events, or gifts or meals worth more than $100 from any one individual in a year. Such restrictions were easily evaded.[5]

Those rules not only led to an increase in registration of lobbyists (which was their intention) but also to an increase in overall lobbying activity. According to data collected by the Center for Responsive Politics, a public-interest group that goes to a great deal of effort to track this sort of information, the number of registered lobbyists increased from 15,000 to more than 20,000 just between 1997 and 1999. The Center estimated that lobbyists spent more than $1.42 billion on behalf of clients in 1998; it calculated that if this amount went just for lobbying Congress, then *each* of the country's 100 senators and 435 representatives would be contacted by an average of 38 paid lobbyists spending $2.7 million on each legislator to do so.[6] It must be understood that this army of largesse-dispensing lobbyists represents every conceivable component of American corporate and private enterprise; no industry is too small, no group too isolated, and no opinion too extreme to forgo paying for its own professional lobbyist. With billion-dollar expenditures, lobbying is a huge industry unto itself. At this point, we can now examine how food lobbies fit into the broader political picture.

INFLUENCING THE AGRICULTURAL ESTABLISHMENT

To understand how food lobbying works, we need to know something about the relationships between Congress and the federal agency most responsible for food and agriculture, the U.S. Department of Agriculture (USDA). By the end of World War II, a period during which government and food producers worked together in the national interest, farmers and food producers had come to view USDA as *their* department and its secretary as *their* spokesman. Food producers, together with USDA officials and members of the House and Senate Agricultural Committees, constituted what was universally understood to be the "agricultural establishment"—an entity so strongly united in purpose that it could ensure that any federal policy related to land use, commodity distribution, or prices would promote the interests of food producers. The control exercised by producer groups over USDA and congressional actions was so complete that this "establishment" virtually excluded the Secretary of Agriculture and even the President of the United States from any significant role in policy decisions. Their jobs, after all, were temporary.[7]

Guaranteeing the perpetuation of this system were congressional seniority and the strong representation on agriculture committees of members from farm states. Membership on such committees gave the appearance of lifetime tenure. Allen Ellender (Dem-LA), for example, chaired the Senate Agriculture Committee for 18 years; his successor, Herman Talmadge (Dem-GA), held the position for 10 more. Most remarkably, Representative Jamie Whitten (Dem-MS) chaired House Agriculture Committees from 1949 to 1992, accumulating so much power during this 43-year period that he was referred to as the *permanent* Secretary of Agriculture.[8]

In the early 1970s, this system began to break down as new constituencies began to demand influence over agriculture policies. Consumers, for example, complained when a combination of bad weather, poor harvests in foreign countries, and massive purchases of U.S. grain by the Soviet Union caused an increase in food costs. Large processing and marketing companies formed as agriculture gained importance in the U.S. economy, and the interests of these new entities differed from those of smaller food producers. Even more, the expansion of food assistance programs following the 1969 White House Conference on Food, Nutrition, and Health meant that an increasingly large proportion of USDA's funding went for Food Stamps and other such activities. Advocates for the poor became a new agricultural interest group. In response to these new demands, the House expanded agricultural committee membership in 1974 to include representatives from urban as well as rural areas. In 1977 Congress gave the agriculture committees of both houses jurisdiction over policies and programs related not only to agricultural production, marketing, research, and development but also to a wide range of new areas: rural development, forestry, domestic food assistance; some aspects of foreign trade, international relations, market regulation, and taxes; and, as we have seen, nutrition advice to the public. These changes stimulated a huge proliferation of lobbying activities related to the expanded functions of federal agriculture committees.[9]

REPRESENTING FOOD INDUSTRY INTERESTS

In the 1950s just 25 groups of food producers dominated agricultural lobbying, but by the mid-1980s there were 84 such groups, and by the late 1990s there were hundreds—if not thousands—of businesses, associations, and individuals attempting to influence federal decisions related to every conceivable aspect of food and beverage production, manufacture, sales, service, and trade.[4] Although the total number of lobbyists and groups working on food and nutrition issues is uncertain, a 1977 study identified 612 individuals and 460 groups in this category.[10] A cursory review of the list of all registered lobbyists suggests that less than 5% might be concerned with such issues—perhaps about 1,000 individuals, law firms, and associations representing widely diverse groups with interests in federal policies on food, nutrition, and agriculture. Advocacy groups, professional societies, and universities with agriculture programs also retain lobbyists to work for them, but these groups are usually acting on behalf of public interest or nonprofit goals.

Like all lobbyists, those for food companies gain access to federal officials and staff in ways that extend far beyond technical expertise, although such expertise provides an excuse for regular contact. Among these ways, two are worth particular attention: (1) the evident and not so evident transfer of funds from lobbyists to federal officials through federally sanctioned donations of "hard" money, legal but unsanctioned "soft" money, and gifts and (2) the frequent job exchanges between lobbyists and federal officials known as the "revolving door." Both practices raise questions about undue influence. Because the revolving door sets the scene for later discussion of more obviously commercial transactions, let's examine that method first.

Recruiting Lobbyists: The "Revolving Door"

Charges of undue influence cannot help but arise from the realization that lobbyists and government officials are not always distinct populations. Today's public servant is tomorrow's lobbyist, and vice versa. The revolving-door transformation of government officials into lobbyists and of lobbyists into government officials is not a new phenomenon. In 1968, for example, at least 23 former senators and 90 former representatives had registered as lobbyists for private organizations. More recently, among congressional representatives defeated in the 1992 election, 40% became lobbyists. So did their staff; from 1988 to 1993, 42% of Senate committee staff directors and 34% of those on the House side became lobbyists. By 1998, 128 former members of Congress were listed as lobbyists—12% of all senators and representatives who had left office since 1970. As an example of what is at stake, the firm to which former senator (Rep-KS) and presidential candidate Robert Dole belonged earned $19 million in lobbying fees in 1997.[11]

In the food industry, job exchanges between lobbyists and the USDA are especially common because as many as 500 agency heads and staff are political appointees chosen on the basis of party affiliation and support. Some examples are especially striking. In 1971, USDA Secretary Clifford Hardin traded places with Earl Butz, who was then director of Ralston Purina; Mr. Butz became Secretary of Agriculture, and Mr. Hardin went to Ralston Purina. The chief USDA negotiator who arranged for private companies to sell grain to the Soviet Union in 1972 resigned to work for the very company that gained the most from the transaction. A report in 1974 listed numerous assistant secretaries, administrators, and advisors who had joined USDA from positions with meat, grain, and marketing firms or, on the other hand, had left the agency to take positions with food producers.[12] Later, in the early 1990s, the appointment of a former president of the National Cattlemen's Association, JoAnn Smith, as chief of the USDA's Food Marketing and Inspection Division, raised questions about two of her decisions that seemed to favor the interests of meat producers over those of consumers: she approved the euphemistic designation "fat-reduced beef" for bits of meat that had been processed from otherwise unusable slaughtering by-products, and she opposed an American Heart Association proposal to put a seal of approval on certain meat products that were low in fat, an action that might suggest that low-fat meats were more healthful.[13] The changing administration in 2001 continued this tradition. The new Secretary of Agriculture, Ann Veneman, appointed a lobbyist for the National Cattlemen's Beef Association as her chief of staff, while the former secretary Dan Glickman, went to work for a law firm that lobbies for agriculture and food companies.[14]

Similar exchanges apply to the Food and Drug Administration (FDA). In the mid-1990s, Dr. John Hathcock, a senior researcher at FDA and an expert on nutritional toxicology, accepted a high-level position with the Council for Responsible Nutrition, a leading trade association for the dietary supplement industry. In 1999 Dr. Fred Shank, former director of the agency's Center for Food Safety and Applied Nutrition, became director of government relations at the Institute of Food Technology, a trade organization for academic and professional developers of food products and ingredients. Also in 1999 Dr. Morris Potter left his FDA position as director of the Food Safety Initiative to work for the International Life Science Institute, an organization that represents concerns and interests of the food industry. In 2000 Joseph Betz, an FDA expert on the pharmacological properties of plants, joined the American Herbal Products Association, thereby ensuring that this organization would "continue to play a leadership role in addressing the unique challenges confronting botanical products."[15]

When officials of regulatory agencies go to work for industry, they are almost certain to be paid better than they were in their government jobs, and they contribute to industry the valuable expertise that they acquired at the expense of taxpayers. The practice of recruiting industry executives to government work raises questions of conflict of interest, even when they accept lower salaries to do so, because it is difficult to imagine that they can make decisions without keeping their former employer's interests in mind. Revolving-door issues are not always easy to categorize, however, as is perhaps best illustrated by the career of Michael Taylor.

Mr. Taylor is a lawyer who began his revolving-door adventures as counsel to FDA. He then moved to King & Spalding, a private-sector law firm representing Monsanto, a leading agricultural biotechnology company. In 1991 he returned to the FDA as Deputy Commissioner for Policy, where he was part of the team that issued the agency's decidedly industry-friendly policy on food biotechnology and that approved the use of Monsanto's genetically engineered growth hormone in dairy cows. His questionable role in these decisions led to an investigation by the federal General Accounting Office, which eventually exonerated him of all conflict-of-interest charges.[16] In 1994 Mr. Taylor moved to USDA to become administrator of its Food Safety and Inspection Service. In this position, he became the *hero* of food-safety activists for his courageous development of the agency's groundbreaking policies for controlling dangerous microbial contaminants in meat and poultry. After another stint in private legal practice with King & Spalding, Mr. Taylor again joined Monsanto as Vice President for Public Policy in 1998. He resigned that position late in 1999 during the height of public controversy over Monsanto's aggressive promotion of its genetically engineered foods. At the time of this writing, he had returned to the private sector, this time to Resources for the Future, a nonprofit think tank on environmental and natural resource issues in Washington, DC.

This example illustrates the dilemma posed by revolving-door issues. Although former government officials provide expertise useful to food companies, it is also true that former food company employees provide expertise that can help government agencies do a better job of regulation. Mr. Taylor's career demonstrates that the revolving door does not *always* favor industry, even though it invariably gives the appearance of doing so.

Funding Elected Officials

Less ambiguous is the role of money in interactions between lobbyists and government officials. One of the most unsettling ways in which lobbyists exert influence over federal decisions is by spending money and, insofar as can be determined, lots of it. Despite reporting requirements, it is difficult to find out precisely how much money lobbyists spend on federal officials. A great deal of lobbying takes place in unreportable gray areas of social transaction, such as dinner parties, receptions, meetings, golf games, birthday parties, and weddings. The Center for Responsive Politics estimates that food and agriculture lobbyists spent $52 million in 1998 on issues other than tobacco (on which they spent another $67 million). For example, lobbyists for the Grocery Manufacturers of America reported spending more than $1.4 million, the National Cattlemen's Beef Association $400,000, the National Pork Producers Council $200,000, Kraft General Foods $120,000, and the Cheese Importers Association $20,000 in 1998.[4] These are reported amounts, required by law to be revealed. Donations are conveniently classified into two categories of money: "hard" and "soft."

Giving "Hard" Money (PACs)   Like other industries, food companies disburse most funds to individual members of Congress through Political Action Committees (PACs). PACs began in the early 1940s when Congress prohibited labor unions from contributing to political campaigns; the unions got around this restriction by collecting *voluntary* contributions from members to support the reelection of President Franklin D. Roosevelt. In 1974, soon after the scandals of Watergate, amendments to the Federal Election Campaign Act authorized formation of PACs by unions, corporations, and other groups for the purpose of collecting and allocating voluntary campaign contributions. These funds are governed by legislation and for this reason are known as "hard"—legally sanctioned—money. Although the law limits the amount of money any one *individual* can contribute to federal candidates to $1,000 each for each election, it permitted PACs to donate up to $5,000 to each candidate. Because the act did not restrict either the number of candidates to whom contributions could be made or the number of PACs to which any one donor could contribute, individuals could contribute quite large amounts of money. Within just one year, 608 PACs formed and contributed $12.5 million to the 1974–1975 election campaigns. The number of PACs grew rapidly. In 1982, 3,400 PACs contributed $83 million, and in 1990, 4,700 PACs contributed more than $370 million. In the 1997–1998 election cycle, about the same number of PACs raised more than half a billion dollars.[17]

Most PACs represent businesses, but in the greater scheme of Washington lobbying, relatively few represent food and agriculture interests. A survey in 1978 identified 82 such PACs, 46 of them representing producer groups.[10] Data from the Center for Responsive Politics indicate that 211 agribusiness PACs contributed $4.3 million to federal candidates in the 1999–2000 election cycle. For example, the American Meat Institute PAC contributed $56,500, PepsiCo $66,825, ConAgra $86,750, and the Food Marketing Institute $113,308 to various candidates. Agribusiness PAC money is remarkable for its unequal distribution among Democrats and Republicans; $1.5 million went to Democrats but $2.8 million to Republicans in that cycle. Although some types of PACs contribute almost equally to Democratic and Republican candidates, most do not. Republican candidates received nearly 64% of the funds from egg and poultry PACs, 78% from livestock producers, and 84% from food processors, which suggests that PAC money preferentially goes to candidates most likely to favor particular corporate interests.[4]

PAC funds also go to where they seem most likely to benefit the donors. Not surprisingly, agribusiness contributions go preferentially to members of House and Senate Agriculture Committees. From 1987 to 1996, 18 of the 25 leading Senate recipients of contributions from meat and poultry processor PACs—and 17 of the 25 leading House recipients—were members of agriculture committees, as were about half of the top 25 recipients of contributions from grocery distributors, wholesalers, and retailers.[18] As just one example, Table 12 provides a partial listing of food and agriculture PACs that made contributions to Richard Lugar (Rep-IN) in 1997–1998 when he chaired the Senate Committee on Agriculture, Nutrition, and Forestry. Mr. Lugar received $316,300 in total PAC contributions, of which 36% came from food and agriculture groups, most of them corporate. Among the few noncorporate exceptions were the American Dietetic Association, which represents nutritionists who hold credentials as Registered Dietitians ($1,000), and the American School Food Service Association, whose members work in school cafeterias that provide federally supported meals to low-income children ($750).[4] In general, PACs that represent consumer, health, or public-interest groups are very much in the minority.

Most of Mr. Lugar's PAC contributions amounted to $1,000 or $2,000 and ranged from $250 (National Confectioners Association) to $5,000 (Archer Daniels Midland)—amounts too small to seem likely to influence anyone, especially compared to the annual income and advertising budgets of food corporations (refer to Table 1). The contributions can add up to substantial amounts, however. In 1997–1998, for example, the ranking minority member of the House Committee on Agriculture, Charles Stenholm (Dem-TX), received $862,000 in PAC contributions—all, as required by law, in amounts no greater than $5,000; to this total, 133 food and agriculture PACs contributed $330,000 (38%).[4]

Because it is not certain whether PAC money goes to candidates who already share corporate interests or to candidates who change their opinions in response to the contributions, observers differ on whether PAC contributions "buy" influence. Some believe the power of PACs to be vastly overrated, whereas others view PACs as an insidious system that makes legislators "more beholden to the economic interests of their committee constituents than to the interests of their district residents or to the President or party."[19]

Although research on the effects of PACs does not prove that they buy influence, it certainly suggests a strong correlation between contributions and desired outcomes. About 95% of the funds from agricultural PACs go to incumbents. Thus PAC money follows voting records and reinforces them. In the 1980s, researchers demonstrated that members of the House of Representatives who received PAC funds from dairy industry groups were almost twice as likely to vote for dairy price supports as those who did not. Legislators who favored price supports received 2.5 times more PAC funds than those in opposition, and the more money the members received from dairy PACs, the more likely they were to back price-support legislation.[20] More recently, a study of the connection between PAC contributions and congressional votes on sugar subsidies indicated that the largest contributions from sugar PACs had gone to members who voted for the subsidies and that the larger the PAC contribution, the more likely the members were to support industry positions. Month-by-month analyses of the history of legislation on sugar and peanut subsidies demonstrate an increase in contributions to both parties just prior to votes. Because PACs give more money to legislators who are more likely to vote for their interests, researchers conclude that PAC

TABLE 12. A partial list of food and agriculture political action committee (PAC) contributors to Senator Richard G. Lugar (Rep-IN), chair of the Committee on Agriculture, Nutrition, and Forestry, 1997–1998[4]

Agricultural Retailers Association	Nabisco Brands
Agri-Mark	National Broiler Council
American Dietetic Association	National Cattlemen's Beef
American Feed Industry Association	Association
American Frozen Food Institute	National Confectioners Association
American Meat Institute	National Food Processors
American Peanut Shellers Association	Association
American School Food Service	National Grain and Feed Association
Association	National Pork Producers Council
American Sheep Industry Association	National Restaurant Association
Archer Daniels Midland Co.	National Turkey Federation
Central Soya Co.	Nestlé, USA
ConAgra	Novartis Corporation
Farmers' Rice Cooperative	PepsiCo
Florida Citrus Mutual	Snack Foods Association
Food Marketing Institute	Sunkist Growers
Grocery Manufacturers of America	United Egg Association
International Dairy Foods Association	United Fresh Fruit & Vegetable
Kraft Foods	Association
Milk Marketing	Western Pistachio Association
Monsanto	

contributions do have a significant effect on voting decisions.[21] Given the costs of election campaigns, the lack of public funding for them, and the resistance of Congress to reform campaign finance laws, it is no mystery why legislators might not want to make decisions that displease PAC contributors.

Giving to National Committees ("Soft" Money)   Provisions of the Election Campaign Act apply to *federal* elections; they do not limit the amounts of money that can be contributed to state or national political organizations. This loophole allows for contributions of "soft" money for administrative and other expenses involved in supporting issues that political parties and candidates might favor. This money supports elections indirectly, can come from any source, is unrestricted in amount, and does not need to be disclosed.[22] Unlike PAC funds, soft-money donations can be substantial; in 1991, for example, several food and agriculture corporations made $100,000 contributions to the Republican Party, and in the 1997–1998 election cycle, agribusiness corporations made soft-money donations of $1.3 million to Democrats and $1.4 million to

Republicans. As just one example, the Flo-Sun Sugar Company and its subsidiaries made 21 donations of amounts ranging from $2,500 to $25,000 to congressional campaign committees in 1997–1999, for a total of $202,500 to Democrats and $147,500 to Republicans.[17]

Flo-Sun is unusual in distributing more money to Democrats than to Republicans—and to good effect, as I shall soon explain. As I mentioned earlier, most food corporations favor Republicans because members of this party are more likely than Democrats to protect and promote business interests. Dole Food, for example, gave $15,000 in soft money to Democratic committees in 1998 but gave $382,000 to Republican committees. In 1997–1999, food retailers gave nearly $1.1 million to Democrats but more than $3.8 million to Republicans—for example, Coca-Cola (Democrats $215,500 versus Republicans $394,000), the American Meat Institute ($4,000 versus $142,000), and the Grocery Manufacturers of America ($30,000 versus $290,000). The tangible rewards of such generosity will be evident throughout this book.

Giving Presents   Election laws have long permitted lobbyists to give members of Congress small gifts such as lunches, books, awards, liquor, samples, and theater tickets. The lobbying reform law that went into effect in 1996 was designed to limit the value of such gifts. It prohibited House members from accepting all but the smallest gifts from lobbyists and firmly excluded meals and entertainment; it allowed Senate members to accept individual gifts worth no more than $50 each and totaling no more than $100 during any one year. As might be expected, this law caused much consternation in Congress over how members might continue business as usual while adhering to the letter—if not to the spirit—of the law.

That lobbyists might be paying for legislators' vacations particularly attracts scrutiny. Under the terms of pre-1996 ethics rules, members of Congress could take trips and accept speaking fees paid for by lobbyists. An analysis of the travel practices of members of the House of Representatives in 1989–1990, for example, found that collectively they had taken nearly 4,000 sponsored trips, two-thirds of them courtesy of corporations or trade associations; they also had accepted more than $500,000 in honoraria. Agriculture interest groups sponsored 390 trips, 239 of them taken by members of agriculture or appropriations committees. Charles Stenholm (Dem-TX), a senior member of the House Agriculture Committee, for example, had taken 50 trips, 37 of them sponsored by agricultural lobbying groups, and had earned $38,250 in honoraria for these efforts.[23]

The 1996 law attempted to bar elected officials and their staff from accepting vacations paid for by special-interest groups, but loopholes remained: members of Congress could take trips paid for by corporate lobbyists if the event was sponsored by a political party, was a fact-finding mission, or was a conference at which the member was an invited speaker. In 1996–1997, 87 senators, 356 representatives, and 2,020 of their staff employees took paid trips worth about $8.6 million. The leading recipient of trips paid for by the meat industry, for example, had gone on 26 of them worth $18,550.[18] Two agriculture concerns—the Florida Sugar Cane League and the Sugar Cane Growers Cooperative of Florida—were ranked 9th (44 trips) and 11th (39 trips), respectively, among the 20 leading sponsors of congressional travel that year.[24]

BUYING ACCESS AND INFLUENCE

Do campaign contributions, trips, and presents buy corporate influence over government decisions? Much evidence suggests that they do, and in proportion to the amounts spent.[25] Here, I present just two especially intriguing examples that involve food companies.

Fighting the Banana Wars

Bananas are the most popular fruit among Americans; per capita consumption is about 75 annually, and nearly all are imported from Central America by Chiquita Brands International. This company, formerly known as United Fruit, has dominated global trade in bananas for a century and has an exceptionally rich history of influence over the U.S. government.[26] The head of Chiquita Brands, Carl H. Lindner, gives generously to both political parties. In 1998, he gave $176,000 in soft money to Democrats and $360,000 to Republicans, ranking him fourth on the *Mother Jones* list of the top 400 political contributors that year.[27] In 1999–2000, his contribution of $500,000 placed him second among the leading donors of soft money to Republicans, but he also gave $250,000 to Democrats. He contributed both donations through the American Financial Group, an insurance business. All told, Mr. Lindner's enterprises were worth at least $14 billion at the turn of the twenty-first century.[4]

In the late 1990s, Chiquita Brands encountered a problem with the European Union (EU). In an effort to strengthen the economies of former colonies, the EU had imposed limits on imports of bananas from everywhere else, a policy that Chiquita Brands believed was responsible for some of its financial difficulties. In response to pressure from Chiquita's sympathetic allies in Congress, the U.S. trade representative filed a formal complaint with the World Trade Organization (WTO), arguing that quotas on bananas violated international trade agreements. When, in retaliation, the United States imposed high tariffs on certain European luxury goods, the WTO supported that action and ordered the EU to comply with trade accords.

The methods through which Chiquita Brands achieved this remarkable victory have been described by investigative reporters for *Time* magazine who "followed the money" and documented how "$5.5 million in campaign contributions . . . bought Chiquita access in Washington" and got the Clinton administration to "mount a global trade war on Lindner's behalf."[28] The reporters noted that the government's decision to wage a trade war over bananas differed significantly from its handling of issues related to other agricultural products and was especially noteworthy because Chiquita *already* controlled 20% of the European banana market, even with the trade restrictions. They considered the unusual intervention an attempt to strengthen the WTO's ability to negotiate international trade disputes. Alternatively, it seemed possible that the White House was engaging in a collegial effort to help the company compensate for having lost $350 million in income from 1999 to 2000 and more than $1.3 billion since the EU imposed the quotas. Late in 2000, the EU offered to drop the colonial preference and establish import quotas, but Chiquita rejected that proposal, blamed the Clinton administration for the company's financial difficulties, threatened bankruptcy, and sued the EU for $525 million. Soon after the Republican administration of George W. Bush took office in 2001, its trade negotiators pushed the Europeans to make concessions to Chiquita, saving it from threatened bankruptcy and, for the moment, ending a nine-year conflict—the latest episode in the company's long history of success in influencing the U.S. government to solve its problems.[29]

Getting Sweet Attention

A second example concerns sugar, a top-of-the-*Pyramid* food that provides calories but no other nutrients. As explained in Part I, government dietary guidelines suggest moderation (meaning limits) in sugar consumption. Nevertheless, for more than 200 years, the United States has controlled the price of sugar, at first to raise revenue but later to protect the economic interests of domestic producers. For this commodity, the relationship between agricultural policy and health is unusually complex. As a result of an elaborate system of price-support programs and import tariffs and quotas codified during the Depression and the early years of World War II, Americans pay artificially high prices for sugar, a practice that cost consumers $1.9 billion in 1998. Since 1985 the price of a pound of raw sugar has ranged from 8 to 14 cents higher in U.S. markets than in world markets, and by the time sugar is sold at retail prices, this difference doubles.[30]

From a nutritional standpoint, higher sugar prices might be a useful disincentive to consuming soft drinks, desserts, and candy, but from a financial standpoint, the policy is highly undesirable. Besides the harm it causes consumers, the windfall benefits a surprisingly small number of sugar producers. In 1991, for example, 1,700 farms raised sugarcane and 13,700 raised sugar beets in the United States, but 42% of the sugar subsidies went to just 1% of these growers.[31] The owners of these few farms give generously to both political parties. The Fanjul family, for example, controls about one-third of Florida's sugarcane production and collects at least $60 million annually in subsidies. The Fanjuls contributed more than $350,000 to the two political parties—more to Democrats than to Republicans—through their Flo-Sun companies in 1997–1998. In 2000, Alfonso Fanjul hosted a dinner attended by President Bill Clinton that raised more than a million dollars for the Florida Democratic party.[32]

Sugarcane production is concentrated in two Southern states, Florida and Louisiana, where working conditions of migrant canefield workers from Caribbean countries have raised human-rights concerns.[33] Environmentalists view the Florida canefields as blocking the free flow of water into the Everglades. Sugarcane companies, in particular those owned by the Fanjul family, have successfully resisted attempts to mandate improvements in working conditions or the return of canefields to marshland in order to protect the Everglades. The same investigative reporters for *Time* magazine who were mentioned in connection with the banana wars also described how the Fanjuls used their political connections to avoid having to pay for cleaning up the Everglades. Even if their account misrepresented the family's actions (as one critical response has claimed), the Fanjuls indisputably have unusual access to the highest levels of government.[34]

The most stunning example of such access is documented in, of all unexpected places, the *Starr Report*—the 1998 account by Independent Counsel Kenneth Starr of the relationship of President Clinton with a young White House intern, Monica Lewinsky. According to Mr. Starr, on the afternoon of the President's Day holiday, Monday, February 19, 1996,

> The President told her [Ms. Lewinsky] that he no longer felt right about their intimate relationship, and he had to put a stop to it . . . At one point during their conversation, the President had a call from a sugar grower in Florida whose name, according to Ms. Lewinsky, was something like "Fanuli." In Ms. Lewinsky's recollection, the President may have taken or returned the call just as she was leaving . . . the President talked with Alfonso Fanjul of Palm Beach, Florida, from 12:42 to 1:04 p.m. The Fanjuls are prominent sugar growers in Florida.[35]

Reportedly, Mr. Fanjul had called the President on a federal holiday because Vice President Gore had just announced a plan to tax Florida sugar growers. The proposed tax would help pay for federal efforts to restore parts of the Everglades that had been polluted by sugarcane runoff. Furthermore, the House was debating whether to phase out sugar subsidies. The *Time* reporters noted that the tax was never passed. Their account concluded, "That's access."

In these two instances, financial contributions bought access to government officials and resulted in policies favorable to donors. Given that level of connection, it is understandable that agency officials would not want to do battle over a matter so seemingly trivial as the use of the verb *moderate* rather than *limit* in guidelines about sugar consumption. The job of food lobbyists is to make sure that the government (1) does nothing to impede clients from selling more of their products and (2) does as much as possible to create a supportive sales environment. We have seen that they accomplish this goal most effectively through personal contacts established through the revolving door, as well as through financial contributions. In the next chapter, we will see how food companies engage food and nutrition professionals in marketing campaigns by encouraging them to emphasize the health benefits of products or to minimize potentially adverse effects.

CHAPTER 5

CO-OPTING NUTRITION
PROFESSIONALS

THE EFFORTS OF FOOD COMPANIES TO INFLUENCE DIETARY advice to the public and to establish an image of their products as nutritious extend well beyond lobbying Congress and government agencies. They go right to the heart of nutrition as a profession. Indeed, co-opting experts—especially academic experts—is an explicit corporate strategy. A guide to such strategies 'explains that this particular tactic "is most effectively done by identifying the leading experts . . . and hiring them as consultants or advisors, or giving them research grants and the like. This activity requires a modicum of finesse; it must not be too blatant, for the experts themselves must not recognize that they have lost their objectivity and freedom of action. At a minimum, a program of this kind reduces the threat that the leading experts will be available to testify or write against the interests of the regulated firms."[1]

Food companies apply this strategy to engage nutritionists as allies in various ways, some evident but some less so. They routinely provide information and funds to academic departments, research institutes, and professional societies, and they support meetings, conferences, journals, and other such activities. Most nutrition professionals depend on such support, and some actively seek it. At issue is whether doing so corrupts academic and professional integrity.

This question is not so easy to address as it might seem. As an academic nutritionist, I cannot fail to recognize that the industry has created a plentiful, varied, readily available, relatively safe, and relatively inexpensive food supply that is the envy of people throughout the world. Many—perhaps most—of my colleagues sincerely believe that the only way to improve the diet of Americans is to work with industry to produce more nutritious food. Nevertheless, although accepting support from a food company does not necessarily mean that we endorse its products, the public may perceive us as doing so. Thus people outside the field who observe partnerships among nutritionists and food companies might wonder how we can possibly maintain objectivity and critical judgment when engaged in alliances with industry—and they would wonder with good reason, as this chapter suggests.

SPONSORING EDUCATION AND RESEARCH

Food companies routinely sponsor the educational activities of nutrition professional societies as well as the research of individual investigators, and nutrition academics routinely consult for food companies on these and more product-oriented matters. In my own experience, it is impossible for nutrition academics *not* to be involved with food companies in one way or another. This issue is not new; a survey by the Center for Science in the Public Interest in the mid-1970s identified frequent payments by food companies to agriculture and nutrition faculty for consulting services, lectures, membership on advisory boards, and representation at congressional hearings; this same group now reveals academics' ties to industry on a Web site that provides hundreds of examples of nutrition researchers and educators who receive funding from food companies.[2] Nor are the apparent conflicts of interest in such interactions confined to the United States; a recent British study found 158 of 246 members of national committees on nutrition and food policy to consult for or receive funding from food companies.[3] Table 13 lists a few examples of food company sponsorship of professional societies. Inevitably, such connections raise questions about the ability of academic experts to provide independent opinions on matters of diet and health.

Journals and Journal Supplements

Nutrition societies publish journals and supplements to journals. These are expensive to produce, and corporate sponsorship helps to defray costs. Thus the *Journal of Nutrition Education* acknowledges 8 "corporate patron friends" and 4 "corporate sustaining friends . . . who make an annual financial contribution to support the goals of the society and its journal." The more research-oriented *Journal of Nutrition* lists 10 food and drug companies as sustaining associates of its parent society, and the

TABLE 13. Examples of food company sponsors of groups that advise the public about nutrition and health

Organization: Activity	Sponsors: Selected Examples
American Cancer Society: promotion campaign	Florida Department of Citrus
American Council on Science and Health: general activities	300 funding sources, including many food corporations and trade associations
American Dietetic Association: fact sheets	Dairy Council, Sugar Association
American College of Nutrition: annual meeting	Quaker Oats, Novartis
American Heart Association: HeartCheck	More than 50 food companies
American Society for Clinical Nutrition: educational activities	Knoll Pharmaceutical, Amgen, BestFoods, Coca-Cola
American Society for Nutritional Science: annual meeting	Mead Johnson, Ross Products, Procter & Gamble
Food and Nutrition Board, Institute of Medicine: Dietary Reference Intakes	Roche Vitamins, Mead Johnson, M&M Mars, Weider Nutrition Group
Society for Nutrition Education: educational programs	Food Marketing Institute, Dole Foods, Nestlé USA
Tufts University: Nutrition Navigator Web site	Kraft Foods (Philip Morris)

American Journal of Clinical Nutrition lists 28 such companies supporting "selected educational activities of the Society." Sponsors of nutrition journals include such companies as Coca-Cola, Gerber, Nestlé/Carnation, Monsanto, Procter & Gamble, Roche Vitamins, Slim-Fast Foods, and the Sugar Association, as well as others that make baby food or formula, vitamin supplements, functional foods, diet products, sugar-sweetened breakfast cereals, and genetically modified crops—virtually all of them products with nutritional attributes considered controversial and currently under debate.

Some journals go to great pains to erect a "firewall" between their editorial and business functions, but this barrier is all too easily breached. One reason for the breach is that advertisers contribute to the financial health of academic as well as popular journals. The American Dietetic Association, for example, reported an income of about $3 million from its journal in 1999.[4] Its April 2000 issue carried 12 full-page advertisements, mainly from companies selling diet supplements or nutrient-analysis software; a separately bound 20-page "educational" insert from the Dannon Institute; and another 8 pages of classified advertisements. An account of the advertising practices of the two leading U.S. medical journals—the *New England Journal of Medicine* and the *Journal of the American Medical Association*—both of which publish the "hottest" of nutrition research, observed that both have business as well as academic functions and "are beholden to drug makers for their economic viability;" each takes in about $20 million annually from drug company advertising.[5] At the very least, this sponsorship causes considerable discomfort to the editorial side of the firewall.

Papers presented at conferences sponsored by food companies are sometimes published as supplements to nutrition journals, and the companies also underwrite the costs of publication. In 2000, for example, companies such as Wyeth Nutritionals, Bristol-Myers Squibb, Mead Johnson, and the International Nut Council helped support publication of supplements to the *American Journal of Clinical Nutrition*. Researchers on drug company sponsorship have shown it to be highly correlated with publication of articles favorable to sponsors' products, and nutrition journal supplements also tend to highlight the benefits of particular foods or diets in which the sponsors have some interest. A rare exception was a supplement to the *Journal of Nutrition* on the role of soy foods in disease prevention and treatment. Although the sponsors included Archer Daniels Midland, Cargill, and a host of other soy producers, product manufacturers, and promotion boards, the editors introduced the supplement with this caveat: "With few exceptions, considerably more research is required before a good understanding of the health effects of soy can be realized . . . [and] there is some lack of confidence about the validity of some of the effects that have been observed . . . [A]lthough most delegates considered soy foods to be absolutely safe, not all were in agreement on this point."[6]

I can speak from experience about the difficulties inherent in sponsored supplements: I edited one for the *American Journal of Clinical Nutrition* in 1995.[7] The papers came from a conference on the health effects of Mediterranean diets for which the principal sponsor was the International Olive Oil Council—a group that might be expected to have much to gain from favorable publicity about the health benefits of diets in which olive oil is the principal fat. After much discussion, the editor and I dealt directly with problems of conflict of interest. We agreed that the sponsors would not participate in the editorial process, pay authors for their contributions, or pay me for my editorial work. The entire supplement was peer-reviewed, and the sponsorship was fully disclosed: "Sponsor: Oldways Preservation & Exchange Trust through a grant from the International Olive Oil Council, Administrator of the United Nations

Olive and Olive Oil Agreement." This journal requires such disclosure; like others, it adds the letter "s" to supplement page numbers—a signal to readers that the articles may not have undergone as rigorous a peer review as is customary. Not all journals are this scrupulous, however.

Conferences

Professional meetings normally take place in hotels; they are expensive to run but can produce substantial income for nutrition societies. The American Dietetic Association, for example, reported revenues of nearly $900,000 from its 1998 annual meeting, a figure that surely must exceed expenses.[4] To generate such income, nutrition societies routinely seek corporate sponsorship, and companies willingly comply. Food, beverage, and supplement companies buy space at exhibits; place advertisements in program books; underwrite coffee breaks, meals, and receptions; sponsor research awards and student prizes; and provide bags, pens, and other meeting souvenirs—for which they are thanked in program books. This phenomenon is not confined to the United States. In 1998 I attended a meeting of the British Nutrition Society where the program book thanked Nestlé UK and Sainsbury's for receptions, Coca-Cola and Mars for refreshments, and the Meat and Livestock Commission for barbecue and banquet meat. I also attended a meeting of the Community Nutrition Society of Spain sponsored by 20 groups representing vitamin supplements, juice, margarine, olive oil, and beer.

In the United States, the annual meeting of a leading nutrition research group, the American Society for Nutritional Sciences, sets aside time for a Kellogg-sponsored breakfast meeting for heads of university nutrition departments; an especially memorable one featured samples from the company's line of psyllium fiber-supplemented foods, which were then undergoing test-marketing. That same conference offered research sessions sponsored by trade associations such as the National Dairy Council and the National Cattlemen's Beef Association. The program book for the American Dietetic Association's annual meeting in 2000 acknowledged session sponsorship by more than 30 food, beverage, or supplement companies, some with commercial interests in the topic under discussion. The Distilled Spirits Council, for example, sponsored a session on the risks and health benefits of alcohol consumption, Slim-Fast sponsored talks on obesity prevention and treatment, the company that makes Benecol margarine underwrote a session on its cholesterol-lowering ingredient, and Quaker/Gatorade supported lectures on athletes' dietary supplements.

Does sponsorship influence the content of conference sessions? In my experience, speakers at sponsored sessions are *offended* by such a question. Sponsorship is so ubiquitous and is considered so helpful that hardly anyone can imagine that it might have harmful consequences. A study of pharmaceutical industry practices, however, has reported that physicians who accept travel funds, meals, or gifts from drug companies, or who attend conferences sponsored by them, are more likely to write prescriptions for the sponsors' medications.[8] Another study described how a drug company used a medical conference as a public relations strategy to generate interest in vitamins as "potent agents of health"; it concluded that if nothing else, critics of the products were excluded from the debate.[9]

Such research suggests that to avoid undue influence, nutritionists should refuse sponsorship or decline invitations to attend or speak at sponsored meetings. Perhaps so, but if we take this ethical high road, we end up talking only to ourselves. To give a personal example: Should I have declined an invitation to debate food biotechnology at a sponsored session at the American Dietetic Association's annual convention? The association offered airfare, meals, and hotel expenses and an honorarium of $1,500—all paid for by Monsanto, the leading U.S. producer of genetically modified crops. Although the company approved the program in advance, it is "innocent" of buying influence; Monsanto's funds go to the association, not directly to the speakers. If I refuse such invitations, I lose an opportunity to explain my views to an influential audience. If I decline the funding, I am out the considerable costs of travel and hotel accommodations. But if I accept the invitation, will my views be compromised by the sponsorship? Will I feel that I am being impolite if I criticize Monsanto for its opposition to labeling of genetically modified foods? This ethical dilemma is not easily resolved, even by people sensitive to the issue.

Research Studies

Whether nutrition professionals are compromised by support from food companies is a troubling issue, but an even more troubling question is whether corporate sponsorship affects the conduct of nutrition research or its results. Research funds are scarce, and researchers are always looking for funding sources. Given the cautious interpretation required for most nutrition research, any study, review, or commentary with conclusions favorable to sponsors may give pause, as indicated by the selected—

but quite typical—examples offered in Table 14. So might the actions of the National Academies' Food and Nutrition Board (FNB) in recommending higher levels of intake of vitamins C and E when the board's work is funded in part through a foundation supported by companies such as Roche Vitamins, Mead Johnson Nutrition Group, Daiichi Fine Chemicals, Weider Nutrition Group, and the Natural Choice Vitamin E Association—all with vested interests in having nutrient standards set so high that people can meet them only by taking supplements. The FNB itself is supported directly by food and supplement companies such as G.D. Searle, Monsanto, NutraSweet, and Nestlé.

Nearly everyone believes that the first step in preventing sponsorship from influencing research is to disclose it. One notable exception is the prestigious British journal *Nature.* Its editors dismiss concerns about research sponsorship and explain that they persist in the "stubborn belief that research as we publish it is indeed research, not business."[10] This view may explain why the journal was "pleased to acknowledge" the financial support of The Roche Group—a company that makes a drug used in obesity treatment—for a "Nature Insight" section containing six scientific papers on this condition. Roche advertisements introduce the Insight section: "There is no doubt that, in addition to lifestyle and behavior changes, innovative new drugs will play an important role in managing obesity. We take pride in sponsoring this special issue." The final Insight article concludes that current drugs have a useful place in the treatment of obesity; one of its authors works for Millennium Pharmaceuticals, a Roche partner "in attempting to understand the underlying cause of obesity and diabetes."[11] Although the quality of the sponsored papers may be excellent, this section cannot help but appear more as advertising than as science.

The most important consideration is whether industry sponsorship influences research results and opinions. This question demands careful consideration if for no other reason than sponsorship by industry is so common. A 1996 survey found that nearly 30% of university faculty members accept industry funding;[12] another found 34% of the primary authors of 800 papers in molecular biology and medicine to be involved in patents, to serve on advisory committees, or to hold personal shares in companies that might benefit from the research.[13]

Some self-selection surely is involved in these relationships. Most research on this question concerns sponsorship by drug or tobacco companies. Those studies demonstrate that investigators who support the use of drug or tobacco products are more likely than neutral or critical

TABLE 14. Quotations from selected research studies, reviews, or editorials supported fully or in part by food, beverage, or supplement companies

---

"High-fibre breakfast cereals may help to reduce risk of cancers that are associated with poor fibre intakes." (The author is employed by Kellogg's, UK.)[a]

"Eating two eggs daily for 12 weeks . . . resulted in no statistically measurable effect on plasma LDL-C [low density lipoprotein-cholesterol, the "bad" kind] in HC [high-blood-cholesterol] subjects" (funded in part by The Egg Nutrition Center).[b]

"Margarine intake compared with butter intake lowered LDL-C levels 11% in adults...and 9% in children." (Sponsors included the United Soybean Board and the National Association of Margarine Manufacturers.)[c]

"The prepared meal plan is a simple and effective strategy for improving dietary compliance and CVD [cardiovascular disease] endpoints." (This study was funded by Campbell Soup, maker of the prepared meals.)[d]

"Scientific findings indicate that the prevalence of lactose intolerance is grossly overestimated." (One of the authors is an officer of the National Dairy Council. Lactose is the principal sugar in dairy products.)[e]

"Zinc gluconate . . . significantly reduced the duration of symptoms of the common cold by 40% compared with placebo." (One of the authors is reported to have earned nearly $145,000 from sale of the product's stock before the paper was published. A later study by the same group found zinc to be ineffective against colds.)[f]

"Substantial evidence indicates that intakes greater than the recommended dietary allowances (RDAs) of . . . calcium, folic acid, vitamin E, selenium, and chromium reduce the risk of certain diseases for some people." (The author of the review is a scientist/official of the Council for Responsible Nutrition, a supplement-industry trade association.)[g]

"The possible risk of pulmonary hypertension associated with dexfenfluramine [an anti-obesity drug] is small and appears to be outweighed by benefits when the drug is used appropriately." (The authors consulted for the drug manufacturer.)[h]

---

authors to have financial relationships with such companies. They also demonstrate that favorable attitudes toward the product are associated with favorable research results, whether or not the companies can be proved to exert influence. Other studies demonstrate an even stronger association with research results that minimize negative effects of these products on health. Researchers on such relationships do not suggest that industry-sponsored research is *always* biased, just that there is a higher probability that it will draw favorable conclusions.[14]

As indicated by the examples given in Table 14, it seems entirely likely that investigations of sponsored nutrition research would arrive at similar conclusions. No matter how carefully the research is conducted, its partisan sponsorship conveys the impression that the results were purchased.

TABLE 14. *(continued)*

"For most patients [with blood cholesterol levels above 130 mg per deciliter] an LDL-lowering drug will be required." (The chair and 5 of 13 other members of the committee responsible for this recommendation consulted for or received honoraria or grants from pharmaceutical companies making cholesterol-lowering drugs.)[i]

"There is reason to be concerned that lowering NaCl [salt] intake may have long-term metabolic risks that have not been fully identified . . . we do not have solid evidence that lower NaCl intake prospectively will prevent or control high blood pressure." (The review in which this appears was funded in part by The Salt Institute, a trade association for the salt industry.)[j]

"A moderate intake of wine (2–5 glasses per day) was associated with a 24–31% reduction in all-cause mortality." (This study was funded in part by The French Technical Institute of Wine.)[k]

"The symposium reviewed . . . the new evidence suggesting that certain cocoa flavonoids may have cardiovascular health effects . . . the research to date suggests that chocolate lovers may obtain more than a sensory benefit from their indulgence." (The journal supplement in which this was published and some of its studies were sponsored by Mars, Inc., United Kingdom.)[l]

SOURCES: [a] O'Sullivan KR. In: Smith G, ed. Children's Food: Marketing and Innovation. London: Blackie Academic & Professional, 1997. [b] Knopp RH, et al. J Am College of Nutrition 1997; 16:551–561. [c] Denke MA, et al. JAMA 2000;284:2740–2747. [d] Metz JA, et al. Am J Clin Nutr 1997; 66:373–385. [e] McBean LD, Miller GD. J Am Diet Assoc 1998;98:671–676. [f] Mossad SB, et al. Annals of Internal Medicine 1996;125:81–88. Hilts PJ. New York Times February 1, 1997:6. Macknin ML, et al. JAMA 1998;279:1962–1967. [g] Hathcock JN. Am J Clin Nutr 1997;66:427–437. [h] Manson JE, Faich GA. N Engl J Med 1996;335:659–660. Hilts PJ. New York Times August 29, 1996:D18. [i] Expert Panel on Detection, Evaluation, and Treatment of High Blood Cholesterol in Adults. JAMA 2001;285:2486–2497. [j] Muntzel M, Drüeke T. Am J Hypertension 1992;5:1s–42s. [k] Renaud SC, et al. Epidemiology 1998;9:184–188. [l] Erdman JW et al., eds. J Nutrition 2000;130(8 suppl)2057s–2126s.

This impression is reinforced when sponsors use the results to advertise or publicize their products. Following publication of the margarine study cited in Table 14, for example, a trade group identified only by its Web site (**www.margarine.org**) placed a full-page advertisement in the *New York Times* (December 8, 2000): "46 families end the margarine vs. butter debate. A groundbreaking study in the *Journal of the American Medical Association* proves that using margarine instead of butter *significantly lowers cholesterol*. The debate is over . . . the results proved once and for all that soft margarine is clearly the healthier choice . . . everyone in your family can feel good about eating it."

The advertisement, of course, says nothing about the caloric equivalence of butter and margarine, nor does it particularly emphasize that the margarine must be soft in order to avoid cholesterol-raising *trans*-saturated fatty acids. Industry publicity about the finding of beneficial flavonoid phytochemicals in chocolate and wine also rarely mention their dietary context. That such publicity adds to public confusion is illustrated by the wry commentary of Mr. Calvin Trillin in *The Nation*, November 27, 2000:

RARE GOOD NEWS

The *Journal of Nutrition* wrote about
Some researchers who tested chocolate out.
It may help stave off heart attacks, they claim.
Red wine, we've known for years, can do the same.
Without the need of any doctor's urging.
I feel a healthy diet plan emerging.

Copyright © 2000 by Calvin Trillin. This usage granted by permission of Lescher & Lescher, Ltd.

Mr. Trillin refers here to the studies funded in part by Mars, Inc., the maker of M&M's, Mars Bars, and other popular chocolate candies.

CREATING PARTNERSHIPS AND ALLIANCES

Collaboration with food companies also poses difficulties for nutrition organizations and individuals, despite the fact that many actively seek such alliances as a means of supporting educational, research, and service projects. All parties engaged in partnerships and alliances justify them in terms of common goals and congruent interest in helping to improve the health of the public, and all invariably maintain that the relationships do not compromise their views or opinions on nutrition issues. Evidence from the following examples, however, suggests otherwise.

Buying Academic Departments: Novartis at UC Berkeley

Nutrition, food science, food technology, and agriculture departments at public and private colleges and universities eagerly seek corporate funding for research, scholarships, equipment, facilities, and buildings. A walk through any major agricultural campus, for example, is sure to reveal buildings and programs named after corporate donors. Such arrangements have a long history in the federal land-grant system through which the U.S. Department of Agriculture (USDA) funds agricultural research and training at certain state universities. More recently, these arrangements have begun to involve *exclusive* contracts between companies and academic departments.

In 1998 the Department of Plant and Microbial Biology at the University of California (UC), Berkeley, concerned about the "crowding out" of funding for public-interest research at land-grant universities, created a new venue for corporate support. Its dean wrote that public research universities "have naively pursued the public interest" and failed to recognize "the integrative evolution of fundamental, applied, exclusive or proprietary research."[15] On the premise that a public–private partnership could form a basis for enhancing "public good" research and that such "complementarities . . . can not be effectively pursued with more than a single partner," the department decided to auction itself to just one company. The new partnership would permit the *industry* partner to

- Select the participating faculty.
- Have free access to all uncommitted research of participating faculty.
- Review research results prior to publication.
- Negotiate for licensing rights to technologies produced by the research.
- Negotiate with faculty for specific projects.
- Veto faculty participation in other projects.
- Place a full-time scientist of its own on the faculty.

With these principles accepted by the faculty, and with the idea that the alliance would "*crowd in* public good research" (translation: promote research in the public interest), a "tactical implementation team" presented proposals to five major biotechnology firms that had responded to an invitational letter.[16]

The department chose Novartis, the Swiss agriculture and drug company (which also owns Gerber Products), as its partner in a deal said to be worth $50 million—$25 million for laboratory support and $25 million for research support over a five-year period, an amount equivalent to one-third of the department's annual research budget. Critics immediately charged that the agreement impinged on academic freedom. They feared that it would take the campus "one step further away from the reality of a publicly funded university, where all ideas rise or fall on their own merit and where tensions exist between the demands of academic freedom and the politics of the state of California—not between the research agendas of faculty and a profit-making enterprise . . . this represents a marked change in the very soul of Berkeley . . . Here the private sector is making research decisions . . . this is a turning point."[17]

The department denied such charges, explaining that "the driving force for this is not the research money, but the training aspect. It will give students opportunities that we couldn't otherwise give them."[18] Furthermore, the dean, who found the controversy "surprising," defended the arrangement on the grounds that "we are, after all, one of the original land-grant universities whose stated purpose was to marry scientific insight with practical knowledge to improve agricultural productivity. This might not sound like commerce, but it was and still is."[17]

Regardless of the accuracy of this interpretation of the land-grant system, some observers viewed the Novartis partnership as an inevitable result—and extension—of the Bayh–Dole Act of 1980. This act permitted universities to patent and commercialize discoveries from publicly funded research, thereby establishing an incentive for industries to enter into partnerships. The act is considered to have succeeded admirably in this purpose. The number of university–industry partnership patents grew from 250 in the years prior to Bayh–Dole to more than 4,800 in 1998.[19] What particularly troubles critics, however, is the idea that companies might dictate the direction of research or unduly influence or delay its publication. Although faculty have reported incidents of intimidation and of pressure on students to work on Novartis-funded projects, the dean of the college reportedly termed such concerns "silly."[20]

Claiming Independence:
The American Council on Science and Health

The American Council on Science and Health (ACSH) is a nonprofit group whose representatives comment frequently on food issues. As its public relations materials explain, "Unlike some so-called consumer-advocacy organizations that misrepresent science and distort health priorities, ACSH has a well-established policy of presenting balanced, scientifically sound analyses of current health topics."[21] Apparently agreeing with this description are the 250 physicians, scientists, and policy advisors on the council's board, many of them quite distinguished. ACSH takes a strong position against cigarette smoking but is infamous for debunking concerns about food safety issues that especially trouble consumers: pesticides, additives, sugar, and food biotechnology, for example. Its executive director, Elizabeth Whelan, regularly writes op-ed pieces for the *New York Times* and articles for former Surgeon General C. Everett Koop's health Web site arguing in favor of the safety of eating red meat or artificial fats like olestra, or taking diet drugs viewed as dangerous by the FDA. What the public relations materials do not reveal is the extent to which the ACSH is funded by the makers of such products. Its Web site does not list corporate supporters, but its long-time nemesis, the Washington, DC-based consumer advocacy group the Center for Science in the Public Interest (CSPI), has noted such connections since 1982, and *Consumer Reports* identified 40% of ACSH's funding as derived from industry sources, some of it for specific projects.[22] I asked a senior nutrition scientist on the ACSH board whether he endorsed the group's relationships with food companies. He said he was unaware of the group's pro-industry positions and that he lends his name, is not paid for his participation, and performs no other service to the organization. Apparently, use of his name is service enough.

Endorsing "Healthy" Foods:
The American Heart Association

In 1988 the American Heart Association (AHA), long a distinguished champion of research and education promoting low-fat and other dietary approaches to prevention of coronary heart disease, decided to raise funds by labeling foods "heart-healthy." The AHA would identify foods that met certain standards for content of fat, saturated fat, cholesterol, and sodium with a logo consisting of a red heart with a white check mark and the words "American Heart Association Tested & Approved." The association planned to collect fees from food companies that made approved products and expected to benefit from company advertising and promotion of the partnership.[23]

This proposal immediately ran into opposition from USDA officials concerned that identifying single foods as heart-healthy distorted basic principles of good nutrition, which depend on overall dietary patterns. FDA officials also were concerned that the "HeartCheck" might interfere with the agency's efforts to develop new labeling rules.[24] Nevertheless, the AHA invited 2,300 makers of margarines, crackers, and frozen foods to apply for endorsement. Each was to pay a nonrefundable fee of $40,000 for testing, as well as an annual educational fee—ranging from $5,000 to $1 million, depending on the size of the company—to cover the cost of public relations. An AHA spokesman explained that the association now had "a chance to reach millions of Americans with a health message," but food companies protested that the program was "an extortion racket."[25] Later, the AHA reduced the fees to $10,000 and capped the educational fee at $600,000 per year. In the meantime, federal agencies charged that the HeartCheck label would be misleading. FDA officials wrote that although they agreed with

> the laudable *objectives* of your program . . . we have serious reservations about the *means* you have chosen to meet those ends. The most significant drawback from our perspective is that your proposed program could very easily result in the endorsement of products . . . that quite simply do not represent the kinds of foods that ought to be promoted to achieve healthy hearts . . . In addition to risking regulatory action, FDA believes that your program will increase consumer confusion and hamper any comprehensive solution to the food labeling problem.[26]

Early in 1990, the first HeartChecked foods appeared on shelves: C&W frozen vegetables, Promise margarine, and Colavita olive oil. Nutrition scientists complained that the program gave "a misleading impression that margarine is a heart-healthy food, and clearly it is not . . . the message is that what is labeled is good food, and what is not is bad food . . . and fresh foods are not going to be labeled at all."[27] In the meantime, the legal staff of seven states and two leading nutrition societies wrote FDA opposing the program on the grounds that promoting the health benefits of single foods was misleading. As a result, nearly two-thirds of the companies that had joined the program withdrew from participation. In April 1990, "besieged by stinging criticism and threats of strong government action," the AHA ended the program and agreed to return the fees it had collected.[28]

The association did not give up on the idea, however, and tried again in 1993—this time successfully. Because its revised criteria generally followed FDA labeling guidelines, the program encountered little opposition and went into effect in 1994. Companies paid an initial fee of $2,500 and an annual renewal fee of $650 for the seal of approval, and more for exclusivity rights. The AHA maintained that the arrangements constituted "food-certification programs or corporate relationships. None of this constitutes an endorsement." Perhaps not, but by 1996, Kellogg's public relations materials were boasting that more than 50 of its products carried the AHA seal of approval and proclaiming that the company was "pleased to provide consumers with guidance on selecting heart-healthy foods," among them such unlikely items as Kellogg's Frosted Flakes, Fruity Marshmallow Krispies, and Low-Fat (but by no means low-sugar) Pop-Tarts.[29] By October 1997, 55 companies were participating, with 643 products certified.

The current program requires a $7,500 fee per product and $4,500 for annual renewals, with a discount if more than 25 products are submitted in one year; these funds are said to be earmarked solely for

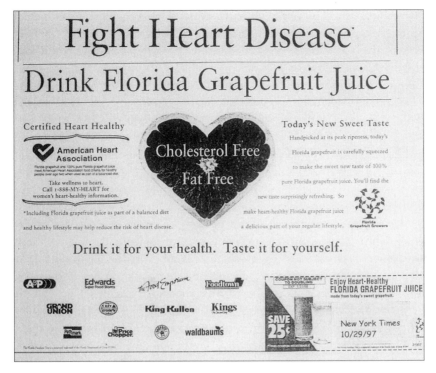

FIGURE 13. The American Heart Association's HeartCheck program requires payment for certification of grapefruit as heart-healthy; this juice would not be expected to be high in fat or cholesterol. The advertisement appeared in the *New York Times* on October 29, 1997.

administration of the program.[30] The rules preclude endorsement of medical foods, dietary supplements, alcoholic beverages, and products owned by tobacco companies, with the result that Kellogg's Cocoa Frosted Flakes—a product famously high in sugar content—is "heart smart" but the Post equivalent is not (the company is owned by Philip Morris). The program also leads to nutritionally absurd advertisements such as the one illustrated in Figure 13. Although the association undoubtedly uses this funding for good purposes, the program cannot help but raise questions about credibility.

Avoiding "Eat Less" Advice: Public–Private Alliances

The food industry willingly enters into alliances with government agencies and professional societies to promote health through dietary "flexibility." In 1993 one such partnership of 70 agricultural producers, processors, and retailers, industry trade associations, scientific foundations, university groups, consumer and media groups, and state and federal agencies endorsed a National Action Plan to Improve the American Diet by eating more "healthy" foods. The plan's "specific benefits for the food industry include enlarging the healthy eating market and, potentially, reducing the fierce competition for the currently rather small consumer segment that is concerned about healthy eating. . . . For everyone involved, the [plan] offers a means of accomplishing vital goals that are achievable only through collaboration."[31] Despite its industry-friendly "eat more" message, the plan never got translated into action and quietly disappeared, perhaps because direct benefits to donors were not obvious.

Public–private partnerships are unlikely to promote "eat less" messages, which may be one reason why they have difficulty dealing with federal *Dietary Guidelines*. In 1997 the USDA and the Department of Health and Human Services announced participation in an alliance formed to develop "science-based and consumer-oriented messages to promote the *Dietary Guidelines for Americans*."[32] The Dietary Guidelines Alliance includes industry groups such as the Food Marketing Institute, the National Pork Producers Council, and the Sugar Association, along with professional organizations such as the American Dietetic Association. The principal message of the alliance's program, "It's All About You," is to enjoy a variety of foods. The alliance says that dietary changes should be small and nonrestrictive: "Go ahead and balance what you eat . . . over several days. No need to worry about just one meal or one day."[33] Its explicit purpose is to counter the "myth" that some foods are bad and should be excluded from healthful diets. Industry partners are more than willing to promote this "anything goes" approach to dietary advice.

Undermining Credibility: The American Dietetic Association

A major player in the Dietary Guidelines Alliance is the American Dietetic Association (ADA), a professional society that represents the interests of 70,000 or so nutritionists who hold credentials as registered dietitians. Many ADA members are employed by food companies, and the association's relations with industry are especially close. The ADA acknowledged donations of $735,000 from groups and individuals contributing $10,000 or more during the 1998–1999 fiscal year, among them 22 food product and trade associations, and nearly 8% of the

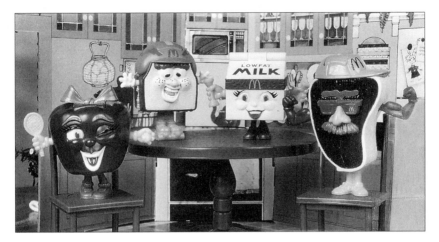

FIGURE 14. The American Dietetic Association collaborated with McDonald's to develop "Food FUNdamentals" toys as part of a shared "commitment to nutrition education." McDonald's featured the toys in a special "Happy Meals" promotion celebrating National Nutrition Month. (McDonald's press release, Oak Brook, IL, February 24, 1993)

association's $25 million annual income came from such grants. Critics charge that ADA's reliance on such funding means that "they never criticize the food industry."[34]

Indeed, ADA's stance on dietary advice is firmly pro-industry; one of its basic tenets is that there is no such thing as a good or a bad food.[35] The association apparently is willing to enter into partnerships with any food company or trade organization, regardless of the nutritional quality of its products. In 1993, for example, the ADA collaborated with McDonald's on a campaign built around Happy Meals and toy food characters representing the major food groups (see Figure 14). The association's journal routinely carries a page of federal nutrition news compiled by the Sugar Association. This blurring of the distinction between food advertising and dietary advice is most evident in the association's 70 or so informational Fact Sheets—each with its own corporate sponsor. Table 15 provides examples of Fact Sheet topics, their sponsors, and typical statements. If these statements give the impression that they were written by the company's public relations staff, it is for good reason: They were. In response to membership complaints about the one-sided content of a Fact Sheet on agricultural biotechnology that was sponsored by Monsanto, the leading U.S. maker of genetically engineered crop

TABLE 15. American Dietetic Association nutrition Fact Sheets: examples of topics, sponsors, and representative statements, 1999–2000[4]

Topic	Sponsor	Sample Statement
Agricultural biotechnology	Monsanto	"The U.S. government has a well-coordinated system to ensure that new agricultural biotechnology products are safe for the environment and to animal and human health."
Aspartame	NutraSweet	"Aspartame makes available a wide variety of food and beverage choices for the person interested in maintaining a healthful lifestyle."
Canned foods	Steel Packaging Council	"Canned food is as nutritious as its fresh and frozen counterparts upon preparation."
Chocolate	Mars	"Chocolate is no longer a concern for those wary of saturated fat, and . . . in fact, chocolate can be part of a heart-healthy eating plan."
Fats and oils	National Association of Margarine Manufacturers	"Margarine products and liquid vegetable oil have little saturated fat and contain no cholesterol."
Olestra	Procter & Gamble	"Fat replacers like olestra are one of the many acceptable ways to help reduce the amount of fat and calories in your diet."
Snacking	Nabisco	"In today's busy world, snacking is part of our daily routine. We enjoy milk and cookies after school . . . and reach for a handful of crackers before bed."
Sodium	Campbell Soup	"The link between the sodium you eat and high blood pressure is unclear."

plants, the ADA president explained that "the first draft of the fact sheet may be submitted by the funder or PR agency staff . . . [but] ADA has final editorial control of the content of all Nutrition Fact Sheets."[36]

This explanation appeared in the same issue of the journal as a Kellogg-sponsored fact sheet on vitamins during pregnancy: "'B' smart for your heart and pregnancy with folic acid and vitamins B6 and B12." Placed directly opposite this page was an advertisement for Kellogg's cereals: "Have you heard the good news? Now many of your patients' favorite Kellogg's cereals are fortified with 100% of the Daily Value of folic acid, B6 and B12." Statements on package labels about nutrients and disease risk are health claims that require FDA approval, but the FDA had not yet approved a claim that B vitamins could prevent heart disease. Thus, in publishing the fact sheet, the ADA became an unwitting participant in Kellogg's strategy to evade FDA restrictions on label statements.[37]

The intermingling of advice and advertising does not mean that the association ignores conflicts of interest with food companies; it just does not seem terribly concerned about them. The ADA's 1988 code of ethics stated: "The dietetic practitioner promotes or endorses products in a manner that is neither false nor misleading." A revision of the code in 1999 retains that statement but adds another: "The dietetic practitioner is alert to situations that might cause a conflict of interest or have the appearance of a conflict. The dietetics practitioner provides full disclosure when a real or potential conflict of interest arises."[38] One editorial on the revised code points out that "in the world of nutrition research, a conflict of interest does not necessarily exist just because scientists receive support from a food/drug company or a government agency as long as the interests of the various groups do not conflict." Another argues that adequate safeguards exist in the form of codes of ethics and peer review.[39] It is not possible to know whether the Fact Sheets—or the association itself—might express more critical views if they were independent of food company sponsorship.

Confusing the Issues: The Tufts Nutrition Navigator

The Tufts "Navigator" is the top-rated nutrition Web site. Produced by Tufts University's School of Nutrition Science and Policy—and underwritten by Kraft Foods (Philip Morris)—it ranks other nutrition Web sites on a 25-point scale according to scientific accuracy, context, and balance; the depth to which they cover nutrition information; how recently they were updated; and their usability. Sponsorship by food companies that might be using nutrition information on their Web sites to sell products is not considered a factor in the rating scale, nor is lack of critical thinking about that issue. Thus the Tufts Navigator gives high rankings to Web sites produced by the ADA (23 points), the International Food Information Council (23), the National Pork Producers Council (22), Campbell's Soup (21), the American Council on Science and Health (20), and the National Cattlemen's Beef Association (20)—all groups directly or indirectly sponsored by food companies. The Navigator says of the ADA's site: "The ADA is one of the best places to go for solid nutrition information . . . [c]onsumers can access 'the good nutrition reading list,' the *Food Guide Pyramid*, and fact sheets on everything from the place for chocolate in a healthy diet to men's nutrition concerns."[40] In contrast, the Navigator ranks the site of the independent, but often sharply critical, Center for Science in the Public Interest (CSPI) as just average (19 points), not because of any problem with scientific accuracy but because "we take issue with [CSPI's] sensationalist and alarmist tone . . . [I]f you are to avoid as many processed foods and additives as they advise, what else is left to eat?"

CSPI has objected to this review and notes that the site's biases reflect its sponsorship by a company that makes margarine, hot dogs, and cheese: "If there is anything worse than unreliable information on the Web, it is raters of Web sites who fail to disclose prominently their rating criteria and potential conflicts of interest."[41]

Struggling to Do Good: 5 A Day for Better Health

By this time, anyone might conclude that no professional society should ever forge an alliance with a food company, but it is time to introduce the one outstanding exception: the National "5 A Day" Campaign for Better Health. This public–private partnership is a joint venture of the National Cancer Institute (NCI), a division of the taxpayer-supported National Institutes of Health, and the industry-funded Produce for Better Health Foundation (PBH). The partnership's purpose is to promote consumption of at least five servings of fruits and vegetables each day on the basis that eating more fruits and vegetables is demonstrably good for overall health and is especially protective against cancer. Because the United States does not produce enough fruits and vegetables to provide five daily servings to everyone in the population, USDA economists have estimated that following this advice would require a doubling in production; dietary intake surveys, which underestimate actual intake (see the Appendix), estimate that consumption would need to increase by one-third.[42] Thus, the 5 A Day program is an ideal "win–win"; the campaign should improve the health of the public while helping the industry sell more food.

The national campaign derived from an NCI-funded project conducted in California in the late-1980s, and during the two years that it was active, consumption of fruits and vegetables increased in that state. On that basis, the NCI took the program to the national level. The elements of the state and national campaigns were based on theories of behavior modification and were thoroughly researched, consumer-tested, and evaluated. From the standpoint of nutrition education, its concept was—and remains—ideal: the 5 A Day message is simple (fruits and vegetables), positive (eat more), measurable (5), credible (NCI sponsorship), and able to reach vast numbers of people through food stores.

In 1991 NCI developed a partnership with a coalition of 60 fruit and vegetable producers, packagers, retailers, and trade associations who formed the PBH Foundation specifically to work on the campaign; PBH now includes 1,000 industry groups representing more than 35,000 supermarkets. The campaign's promotional, education, and research programs began in 1992 with an initial five-year grant of $27 million from NCI and a contribution of $415,000 from PBH.[43]

Although this level of funding appeared generous, the NCI soon reduced its contribution by $6 million. Furthermore, its leadership insisted that most of the remaining funds go toward research rather than education or outreach. As a result, 89% of NCI's first-year allocation of $5 million went toward demonstration research projects. From 1993 to 1999, NCI's funding for 5 A Day ranged from a high of $6.2 million (1996) to a low of $4.3 million (1997), with about 80% going for research and evaluation. NCI was decidedly less interested in the educational components of 5 A Day, and its annual funding for that purpose ranged from just $750,000 to $1.1 million. The agency assumed that the industry partners would take care of the promotional aspects of the campaign.

Insufficient funding also affected the PBH side of the partnership, however. Although industry contributions have increased over the years, they barely reached $1.2 million in 1999, and funding from all sources combined was just under $2 million. PBH raises about 12% of its funds from catalog and Internet sales of licensed logo items such as sweatshirts, magnets, and golf tees—the modern equivalent of bake sales. At issue, therefore, is why 5 A Day is not better supported by industry. Unlike meat, dairy, and other commodity producers who lobby the government to force their industries to support generic advertising (as discussed in the next chapter), fruit and vegetable producers view each other as *competitors*, a contest of peaches versus apples or carrots versus broccoli. Although grain producers might be expected to join alliances to promote plant-based diets, they do not; most grain is fed to animals. NCI's research focus and PBH's limited contributions mean that the educational aspects of 5 A Day have never been adequately funded. The total funding available for public communication was under $3 million in 1999—minuscule in comparison to the advertising budget of any single candy bar, soft drink, or potato chip. At this level, 5 A Day cannot compete.

The inadequacy of funding is especially disappointing because the results of the initial demonstration projects and subsequent evaluation studies of state and industry 5 A Day projects gave much reason to think that greater outreach would be highly effective. Taken together, the various studies—many of them now published—demonstrate that when funding was at its peak and the programs were most active, participants increased their average intake of fruits and vegetables (and not just potatoes) by about half a serving a day—a huge amount in population terms. When the funding declined, however, this gain disappeared.[44] Thus the 5 A Day partnership illustrates the underlying problem with such alliances: unless they result in demonstrable and immediate benefits to the industry partner, they will not receive more than token industry support.

HANDLING A DIFFICULT SITUATION

From this discussion it should be evident why food corporations envision funding the professional activities of nutritionists as a worthwhile enterprise. It should be equally evident why nutrition professionals welcome such funding and have grown to depend on it. Thus the issue becomes one of principles and safeguards—establishing guidelines for acceptance of industry funding that preserve independence and integrity to the greatest extent possible.

Despite the need for such guidelines, professional soul searching on this issue has been rare in the nutrition community. Indeed, the last serious debate about food industry sponsorship of nutrition professionals occurred in 1980 when the Food and Nutrition Board (FNB) issued its controversial report *Toward Healthful Diets*. As I noted in Chapter 1, that report chided government agencies for releasing dietary guidelines that the board thought lacked a sound scientific foundation, especially with respect to the effects of dietary cholesterol on heart disease risk. Critics immediately charged that members of the FNB had close ties to food companies; two were company executives, one consulted for the American Egg Board, two had conducted research financed by the egg industry, and at least one other was a consultant to other food industries. At the time, the FNB was entirely supported by an 80-member industry liaison advisory committee, which had paid for the report. These revelations so embarrassed the National Academy of Sciences, the FNB's parent body, that it eliminated the industry panel and restructured the board to include new members with fewer ties to food companies.[45]

Everyone is quick to say that sponsorship does not prove or necessarily cause bias, but most—though by no means all—experts who offer opinions on the matter say that disclosure of financial relationships is essential.[46] In the past, even if nutrition researchers and departments were willing to disclose industry connections, they were rarely required to do so. This situation is beginning to change. The FDA, for example, now asks members of its review committees to state whether they have received stock, consulting fees, or other financial support from companies with interests in the agency's regulatory decisions, a requirement that many consider long overdue. Major science and medicine journals, eager to head off embarrassing incidents, began to require financial-disclosure statements in the 1990s. *The Lancet*, for example, now instructs authors that "the conflict of interest test is a simple one . . . Is there anything . . . that would embarrass you if it were to emerge after publication and you had not declared it? The Editor needs to be informed." Some nutrition journals also request disclosure, for example:

· Authors must inform the Editor in writing of any financial arrangements, organizational affiliations, or other relationships that may constitute a conflict of interest. (*Journal of the American Dietetic Association*).

· Any existing financial arrangement between an author and a company whose product figures prominently in the submitted manuscript [must be] brought to the attention of the editor. (*Journal of Nutrition*).

· Authors should disclose, at the time of submission, any financial arrangement they may have with a company whose product figures prominently in the submitted manuscript or with a company making a competing product. (*Nutrition in Clinical Care*).

The *British Medical Journal* requires authors to submit an elaborate check list, some of which is summarized in Table 16. Its editors explain that they need to know about the items on that list not because they are trying to eliminate competing interests—such interests are almost inevitable—but because they decided to restrict inquiries to *financial* interests. They viewed this decision as a tactical move designed to "increase the number of authors who disclose competing interests. Our experience, supported by some research data, was that authors often did not disclose them."[47]

The research to which they were referring demonstrates that many scientific authors have conflicting interests, but few editors require

TABLE 16. Selected elements of *British Medical Journal* guidance for authors on "competing" interests, 2000 [47]

During the past five years, have you:
  A. Accepted the following from an organization that may in any way gain or lose financially from your study or opinion:
      · Reimbursement for attending a symposium?
      · A fee for speaking?
      · Funds for research?
      · Fees for consulting?

  B. Been employed by—or held stocks or shares in—an organization that may gain or lose financially from your study or opinion?

  C. Held any other competing interests that might prove embarrassing if discovered after publication, such as:
      · A close relationship with, a strong antipathy to, or an academic link or rivalry to a person whose interests may be affected by publication of your paper?
      · Membership in a political party or special interest group whose interests might be affected by publication of your paper?
      · A deep personal or religious conviction that may have affected what you wrote and that readers should be aware of when reading your paper?

---

disclosure and few authors disclose. Researchers who surveyed nearly 1,400 leading scientific journals in 1997 found less than 16% to have disclosure policies. Among such journals, nearly 70% had no disclosures whatsoever, and only 0.5% of 61,000 articles mentioned financial conflicts of interest related to their research. The investigators into this matter suggest that the low levels of disclosure are most likely to be due to poor compliance of authors to the journals' policies rather than the absence of financial sponsorship.[48] Despite such findings, virtually all researchers of my acquaintance believe themselves incorruptible and firmly deny that industry support might affect their views. Others charge that disclosure requirements so unfairly taint good work as to constitute a new form of McCarthyism.[49]

A British pediatric society, wrenched by controversy over sponsorship by infant-formula companies, developed guidelines that extend beyond disclosure. The society's premise is that the products themselves are neither ethical nor unethical but that the ways in which they are used, produced, or marketed could raise ethical issues. Thus it chooses to *refuse* sponsorship from makers of guns or tobacco; to be *cautious* about alcohol, soft drinks, junk foods, and infant formulas; but to be willing to *accept* sponsorship from companies that make pharmaceutical products,

TABLE 17. Recommendations of the Royal College of Paediatrics and Child Health (London) on accepting commercial sponsorship: selected examples[50]

Sponsorship of societies
- Should not be accepted from companies that produce tobacco or firearms or exploit children.
- Should only be accepted from companies that can demonstrate unequivocally that their conduct does not breach any relevant code or practice.
- Should be fully and transparently disclosed.

Sponsorship of individual researchers
- Must not be lavish; the guiding principle should be whether individuals would be willing to have these arrangements generally known.
- May be accepted when convinced that doing so will benefit work without doing harm.
- Must be under the full control of the investigator.

---

medical equipment, or mineral water, products assumed to be effective or at least neutral.[50] Table 17 summarizes some of these guidelines. Whether they will prove effective in practice is not yet known.

AN OUNCE OF PREVENTION

Nutrition professionals are connected to food companies in ways no less complicated than those that connect food lobbyists to elected officials and government regulators. Although it may be tempting to believe that nutrition educators and researchers share common goals with food companies, the goals necessarily differ. And although the public may assume that nutrition professionals and their associations act in the public interest and provide unbiased, objective information about diet and health, the mere existence of alliances with food companies is enough to create doubt about their objectivity.

What, then, is the remedy? Should researchers, practitioners, professional societies, and academic departments refuse corporate funding? This is the advice of a distinguished former editor of the *New England Journal of Medicine*, who was fired for his concern about pressures to increase commercial exploitation of that most prestigious journal. Stating that most doctors in training "have not been challenged to consider that their relations with pharmaceutical companies might compromise their judgment," he called on deans and directors of medical programs to pay more attention to issues related to conflict of interest: "Where professionalism is concerned, they must teach that there is no free lunch. No free dinner. Or even a ballpoint pen."[51]

No such just-say-no solution is likely to happen; the benefits of such "free lunches" are too attractive for most mere mortals to ignore. A more pragmatic compromise is to identify the extent of conflict between the goals of food companies and the goals of individuals or professional societies, to balance risks and benefits, and to disclose all sponsorship relationships no matter how seemingly benign. Most U.S. colleges and universities, for example, now require faculty to file annual conflict-of-interest statements in which sponsorship relationships must be disclosed, and some take these statements seriously.[52] Such requirements are a step in the right direction, though they are difficult to enforce.

Another compromise is to argue that industry contributions in the form of travel, meals, honoraria, and conference sessions pose minimal problems but that the potential for conflicts increases when companies contribute to educational or research programs.[48] In all cases, the challenge facing individuals as well as professional societies is to be wary of gifts from food companies, to pay attention to the potential for conflicting interests, and to take steps to minimize such conflicts. The fact that meeting this challenge is not easy is illustrated by the examples given in the next chapter.

CHAPTER 6

WINNING FRIENDS, DISARMING CRITICS

WE HAVE SEEN HOW FOOD INTEREST GROUPS GAIN ACCESS AND exert influence upon elected officials through donations of money, both hard and soft. Such transactions are legal, publicly disclosed, painstakingly tracked by advocacy groups and investigative reporters, and readily apparent to any interested person with access to the Internet. Far less visible are more subtle lobbying activities directed toward officials of federal agencies and other people likely to wield influence. Such activities do not necessarily involve money or other "things of value." Even when they do, the amounts can be quite small. This kind of lobbying involves forming friendships, doing favors, providing useful information, building commodity coalitions, and managing the image of products through public relations. This chapter describes three examples of "softball" methods that food companies use to promote product sales and discourage unfavorable regulations or perceptions. Only when such efforts prove insufficient do companies resort to the "hardball" methods described in the next chapter.

MAKING FRIENDS WITH FEDERAL OFFICIALS: THE USDA SECRETARY

Friendships between people in the private sector and federal officials are likely to form as a natural consequence of frequent contact. One equally natural consequence of friendship is the exchange of gifts. Because the motivation for making friends could be to win influence, gifts from corporate representatives to federal officials raise questions about propriety.

Congress holds officials of federal regulatory agencies to more restrictive rules about gifts than it imposes on its own members. Thus a member of Congress who takes a position in a regulatory agency must conform to a stricter set of ethical guidelines and must handle friendships with greater discretion.

Although congressional representatives allow themselves to accept funds and favors of various kinds from lobbying groups, they forbid agency officials to do so. Favors from special-interest groups that are considered routine by members of Congress are unacceptable when given to staff of regulatory agencies such as the USDA or FDA. Therefore, food industry representatives must learn to deal differently with agency officials and staff than they do with members of Congress. They can freely disburse to agency officials information, materials, and testimony, but nothing of monetary value: no lunches, no parties, no trips, no honoraria, and no presents. When I worked in a support staff position with the Department of Health and Human Services, for example, I could accept research articles, press releases, and public relations materials from representatives of food companies and trade associations, but the office paid my travel expenses to any conference where I might be likely to meet such people—even when I was an invited speaker—and I was expected to pay for my own meals unless granted special advance dispensation. The potential conflict not only was recognized but also was governed by explicit rules and regulations. In my case, it was not worth the price of a lunch to jeopardize the integrity of the *Surgeon General's Report on Nutrition and Health* by exposing it to the slightest charge of favoritism.

The well-publicized case of former USDA Secretary Mike Espy illustrates how the sharp disparity in ethical standards can wreak havoc when someone steeped in the permissive culture of Congress takes a job in a federal regulatory agency. The roots of Mr. Espy's downfall reach back to the Meat Inspection Act of 1907 (Public Law 59–242), which aimed to eliminate unsafe practices in the meat industry, and prevent the corruption of meat inspectors employed by the USDA. The act made it a federal crime for industry employees to do anything that could be construed as an attempt to unduly influence inspectors. Later, the wonderfully named Bribery, Graft and Conflicts of Interest Act of 1962 (Public Law 87–849) established penalties for any citizen who offered or promised "anything of value" with the *intent* to influence a public official. It also set penalties for any public official who "directly or indirectly, corruptly asks, demands, exacts, solicits, seeks, accepts, receives, or agrees to receive anything of value for himself or for any other person or entity, in return for . . . being influenced in his performance of any official act." The penalties included fines (up to $20,000), imprisonment (up to 15 years), and disqualification from "holding any office of honor, trust, or profit under the United States." Although intention was the critical issue in this context, the law could be—and was—interpreted to mean that USDA officials should not accept *any* gifts from companies or individuals with interests related to the agency's regulatory mission.

In 1993 President Clinton appointed Mr. Espy, then serving his fourth term as a member of the House of Representatives (Dem-MS), as USDA Secretary. Mr. Espy took his new job seriously. Aware that bacterial contaminants of meat and poultry products were causing outbreaks of illness, he immediately attempted to reverse long-standing USDA policies that permitted meat and poultry companies to avoid responsibility for controlling potentially dangerous microbes in their products. In the debates about how to reduce and control microbial pathogens, beef producers had accused the USDA of favoring chicken producers by allowing less stringent safety standards. In response, the USDA proposed that poultry be treated with antimicrobial washes (with trisodium phosphate and organic acids) before chilling; the department also was working on proposals to require poultry companies to do their own testing for microbial pathogens. The poultry industry opposed both suggestions.

Reportedly, USDA staff had warned Mr. Espy—who was accustomed to the freewheeling political climate in his home state and in Congress— to be careful not to take gifts from representatives of companies with regulatory matters under review by the Department.[1] Despite these warnings, Mr. Espy accepted a variety of favors from lobbyists for Tyson Foods, the world's largest chicken-processing company. Early in 1994, federal investigators began examining whether Mr. Espy had violated the Meat Inspection Act by accepting—or permitting a companion to accept—airline travel, tickets to sports events, a $1,200 scholarship, and other gifts worth about $12,000 from that company, and gifts of similar magnitude from other meat and poultry producers. This investigation resulted in Mr. Espy's forced resignation and the appointment of a special prosecutor. The ensuing 4-year, $17 million investigation (which some commentators considered excessive) led to more than a dozen convictions and collection of $12 million in fines. It also led to Mr. Espy's indictment by a federal grand jury. Eventually, Mr. Espy was acquitted of all charges, largely because the prosecutor had not convinced the jury that the gifts had been *intended* to influence the USDA. Although it is difficult to imagine what other purpose they might have had, the Supreme Court also ruled that the gifts to Mr. Espy were acceptable because they were not directly linked to regulatory matters.[2]

When first threatened with investigation, Mr. Espy said that the allegations against him must have been "drummed up by Republicans and political opponents opposed to his efforts to toughen meat and poultry inspection rules" and that he was far too involved in his new duties to pay much attention to the ethical standards that applied to him now that he had moved from Congress to the cabinet.[1] Reporters quoted him as saying that the gifts had come from personal friends, that he was unaware that the lobbyists had billed the cost of the gifts to the companies, and that the ethics rules for agencies were "a bunch of junk."[3]

The investigation revealed that "friends" from other companies with matters under USDA regulatory review also had done some favors for the secretary. One asked the chairman of Quaker Oats to give Mr. Espy two tickets, worth $90, to a football game. When questioned about this gift, Mr. Espy quickly made restitution and called the matter an oversight; his lawyer dismissed concerns by saying, "never has so much been made of so little."[4] Another lobbyist/friend was reimbursed by Sun-Diamond (a California cooperative of 4,500 companies producing nuts, dried fruit, and other foods) for giving Mr. Espy luggage worth $2,400, meals worth $2,100, and expenses of $8,400 incurred while taking Mr. Espy and his companion to the U.S. Open tennis matches. Sun-Diamond received USDA funds under an export-promotion program and also had an interest in delaying a proposed ban on an ozone-depleting fungicide. A third individual, this one also a lobbyist for Sun-Diamond, asked the Mondavi wine company to give Mr. Espy six bottles of wine for his personal use and to pay for a dinner at Kinkead's, a well-known Washington, DC, restaurant frequented by politicians; during the dinner, a Mondavi official gave a speech about the health benefits of drinking wine. Reporters noted that Mr. Espy had promised to help the wine industry by encouraging the USDA to "get moving" on dietary guidelines that would mention the health benefits of drinking moderate amounts of wine.[5]

Other charges involved Mr. Espy's chief of staff, Ronald Blackley, who, before he joined Mr. Espy's congressional staff, had worked for a firm that helped food producers obtain subsidies from the USDA. Reports noted that during his first year at the USDA, five firms representing former clients had successfully obtained help from the agency and that Mr. Blackley had failed to disclose income from two that had received subsidies of $63,000 and $284,000, respectively.[6] Investigators also accused him of interfering with the department's efforts to regulate poultry safety. The *New York Times* quoted a USDA staff member as saying that Mr. Blackley had been surprised to learn that the agency was working on poultry rules: "He said to take it out of the computer . . . We were a little shell shocked . . . wondering if we had all heard what we thought we'd heard. We put a stop to all poultry activity."[1]

In reports of the investigation, the relationships of lobbyists to agencies and to Congress were constantly recurring issues, as was the low cost of "buying" influence. *The New Yorker* said, "The spectacular fall from grace of Secretary of Agriculture Mike Espy raises a delicate question: Is Don Tyson the Devil? . . . What is interesting about all this . . . is how *cheap* it is to tempt a Washington official."[7] An editorial in the *New York Times* pointed out that Mr. Espy's department had always been too close to food producers and that President Clinton had promised to end such "snug relationships" but that Mr. Espy appeared not to have heard him. The *Times* characterized Mr. Espy's behavior as "colossally stupid."[8]

The scandal, of course, made the USDA's ongoing efforts to improve poultry safety much more difficult. Critics viewed a proposed policy on poultry inspection simply as "an effort to prove that . . . Espy was not beholden to poultry interests."[9] When the agency decided not to go forward with the plan, officials had to deny that they had made this decision just to please the poultry industry. The favorable Supreme Court decision that exonerated Mr. Espy meant that the net result of the entire tawdry affair was to make it legal for food companies to give presents to agency officials as long as the gifts were not used explicitly as bribes.

Making connections and doing favors are such common practices in Washington that they would hardly be worth mentioning were they not so insidious. The Espy case is unusual only in that the favors were so visible and the stakes so high; this USDA secretary was poised to modernize his agency's century-old policies on meat safety. The donation by Tyson Foods of tickets to sporting events demonstrated that even small favors are useful to companies if given at the right time—in this case, when the USDA was proposing to require poultry producers to test for *Salmonella* and other disease-causing microbial contaminants. At the very least, it was to Tyson's advantage to keep Mr. Espy preoccupied with responding to legal challenges from a special prosecutor. That Washington politicians consider favors and small gifts to be trivial matters was indicated by one of President Clinton's last official acts: presidential pardons for Mr. Blackley and six other food company executives and lobbyists convicted of attempting to corrupt Mr. Espy. Reportedly, the White House *invited* the defense lawyers to ask for pardons and granted them just hours before the January 2001 inauguration of President George W. Bush.[10]

LEGISLATING COOPERATION: "CHECK-OFFS"

A second example of the friendlier forms of influence exerted by food companies occurs through "check-off" programs that can only be interpreted as federally sanctioned and administered public relations enterprises to benefit certain food commodities. To promote sales, food companies induced Congress to pass a collection of laws that *require* the producers of certain commodities—among them beef, dairy products, milk, eggs, and peanuts—to deduct, or "check off," a fee from sales to be used for generic advertising and promotion. By 1986, U.S. food producers were contributing more than $530 million annually to promote farm commodities through such programs. The three largest check-off funds are for dairy, beef, and soybeans; in 1994 these generated $228 million, $81 million, and $48 million, respectively, for national and state promotional activities.[11] The dairy check-off, for example, funds the $100 million or greater annual cost of the milk mustache campaign illustrated in Figure 12.

These programs have an especially interesting history. The beef check-off, for example, began as a voluntary program that generated $31,000 in 1922. In the 1970s, as beef consumption began to decline, the National Cattlemen's Association started lobbying for a compulsory program through a campaign that involved political action committees, letter writing, and personal visits to members of Congress by hundreds of beef producers. This lobbying was especially effective because cattlemen, who tend to be generous with campaign contributions, are distributed among a great many states—each, of course, with two senators and several representatives.

Although the check-off legislation expressly prohibits use of the funds for lobbying, the distinction between promoting a product to consumers and promoting it to lawmakers can be subtle. Some of the boards are so closely affiliated with lobbying groups that they share office space. For many years, the Cattlemen's Beef Promotion and Research Board (a check-off organization) shared an address with the National Cattlemen's Association (a trade association lobbying group); in 1996, these groups merged to form the National Cattlemen's Beef Association. The National Pork Board (check-off) also shared offices, staff, and telephone services with the National Pork Producers Council (lobbying). Even cozier, the legislation specifies that a certain percentage of the funds must be allocated to the commodity groups responsible for nominating the board members who run the programs; these members are officially appointed by the USDA.[12]

Check-off funds are supposed to be used for research as well as advertising, but only a small fraction is used for that purpose. In the mid-1990s, 8% of the beef check-off's $80 million or so went to research, while the rest was spent on promotion and "information." Research percentages for dairy, egg, potato, and soybean check-off programs were slightly higher. Regardless of level, nearly all of the research is designed to promote the commodity. Beef check-off research is designed to "dispel negative perceptions about beef" and to develop a factual basis for viewing beef products as "part of a varied, convenient, and healthful diet." Egg check-off funds support research designed to link eggs with positive images of taste and to demonstrate that the cholesterol in eggs does not increase the risk of coronary heart disease; the Egg Board paid university researchers $1.5 million for such projects from 1991–1994.[11]

The great majority of the funds are spent to convince consumers to choose one type of food product over another. The meat and beef boards, for example, design campaigns to boost demand for red meats and meat products; encourage consumers to view beef as wholesome, versatile, and lower in cholesterol; and educate doctors, nurses, dietitians, teachers, and the media about the nutritional benefits of beef. A typical advertisement aimed at nutrition professionals is shown in Figure 15. Similarly, the dairy boards promote consumption of cheese, milk, butter, and ice cream as the best sources of calcium and other nutrients. For a wide range of commodities, studies have shown a positive relationship between such campaigns and sales. For example, USDA economists estimated that from 1984 to 1997, the campaigns raised milk sales by about 6% and sales of cheese by even more, and that each dollar spent on generic advertising generated $3.44 in increased sales.[13]

Check-off supporters maintain that these programs benefit farmers at virtually no cost to the USDA and provide useful information to consumers. Critics, however, view the programs as increasing food prices by passing the promotional costs on to consumers, and by causing unnecessary competition among commodity groups. From a nutritional standpoint, check-off programs promote products high in fat, saturated fat, and cholesterol, and the funds are used to influence food and nutrition policies favorable to industry. Smaller growers and those producing specialty commodities believe that the programs favor large food producers

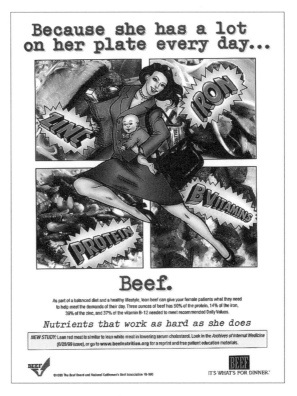

FIGURE 15. This full-color advertisement, paid for through the beef check-off program, suggests that women will have more energy if they eat beef. In small print, it notes that women also should follow a balanced diet and healthy lifestyle and should eat lean beef. Aimed at nutritionists, the advertisement appeared inside the front cover of the *Journal of the American Dietetic Association* in December 1999.

and are no help. Thus peach, plum, and nectarine growers in California sued to opt out of generic fruit-promotion programs on the grounds of free speech; they viewed the advertisements as useless and more likely to benefit producers of more commonly consumed fruits such as apples and bananas.[14] Mushroom growers have objected on similar grounds. The U.S. Supreme Court, however, ruled that the programs are constitutional and an "unexceptional" form of economic regulation: "The mere fact that objectors believe their money is not being well spent does not mean that they have a First Amendment complaint."[15]

Other cases now under litigation may challenge this view. Pork producers, for example, alarmed by overproduction and declining prices in their industry, obtained the right to hold a referendum on the check-off program. Late in 2000 opponents of the mandatory fees (45 cents on each $100 obtained from pig sales) narrowly won the vote to discontinue the program. The National Pork Producers Council, which represents large "factory" hog farms, challenged the vote on the grounds that "the other white meat" campaign had been one of the most successful in American agriculture. When President George W. Bush took office in 2001, his new secretary of Agriculture overturned the referendum, saying it was "procedurally flawed."[16] If nothing else, this action revealed how USDA polices continued to favor the interests of large corporations.

USING PUBLIC RELATIONS:
INFANT FORMULA VERSUS BREAST-FEEDING

A third form of softer influence used by the food industry to promote "eat more" is public relations. Although all kinds of businesses use these strategies as a means of increasing sales, our concern here is the way multinational as well as American food companies use public relations to divert criticism and to convince people that their products promote health or are—at worst—harmless.[17]

Public relations uses advertising only as the most evident of its methods, and unlike advertising, its other aspects are conducted behind the scenes and are largely invisible to the public. Although several chapters in this book describe aspects of public relations campaigns, the example I present here is unusually well documented: that conducted by the Nestlé company (to which I am not related) to defuse worldwide criticism of its promotion of infant formula as a substitute for breast-feeding. The company designed that campaign to counteract antiformula activism and to convince government officials and health professionals to accept its typical marketing practices—even in developing countries where use of infant formula can do more harm than good. To understand the larger significance of this campaign, we need to start with three undeniable premises: (1) breast milk is superior to any other food for infants, (2) nearly all mothers are fully capable of breast-feeding, and (3) even the slightest effort to promote use of formula undermines their ability to breast-feed.[18]

Milk from cows and other animals contains nutrients in too high a concentration to be digested and absorbed by human infants. Prior to the development of successfully diluted formulas in the 1800s, an infant who could not be breast-fed had little chance of survival. Once companies figured out how to make a successful formula, they—in alliance with physicians—began marketing the products not only to mothers who needed them but also to those who did not. By the late 1920s, medical researchers had demonstrated that infants who were fed formulas made with condensed evaporated milk attained levels of physical growth similar to those who were fed breast milk. On that basis, early public relations efforts convinced doctors and mothers that formulas were as good as—or better than—breast milk. Despite overwhelming evidence that breast milk confers significant health advantages, bottle-feeding became a common practice in industrialized countries.[19] In the 1950s, U.S. formula companies began to market their products more aggressively, and by the 1970s, the U.S. market was dominated by just two companies, Ross (Abbott Laboratories) and Mead Johnson (Bristol-Myers). The before-tax profits of the two companies were said to be 15 to 20% of sales, perhaps because they had successfully defeated attempts by Borden, Carnation, Gerber, and Baker/BeechNut to enter the formula market.

The sales practices of formula companies elicited criticism, particularly as applied in developing countries where bottle-feeding is associated with an *increase* in infant mortality. Infant formulas contain cow's milk or soy proteins with added sugars, vitamins, and minerals. Because their composition is determined by law, formula products are virtually identical and the only significant differences are in packaging. Formulas reproduce most of the characteristics of breast milk, but not all; most critically, they lack immune substances that confer protection against microbial diseases. Appropriate use of formula requires adequate income (to pay for it and for the feeding bottles), education (to understand how to dilute it correctly), a clean water supply for the dilution (to avoid contamination with infectious bacteria), and refrigeration (to prevent bacteria from growing in stored formula). Otherwise, contamination of bottles, nipples, and products can cause diarrhea that, in turn, leads to the nutrient deficiencies and overall malnutrition that constitute the leading causes of death and stunted growth among children in developing countries.

The relationship between formula feeding and infant death first came to public attention in the 1930s. Dr. Cicely Williams, a pediatrician who spent most of her working career in Africa, viewed promotion of infant formulas to mothers in developing countries as deliberate infanticide:

> There is no possible doubt, and every sentient being in the world agrees, that the best possible food for a baby is its mother's milk. Nothing has yet been invented that provides a satisfactory substitute. Statistics have been collected to show that the death rate among artificially fed babies is much greater than that among breastfed babies. And this is a death rate that shows a very marked class prejudice . . . [if] your lives were embittered as mine is, by seeing day after day this massacre of the innocents by unsuitable feeding, then I believe you would feel as I do that misguided propaganda on infant feeding should be punished as the most criminal form of sedition, and that these deaths should be regarded as murder.[20]

Although Dr. Williams and her colleagues in developing countries repeatedly made such charges, formula companies increased their marketing efforts. By the late 1970s, they were distributing 50 brands and 200 varieties of infant formulas in 100 countries, with the result that "commerciogenic malnutrition"—the "thoughtless" promotion of products totally beyond the economic resources of those to whom they were advertised—had become rampant.[21] The pediatrician D. B. Jelliffe, then working in Jamaica, framed the problem as a *moral* issue: "Is it ethical to advertise, using modern techniques of motivation and persuasion, infant foods in a population that has no chance financially or hygienically of being able to use them in adequate quantities? Should infant milk foods be widely advertised in regions where breast feeding is currently practiced?" He recognized that nutritionists must realize "that commercial concerns live in a hard, competitive world and that a successful industry is a profitable one," and he urged nutritionists and formula makers to "engage in dialogue."[22]

To create that dialogue, advocates began developing pamphlets, books, and films documenting the tragic effects of formula misuse among infants in developing countries. They accused the industry of using advertising and public relations to make formulas appear superior to breast milk. They criticized the companies for colluding with birth centers to distribute free samples, dressing "milk nurses" in white uniforms and paying them to promote formula or sell it on commission, convincing health professionals to advise mothers to use formula, and targeting illiterate women through word of mouth, billboards, and picture books. They were particularly troubled by the ways in which company advertisements implied that formula might be superior to breast milk. Typical

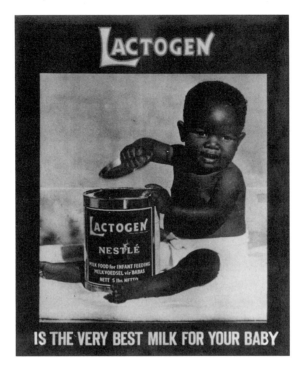

FIGURE 16. Advertisements like this 1975 example from South Africa promoted the use of infant formulas but also led to an international boycott of products made by the Nestlé corporation. (Courtesy Leah Margulies)

advertisements showed photographs of women nursing their babies with statements like "Breast-feed your baby, but when your baby needs a supplement, use our brand of powdered milk."[23] Figure 16 shows a more subtle advertisement of the superiority of formula.

Over the years, the infant-formula controversy has engaged the attention of numerous authors who have documented inappropriate marketing practices and the actions of advocates, government, and industry. They have reviewed events leading to the boycott of Nestlé products and the company's ensuing campaign to defuse opposition and undermine the International Code of Marketing of Breast-Milk Substitutes ("the Code"). To this day, an Internet Web site continues to track events in the ongoing controversy.[24] These accounts are rich in drama and detail, and they demonstrate beyond question that the infant-formula controversy reflects broader societal issues involving no less than "the politics of transnational corporations, international trade agreements, poverty, the

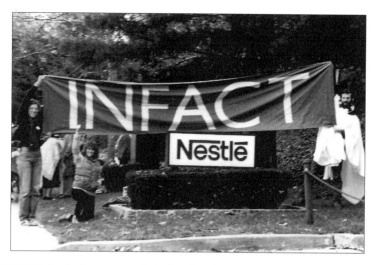

FIGURE 17. In the late 1970s, the Infant Feeding Action Coalition (INFACT) began holding boycott demonstrations at Nestlé headquarters in White Plains, New York. (Courtesy Leah Margulies)

media, the status of women, and the power of industrial capitalism."[25] This brief summary cannot possibly do justice to these authors' work, and its focus is restricted to public relations aspects.

In 1977, American activists singled out the Swiss company, Nestlé, as the object of a worldwide boycott. The company did not market infant formula in the United States, but it held 49% of the international market, nearly all of it in developing countries. The boycott organizers urged the American public not to buy Nestlé products until the company ceased marketing practices that favored bottle-feeding. Church, university, union, women's, and health care groups quickly joined the boycott, as did celebrities and politicians, and the campaign soon spread internationally. A public demonstration for the boycott is illustrated in Figure 17.

The resulting effects on corporate image and loss in sales were sufficient to induce Nestlé to invest heavily in a public relations campaign to control and correct the damage. The principal elements of that campaign are outlined in Table 18. With the help of a succession of public relations firms, Nestlé's first strategy was to attack critics on the grounds that they—to put it bluntly—were communists. Because the company did not sell infant formula in the United States, it sent Dr. Oswaldo Ballarin, chairman of the board of Nestlé-Brazil, to testify at a congressional hearing chaired by Senator Edward M. Kennedy (Dem-MA).

TABLE 18. Selected elements of Nestlé's public relations campaign to counter opposition to its infant-formula marketing practices and the boycott of its products, 1977–2000

1977 Establishes Office of Corporate Responsibility.
Hires Hill & Knowlton, a leading public relations firm, to improve company's image.
Mails information kit to 300,000 clergy.
Issues leaflet criticizing the film *Bottle Babies*.
Recruits succession of other public relations firms.
Releases favorable film, *Feeding Babies—A Shared Responsibility*.

1978 Sends representative to testify at congressional hearing.
Induces Senator Edward Kennedy to refer issue to World Health Organization (WHO).
Issues paper explaining company position.
Meets with boycott activists and church officials.
Sponsors International Nutrition Congress in Rio de Janeiro.

1979 Agrees to abide by international recommendations (but threatens to withdraw).
Insists on statement that infant formulas be provided to those who need them.
Urges writer for *Fortune* magazine to write favorable article.

1980 Gives $25,000 to an "independent" group to reprint the *Fortune* article.
Issues memorandum urging use of academics and the media to create support for ending the boycott.
Lobbies against the International Code of Marketing of Breast-Milk Substitutes.

1981 Establishes Coordination Center in Washington, DC, to control damage, restore credibility, and end boycott.
Announces support for the Code.
Grants research funds to universities; sponsors professional conferences.

DR. BALLERIN: I am aware of the specific charges made by these [boycott] groups, and can state, based on my personal experience in many developing countries, that they are quite misleading and inaccurate. The U.S. Nestlé company has advised me that their research indicates that this is actually an indirect attack on the free world's economic system. A worldwide church organization, with the stated purpose of undermining the free enterprise system, is in the forefront of this activity.

SENATOR KENNEDY: Now, you cannot seriously—[laughter and applause] . . . you do not seriously expect us to accept that on face value . . . 14 Protestant denominations, including the Presbyterian Church, the Episcopal Church, the Lutheran Church, the Baptist Church, the Methodist Church,

TABLE 18. *(continued)*

1982   Announces company will implement the Code.
Establishes newsletter, *Nestlé News*, to promote resistance to the boycott.
Funds Nestlé Infant Formula Audit Commission (NIFAC) to evaluate company compliance with the Code.

1983   Prepares, with critics, a "Statement of Understanding" aimed at ending the boycott.
Offers to donate $1 million to the Save the Children Fund (refused).
Forces the National Institutes of Health to withdraw a panel on infant formulas from an ethics symposium.
Pressures a television station in the Philippines to cancel an unfavorable program.
Convinces church, education, and union groups to end boycott participation.
Convinces UNICEF to mediate the boycott.

1984   Joins 32 other companies from 17 nations to establish common industry policies on the Code.

1988   Sponsors the book *Infant Feeding: Anatomy of a Controversy* to present its version of this history.

1989   Proposes formula-feeding as a way to protect infants against transmission of AIDS through breast milk.

1990   Advertises Carnation formulas directly to parents.
Gives $500,000 in gifts to U.S. universities.
Gives $1 million to establish Nestlé Foundation for Nutrition and Health (Cleveland, OH).

1993   Sues the American Academy of Pediatrics for conspiring with U.S. formula companies to exclude its products from American markets

2000   Reports few violations of the International Code.
Pressures UNICEF to promote infant formula as a way to prevent maternal AIDS transmission.

the United Church of Christ, as well as 150 orders of the Roman Catholic Church, that they are involved in some worldwide conspiracy to undermine or attack the free world's economic system? . . .

DR. BALLERIN: . . . I was led to [these comments] because I was surprised with two things: One, the boycott which is made against one company which does not manufacture these products in the United States; and second, because of the film which has been distributed, under the title of "Bottle Babies," to many local churches and schools . . . and this film has hurt, really, those who fight in a world of free enterprise.[26]

When such statements succeeded only in increasing public recognition of the boycott and recruiting more people to it, the company asked Senator Kennedy to take the matter to two relevant agencies of the United Nations—the World Health Organization (WHO) and UNICEF (United Nations Children's Fund)—and ask them to call a meeting to establish guidelines that the company could live with. Nestlé also flatly denied the charges, arguing that the issues were complex and were misunderstood by opponents: "All consumer advertising of formula products has been suspended in developing countries . . . Nestle medical representatives are qualified nurses or midwives . . . They are not permitted to give samples to mothers and are not salespeople . . . We believe it is time to turn away from negative efforts, such as boycotts."[27]

Instead, the company issued a position paper: Mothers in developing countries produce inadequate supplies of breast milk; infant formulas are necessary to *save* their babies; infant mortality is *declining* in developing countries; no scientific evidence links formula-feeding with higher mortality rates; poverty and lack of clean drinking water are the problem, not formula; mothers' need to work (not company practices) is responsible for the decline in breast-feeding; and it is not Nestlé's fault if uneducated mothers use bottles to feed babies animal milk rather than commercial formulas. The Nestlé paper concluded, "It is obvious that the problems of infant nutrition in the developing countries are ones of great complexity. They cannot be solved or probably even affected in any meaningful way by the simplified solutions proposed by the activists . . . An international forum can provide the proper answers and sound guidelines for the sale of infant formulas . . . The announcement of the WHO forum and its widespread support makes the current move to boycott Nestle products in the United States an inappropriate measure whose symbolic significance has disappeared."[28]

During the time leading up to the WHO/UNICEF meeting, Nestlé worked behind the scenes to convince delegates that restrictions on infant-formula marketing practices would not be in their countries' best interest. Nevertheless, delegates passed the Code in 1981. The Code said that governments should provide information about the superiority of breast-feeding and the risks of infant formulas, and it outlined measures that would control use of inappropriate marketing practices.[29] The delegates adopted the Code with only one dissent—that of the United States. The U.S. State Department's official rationale for this dissent was that the Code's provisions might violate the U.S. Constitution. In as much as this explanation strains credulity, it seemed more likely that the State Department instructed U.S. delegates to vote against the Code in response to extensive lobbying by U.S. formula companies. More understandable—though equally indefensible—was the State Department's concern that the Code would set a precedent for controlling drug company practices. Although two U.S. delegates resigned in protest and a huge public outcry followed, the dissenting vote sent a message to formula companies that they could count on the U.S. government to look the other way if they continued to violate the Code.

At this point, Nestlé organized a unit in Washington, DC—the Nestlé Coordination Center for Nutrition (NCCN)—to restore the company's credibility, improve its public image, and end the boycott. Its public relations efforts shifted to a less aggressive approach, beginning with an announcement that the company fully intended to adhere to the aims and principles of the Code and had so instructed its employees. It began publishing a newsletter, *Nestlé News*, to publicize information about groups that were refusing to join the boycott or had withdrawn from it and to tout the company's socially responsible activities in developing countries. As part of this effort, Nestlé formed alliances with other formula manufacturers and with national and international health organizations in industrialized and developing countries. Along the way, it gathered intelligence reports on advocacy groups, suppressed public discussions of the issue, and worked to exclude critics from decision-making processes.[30]

Its most effective public relations maneuver, however, was to create and fund the Nestlé Infant Formula Audit Commission (NIFAC) to collect and evaluate complaints about the company's potential violations of the Code. The company induced former Senator (Dem-Me) and Secretary of State Edmund Muskie to chair the commission and persuaded distinguished church officials and academics to join it. Although Nestlé was reported to be paying him the same hourly rate that he had been receiving as partner in an international law firm, Mr. Muskie maintained that the commission would be completely independent. When he announced in 1983 that the commission had found Nestlé largely to be complying with the Code, and that the Code was an imperfect compromise because it did not address the root cause of misuse of formulas—poverty—many individuals and groups accepted these statements from such a credible source at face value. Activists, however, remained skeptical and interpreted the data collected by the commission as demonstrating precisely the opposite: continued violations of the Code. Their analysis carried far less weight in the popular press than did that of the Muskie Commission. The public relations efforts succeeded in convincing most people that Nestlé had complied with the Code, and groups began withdrawing from the boycott. Its leaders ended the boycott in 1984, when Nestlé agreed to stop promoting infant formulas to doctors and hospitals and to place warning labels on the company's products and literature.

Despite ending the boycott, activist groups continued to argue that Nestlé was engaging in Code-violating practices. When observations convinced them that the company merely had replaced advertising as its principal marketing strategy with placement of free formula in maternity facilities, the groups reinstated the boycott in 1988. Also in 1988, Nestlé introduced Carnation formulas into the U.S. market by advertising the products directly to the public rather than working through pediatricians. The American Academy of Pediatrics (AAP) strongly objected to this approach on the grounds that direct advertising would encourage new mothers to use formulas rather than breast-feed. Understandably, the company countered that the true purpose of AAP protests was to protect the economic interests of its members.

That year also witnessed publication of a book, *Infant Feeding: Anatomy of a Controversy*, containing chapters written by prominent international experts who supported Nestlé's version of this history.[31] The contributors portrayed the company as genuine in its attempts to adhere to the Code and as unjustly targeted by activists. Knowledgeable critics, however, referred to the book as "Nestlé-sponsored," as "blatantly one-sided," and as a "deplorable" demonstration that the company's "old guard is still trying to rewrite history and defend its activities."[32] Others pointed out that the book's editor and the author of its foreword were consultants to Nestlé and to its U.S. subsidiary, Carnation. Nowhere in the book are such connections noted beyond the editor's acknowledgment of the company's cooperation.

In 1993, when it became clear that Carnation formulas were not succeeding in U.S. markets, Nestlé accused the AAP and the leading formula companies of conspiring to stifle competition through price fixing (an illegal sales strategy discussed in the next chapter). The AAP admitted that it had accepted about $1 million annually in donations from other formula companies but had refused donations from Nestlé-Carnation because of the direct advertising to the public. Eventually, Nestlé settled the case against one of the companies but another case went to a jury that decided in favor of the AAP.[33]

With a change in administration, the United States finally joined the rest of the world when it signed the International Code in 1994. Two years later, activists noted that Nestlé and other companies again had shifted strategies and were now marketing infant formula and similar supplements to *pregnant women* in developing countries through advertisements just as misleading as those that had targeted infants ("What's good for mom . . . is better for baby"). The Interagency Group on Breast-feeding Monitoring, an international coalition of church organizations and activist groups, published annual reports called *Cracking the Code,* in which they demonstrated persistent Code violations; the 1997 edition featured violations by companies marketing formulas in four countries: Poland, Bangladesh, Thailand, and South Africa. The Monitoring Group stated that Nestlé representatives were continuing to provide free formula samples and information to health care facilities.[34] The following year, the International Baby Food Action Network carefully documented the continued actions of formula companies to give free samples to mothers, health care workers, and hospitals: to use posters, clocks, calendars, gifts, and educational materials to promote products; and to extend the product range to include pregnant women and preschool children—in dozens of developing countries throughout the world.[35]

At a Montreal meeting of the International Congress on Nutrition in 1997, I heard UNICEF deputy director Stephen Lewis berate conference organizers for their ready acceptance of sponsorship from makers of infant formulas and for their pandering to the

> obdurate self-interest of infant-formula companies who continue to ply their activities we know are essentially hostile to breast-feeding . . . there is no justification for nutritionists, of all people, taking money from companies that peddle milk powder for babies—period. . . . This congress consists of believers in nutritional excellence. It seems therefore to us that it is somehow antithetic to receive money from interests that are hostile to good nutrition and whose marketing practices or commercial interests run counter to the nutritional excellence everyone in this room would want to achieve. . . . The congress should find other sponsors.[36]

The director of Nestlé Canada termed Lewis's statement "ridiculous" because improper preparation was the problem, not nutrition: "You've got to promote breast-feeding . . . where appropriate . . . but you can't be dogmatic about these things. . . . There will always be exceptions to the rule." The "few" exceptions were noted in a Nestlé-commissioned audit of its marketing practices in Pakistan; this audit identified only three

Code violations, leading the company to conclude that it was in compliance with both the letter and the spirit of the WHO Code. A study of practices in 33 cities and towns in Pakistan, however, came to precisely the opposite conclusion: "Not a single company marketing infant food or feeding products in Pakistan was abiding by the International Code in its entirety; also, of the 662 mothers interviewed nearly every fourth mother was buying milk made by the infant formula industry."[37]

Although this controversy may seem like old news, its issues remain current—and not only because of the ongoing boycott. Recent events have presented Nestlé with a new public relations opportunity: the virus that causes AIDS (acquired immunodeficiency syndrome) can be transmitted from infected mothers to their infants through breast-feeding. AIDS affects up to 45% of pregnant women in certain countries in Africa and is transmitted to as many as half of their children. About 590,000 children were infected with the AIDS virus in 1998, 90% of them in Africa.[38]

The proportion of children who were infected as a result of breast-feeding, however, is a matter of considerable debate. Transmission through breast milk depends on such factors as viral load, immune status, age, and the length of time that breast-feeding continues. It also depends on the exclusivity of breast-feeding; rates of transmission are *higher* among infants of infected mothers who supplement breast milk with bottle-fed water or formula. Most estimates of the rate of transmission through breast milk are in the range of 15% to 25%, but some investigators consider estimates of 10% to be too high.[39] Because *appropriate* use of substitutes for breast milk can prevent nearly half of such infections, a decision about whether to breast-feed or bottle-feed becomes an agonizing dilemma for women too poor to obtain prenatal diagnosis or treatment for AIDS, let alone buy formula and use it properly.

Comparative studies of breast- and bottle-feeding in developing countries show that bottle-fed infants of uninfected mothers are six times more likely to die from diarrheal diseases; they also show that the protective effects of breast-feeding are particularly strong among infants of mothers with the least education. On this basis, researchers conclude that "it will be difficult, if not impossible, to provide safe breastmilk substitutes to children from underprivileged populations."[40] Nevertheless, Nestlé began mentioning AIDS as a justification for formula feeding as early as 1989.[41]

It is nothing if not ironic that some individuals and the U.N. agencies once active in promoting the International Marketing Code are now forced to work with Nestlé to provide formulas for infants at risk of

AIDS. In 1998, after "several years of internal debate," the U.N. directed that women infected with the AIDS virus be advised of the risks of transmitting the disease to their infants through breast-feeding, as well as the risks of not breast-feeding. Advocates were troubled by suggestions that the formula industry might have influenced the directive in some way, because they viewed the formula approach as excessively costly and risky.[42] Defending her agency against such charges, Carol Bellamy, the director of UNICEF, explained,

> When we think that a company—any company—may offer a compelling solution to a crucial child health problem such as HIV/AIDS, we will explore how to get that company working on behalf of children and women . . . Are the issues complex? Yes. Is the growing calamity of HIV/AIDS forcing us all to consider new approaches to our work? Absolutely . . . regardless of our soul searching on how best to navigate through the sometimes conflicting policy issues raised in part by AIDS, Unicef remains resolutely committed to breast feeding and the many benefits it provides to both mother and child.[43]

Pressures on UNICEF, however, also came from formula makers and the business community eager to convince the agency to embrace formulas as *the* solution to the childhood AIDS crisis. Such pressures must have been intense and unrelenting, as revealed late in 2000 in a lengthy article in the *Wall Street Journal*. The article attacked UNICEF for blocking what the authors viewed as the only reasonable approach to preventing infant deaths caused by transmission of AIDS through breast milk. An editorial in the *Journal's* European edition expressed even greater sympathy with the plight of formula companies. It began, "Makers of infant formula have long known that no good deed goes unpunished. Offers to donate millions of dollars worth of nutritious baby formula are regarded as 'suspicious' by United Nations Children's Fund officials. In fact, UNICEF has been waging a feud against the industry since the 1970s."[44] Here, public relations efforts achieved press coverage favoring corporate interests in exploiting a difficult and complex situation.

The wicked complexity of dealing with AIDS transmission by breast-feeding mothers is illustrated by the results of recent studies. Among African women with AIDS, for example, drug therapy at birth can reduce transmission rates by about half, but some of the protective effects disappear if breast-feeding continues. Thus, even if women can obtain the drugs, short-term therapy is only partially effective. Pregnant women who are able to obtain a diagnosis and are found to be infected with the AIDS virus, therefore, have two decisions to make: (1) whether to breast-feed, and (2) if not breast-feeding, whether to use formula or other feeding options (cup-feeding, for example, is less likely than bottle-feeding to transmit microbial infections).

Further complicating this issue are debates about whether breast-feeding by mothers with AIDS compromises their own health and longevity.[45] For infected women who have the resources to use formula appropriately, there is little question that bottle-feeding is a viable option for preventing viral transmission. But for women in the more typical situation—lacking adequate health care, sanitation, and education—exclusive breast-feeding may well remain a better option than formula feeding. Given such choices, the best long-term approach is to find ways to improve the safety of breast-feeding. Finding resources to do so, however, is itself a challenge, because there is little financial incentive for private companies to seek approaches that will not lead to the development of marketable drugs or formulas. One possibility is that improved maternal nutrition might help reduce AIDS transmission rates, as suggested by studies using vitamin supplements, but the benefits of this approach have yet to be confirmed.[46] Nevertheless, advocates, international agencies, and formula companies might do the most good by making sure that pregnant women and nursing mothers are adequately nourished and by encouraging women who choose to breast-feed to do so exclusively. In the meantime, the companies are likely to continue public relations efforts to convince international agencies to view formulas as the *only* viable solution to the pediatric AIDS crisis.

Nestlé, the largest food company in the world, has vast resources for influencing the opinions and actions of people who work for national and international agencies. Because the company has such strongly vested interests in selling infant formula to mothers who may not need to bottle-feed and to those whose infants may be harmed by doing so, its offer to "solve" the childhood AIDS problem is not free of conflict. Its use of public relations may be an extreme example of economic motives overriding health considerations, but it illustrates the reasons why softer marketing strategies sometimes reassure skeptics and make any criticism of a food product seem ideologically motivated or overly simplistic. In the next chapter, we will examine far less ambiguous strategies—those that involve direct court challenges to protect the image of food products or conspiracies to reduce competition in their pricing.

CHAPTER 7

PLAYING HARDBALL

LEGAL AND NOT

WHEN ADVERTISING, PUBLIC RELATIONS, ARRANGEMENTS WITH experts, outright lobbying, and the other efforts discussed in previous chapters are insufficient to protect the sales environment, food companies resort to more heavy-handed methods. This chapter illustrates two ways in which companies use "hardball" strategies. To counter suggestions that their products might have adverse health, safety, or environmental consequences, food companies engage in litigation: they sue critics for libel or other reasons. And to avoid the unwanted consequences of free-market competition, some companies use a strategy that crosses the line from legal to illegal: they conspire to fix prices. This chapter presents some examples of this harsher side of food industry action.

USING THE COURTS TO SUE CRITICS

When all else fails, competition for sales sometimes drives food companies to turn to the courts. In later chapters, we will see many situations in which food companies have gone to court to force government regulatory agencies to develop policies more congenial to their interests. What follow are examples of legal challenges *to private citizens* who made critical comments about such things as the way hamburgers are produced or bananas are sold. In the case of hamburgers, the legal challenges appeared so frivolous that it was difficult for observers to take them seriously. For the people who were sued, however, the charges were an extremely serious matter, and although they defended themselves with reasonable success, they did so at enormous financial and personal cost.

As we will see, the banana case raised broader and more fundamental issues involving freedom of the press. More important for the purposes of this discussion, the effect of the lawsuits was intimidation—to ensure that people would think twice about the unpleasant consequences of publicly expressing reservations about the health attributes of foods or the way they might have been produced.

McDonald's versus London Greenpeace: McLibel

In the late 1980s, London Greenpeace, a small activist group with no connection to Greenpeace International, began handing out leaflets titled *What's Wrong with McDonald's? Everything They Don't Want You to Know.* The leaflet said that "the more you find out about McDonald's processed food, the less attractive it becomes . . . [and] the truth about hamburgers is enough to put you off them for life." The leaflet charged McDonald's with exploitation—of food producers in developing countries, children, and employees—and with destroying rain forests, producing unhealthful food, and torturing and murdering animals used for food. Meat, the leaflet said, was responsible for 70% of all food-poisoning incidents, and antibiotics, hormones, and pesticides in animal feed damaged the health of "people on a meat-based diet." The point, it continued, was "not to change McDonald's into some sort of vegetarian organization, but to change the whole system itself. Anything less would be a rip-off."[1]

One might think that a company as large, popular, and successful as McDonald's would view the leaflet as representing an animal-rights agenda and forget about it, but the company's officials chose instead to interpret the charges as libelous. McDonald's sued five members of London Greenpeace in a case that quickly became known as "McLibel."[2] Under Britain's stringent libel laws, the defendants are required to prove that their accusations are true. This task is usually so overwhelmingly difficult that most people charged with libel quickly confess to wrongdoing and settle the case. On this basis, three members apologized and McDonald's dropped the charges against them. "The McLibel Two," however, chose to take on the company. Furthermore, because neither had more than minimal income, they chose to act as their own legal counsel.

The trial began in 1994 and lasted a record-setting two and one-half years. After hearing from 180 witnesses, among them many of Britain's leading nutrition researchers, and reviewing 60,000 pages of transcripts, the judge ruled that the defendants had indeed libeled McDonald's: they had not proved that the company destroys rain forests, discriminates against employees, or poisons customers. In the judge's British legalese, "With all these matters in mind I find that the message and meaning of the leaflet that the First and Second Plaintiffs [McDonald's companies in Great Britain] sell meat products which, as they must know, expose their customers, to whom they promote their meals, to a serious risk of food poisoning and poisoning by the residues of antibiotic drugs, growth-promoting hormone drugs and pesticides, is not justified. It is not true."[1] The judge also ruled that the charge of "a very real risk of heart disease or cancer of the breast or cancer of the bowel simply from eating at McDonald's more than just occasionally, and of a cover up of that fact, is not justified."

To the great pleasure of the defendants and their supporters, however, the judge found *not* libelous the leaflet's assertions that McDonald's is cruel to animals, exploits children in its advertising practices, and depresses wages in the British fast-food industry. He said, for example: "In my judgment McDonald's advertising and marketing makes considerable use of susceptible young children to bring in custom [business], both their own and that of their parents who must accompany them, by pestering their parents . . . [T]his is an inevitable result of advertising at all to children who cannot buy for themselves. So be it."[1]

As might be expected, the press had a wonderful time with this trial. Commentators could not help but note that McDonald's was selling about $30 billion of burgers annually, that it operated 21,000 restaurants in 101 countries, and that the trial surely had to be "something of a nadir" in the company's history of public relations.[3] Some writers could barely contain their sarcasm, as illustrated by this "quiz" question to readers of *The Nation:*

> The leaflet says that workers in the burger chains are paid low wages and accuses you of tempting your customers with food too high in fat, sugar and salt and too low in vitamins to be healthy. Do you: (a) ignore your critics . . . ; (b) hire private detectives to infiltrate their meetings and spy on their private lives; or (c) sue for libel, spending $15 million trying to silence two people with a combined income of $12,000 a year? In McLibel, the legal farce that just closed in London, the correct answers are (b) and (c).[4]

By the time it ended, the trial had become "one of the greatest David and Goliath stories in the history of common-law jurisprudence."[5] Not only had the trial focused public attention on ethical issues related to McDonald's marketing to children of diets high in calories, saturated fat, and sodium, but it also had illustrated the time and expense to which a food company was willing to go to stifle criticism of such practices.

Cattlemen versus Oprah Winfrey

The McLibel trial established a precedent for dealing aggressively with critics. Rather than picking on a David, the next such trial pitted Texas cattlemen against a media-star Goliath; the celebrated television personality Oprah Winfrey. As one commentator explained, "You would have to live under a rock in a particularly desolate stretch of the Sahara to not know who Oprah Winfrey is. The talk show she started in 1985 . . . is seen by 22 million viewers a week in the United States and is broadcast in 119 countries."[6] Nevertheless, the Texas cattlemen chose to sue Ms. Winfrey in 1996 for violating the state's recently passed food-disparagement ("veggie-libel") law.

So that we can better understand the significance of this case, a brief historical digression is in order. Veggie-libel laws emerged during the 1990s in response to an herbicide scare that had affected sales of apples in 1989. Early that year, the Environmental Protection Agency (EPA) proposed to ban the use of Alar, a chemical applied by apple growers to keep fruit on trees until ripe; tests had demonstrated that Alar decomposed into a potent carcinogen when tested in mice. At the same time, the Natural Resources Defense Council (NRDC), an advocacy group for environmental issues, released a report on the "intolerable" risks that chemical pesticides pose to children. The NRDC claimed that Alar was likely to increase the risk of cancer in children who are frequent consumers of apple juice and that EPA standards failed to consider the greater vulnerability of children when setting tolerance limits.[7] When the CBS television program *60 Minutes* aired the report, the reaction was immediate and profound. Schools and supermarkets removed apples from use, and Uniroyal, the maker of Alar, stopped selling it. Uniroyal also mounted a public relations campaign to demonstrate that claims of harm were overstated: "A child would have to drink 19,000 quarts of apple juice a day to equal the excessive dosages fed to the mice that developed vascular tumors."[8] On that basis, apple growers in Washington state filed lawsuits against CBS and the NRDC. Although the Supreme Court refused to hear the case, food companies learned a lesson; statements suggesting that a product was unsafe could reduce sales—and badly.

Two years later, in an account so unimportant that it did not even merit a byline, the *New York Times* reported that the governor of Colorado had vetoed a bill sponsored by an apple grower still reeling from the effects of the Alar scare. The bill would have permitted food producers to sue people who falsely disparaged their products. To many people, such a law seemed too silly to be worth attention. It immediately brought to mind the infamous comments of former President George Bush about his least favorite vegetable: "I do not like broccoli. And I haven't liked it since I was a little kid and my mother made me eat it. And I'm President of the United States, and I'm not going to eat any more broccoli!"[9] In vetoing the bill, the Colorado governor recognized that such comments might adversely affect food sales but acknowledged that "constitutional protection gives individuals as well as consumer groups and researchers the guaranteed right to raise legitimate questions about food safety and quality."[10]

Between 1991 and 1997, however, food industry lobbyists representing chemical and pesticide companies succeeded in inducing 13 states to pass veggie-libel laws and more than 30 others to consider them. From the standpoint of consumer groups, the laws were part of the public relations industry's "secret war on activists . . . [T]he food, pesticide, and agribusiness industries have a common vested interest in silencing criticism of their products."[11] Texas, for example, passed the "False Disparagement of Perishable Food Products Law of 1995," which prohibited people from giving out information that a food is unsafe unless that charge was based on reasonable and reliable scientific inquiry, facts, or data. A South Dakota law specifically prevented people from saying that generally accepted agricultural practices (such as the use of pesticides, no doubt) might make foods unsafe. Most such laws required the people who were being sued for disparagement to prove that their statements were true, just as in the British system. Others, like the law in Texas, placed the burden of proof on the people who filed the lawsuits. Nevertheless, commentators believed that laws such as these would have prevented Upton Sinclair from publishing *The Jungle*, his 1906 muckraking novel on the Chicago stockyards.

With this background, we can return to the case at hand. On April 16, 1996, Oprah Winfrey invited Howard Lyman, a "vegetarian activist" from the Humane Society of the United States, to discuss his concerns about the implications for Americans of the epidemic of mad cow disease then rampant in Great Britain. Here is the critical moment in their conversation:

> LYMAN: . . . we're following exactly the same path that they followed in England . . . One hundred thousand cows per year in the United States are fine at night, dead in the morning. The majority of those cows are rounded up, ground up, fed back to other cows. If only one of them has mad cow disease, [it] has the potential to infect thousands . . .
>
> WINFREY: . . . How do you know for sure that the cows are ground up and fed back to the other cows?

LYMAN: Oh, I've seen it. These are USDA statistics. They're not something we're making up.

WINFREY: . . . It has just stopped me cold from eating another burger! I'm stopped!

AUDIENCE: Yeah![11]

Prices for cattle futures were said to have fallen by more than 10% in the moments following the broadcast and to have taken weeks to recover. One Texas cattleman told a reporter that his company lost $7 million as a result of the show and that "We're taking the Israeli action on this thing . . . Get in there and just blow the hell out of somebody."[12] He and other Texas cattle ranchers instituted a $10.3 million class-action suit against Ms. Winfrey for inciting fear of beef in the minds of consumers. Commentators, however, considered the suit to be "mad litigation disease." Attacking one of the most popular television performers in America seemed so unproductive a way to challenge First Amendment rights that it suggested lawyers had been given "a bum steer."[13]

The trial began in January 1998. Ms. Winfrey argued that she had not intended the segment to be inflammatory, although her principal concern was for viewers, not the beef industry: "I do the show with the people in mind . . . I don't do it for corporations."[14] Her lawyers presented evidence that beef futures had been falling *before* the broadcast took place. Without saying anything about whether food-disparagement laws are constitutional, the judge decided that the cattlemen could not use them as a basis for the suit but would have to use business-disparagement laws instead; this meant that the cattlemen would have to prove that Ms. Winfrey *deliberately* set out to defame the beef industry.

As might be expected, the jury cleared Ms. Winfrey of that charge and granted her a "smashing legal victory."[15] The Humane Society celebrated the decision in a full-page advertisement in the *New York Times* on February 27: "They tried to muzzle the Humane Society of the United States and Oprah Winfrey: they failed." Two years later, a federal appeals court ruled that Ms. Winfrey might have overly dramatized the effects of mad cow disease but that she had not given false information or defamed cattlemen.

With this victory, Ms. Winfrey had defeated the suit, but at enormous cost; her legal fees were said to have exceeded $1 million. In this way alone, the cattlemen achieved their real purpose: to "make reporters and journalists and entertainers—and whatever Oprah considers herself—

more careful."[16] Although they lost the suit, the cattlemen succeeded in demonstrating that the threat of a lawsuit could chill debate about controversial practices of food companies.

Chiquita Banana versus the Cincinnati Enquirer

In the banana wars described in Chapter 4, a different but particularly nasty battle took place over a newspaper investigative report. In 1998 the *Cincinnati Enquirer* published a lengthy account of a year-long investigation it had sponsored into the Cincinnati-based Chiquita company's "unsavory" practices in banana-producing countries. The reporters who wrote the account accused the company of creating secret business entities to avoid local land and labor laws, bribing local officials, using pesticides in irresponsible ways that harmed workers and the environment, and moving plantation residents without their permission. The investigative reporters freely stated that they had used company voice-mail recordings as one source for these allegations.[17]

Rather than dealing with these charges, Chiquita lawyers accused the reporters of obtaining the telephone recordings through illegal means and threatened a lawsuit. Rather than defending its reporters and their account, the newspaper quickly conceded that the reporters had acted inappropriately, fired them, published an apology, and paid a $10 million settlement fee. Chiquita then sued one of the reporters for defamation. Later accounts revealed that the judge who assigned himself to the defamation case had received campaign contributions from Chiquita executives as well as from the special prosecutor who was investigating the charges.[18] To the distress of commentators concerned about journalistic ethics, the reporter—as part of a plea bargain—revealed the name of the person who had given him the voice-mail records. This well-publicized drama, in which the behavior of the newspaper, that of the company, and that of the reporters all raised ethical concerns, thoroughly distracted attention from the content of the investigative report itself. Although Chiquita denied the accusations, neither the company nor anyone else produced evidence to suggest that the reporters' findings were false.[19]

Because Chiquita is based in Cincinnati and might be expected to have close connections with other Cincinnati-based institutions, such as the newspaper and the judiciary, we can only wonder why the newspaper agreed to fund the investigation in the first place. Such investigations take courage, deep pockets, skill, and a commitment to make sacrifices to uphold ethical principles—in short, resources well beyond those of most hometown newspapers. Chiquita's aggressive actions and the newspaper's hasty retreat revealed how high the stakes are in such investigations, perhaps convincing other editors that probing the practices of food companies cannot possibly be worth the price.

CROSSING A LEGAL LINE: FIXING PRICES

As we have seen, most of the methods used by food companies to obtain sales advantages for their products meet the letter (if not the spirit) of the law. Price fixing, however, does not. Although anyone who notes the similarities in the prices of competing brands of cereals, soft drinks, margarines, or candy might be surprised to learn that they are *not* arranged in advance by their various makers, price fixing is indeed against the law; it defeats the benefits (in lower costs and higher profits) of competition in a free-market economy. The following three examples reveal what happens when companies get caught in price-fixing activities. These examples suggest that other food industries may also be engaged in fixing prices, or might consider doing so, if they think they can get away with it.

Infant Formulas

In 1990 the Federal Trade Commission (FTC) responded to complaints from welfare officials and consumer groups that three manufacturers of infant formulas had been engaging in "frequent, substantial, and parallel price increases" for more than a decade.[20] From 1980 to 1993, the prices of infant formulas had increased by more than 200%, a factor six times higher than the increase in the price of cow's milk, their basic ingredient. FTC investigators noted that the companies were dealing with a captive market—infants whose mothers could not or did not want to breast-feed. They observed that the standard marketing practice was to encourage physicians and hospitals to recommend formulas or give samples to new mothers. The American Academy of Pediatrics (AAP), a professional society that accepted large contributions from American formula companies, opposed public advertising, ostensibly on the grounds that it might discourage mothers from breast-feeding. The FTC investigators countered that the real purpose of opposing advertising was to prevent Nestlé from entering the U.S. formula market until 1988.[21] As we saw in the previous chapter, Nestlé advertised its products directly to consumers in developing countries as well as industrialized countries, and pediatricians had objected when Carnation (a Nestlé subsidiary) and Gerber began public advertisements at that time.

Infant formulas have always been enormously profitable for two reasons, both of which involve government policies. The cost of the main ingredient—cow's milk—is low thanks to federal subsidies. Furthermore, government purchases for WIC, the food assistance program for low-income women, infants, and children, account for as much as 40% of the formula market.[22] As we shall see, this second factor led to the price fixing. Because the WIC program is not an entitlement (state programs serve only the number of eligible mothers and children for which funds are available), any rise in the cost of formula forces a reduction in the number of participants. During the Reagan administration, a time of relaxed regulatory control, WIC directors were required to pay retail prices for formula purchases. When formula prices started to rise, they demanded competitive bids in order to serve a larger proportion of the eligible population.

The formula companies resisted that effort. They lobbied legislatures and physicians, arguing that competitive bidding might place children's health at risk by preventing doctors from prescribing certain brands. This argument raised credibility issues; the content of infant formulas is tightly regulated, and all are pretty much the same. A more plausible concern was that unscrupulous companies might "dump" batches that were improperly made or had been held past their "sell dates."

The extent of lobbying by formula companies over competitive bids was so intense that some states began to investigate the industry's pricing methods.[23] Eventually, some states adopted bidding systems, and companies were forced to compete for business. As a result, costs to the state WIC programs dropped. When the companies again raised formula prices, advocates pressed for federal intervention. Formula companies were reported to be concerned that the price-fixing investigation and the requirement for competitive bidding would cut into their profits, but industry analysts believed that infant formulas would still remain highly profitable. Settlement of the case also was considered to mean relatively little with respect to industry profits, because the market for infant formula would always be strong. In 1996 Abbott Laboratories, the maker of Similac and Isomil formulas, agreed to pay $32.5 million in cash and other forms of compensation to settle lawsuits in 17 states.[21] Whether these fines were enough to discourage further price fixing remains to be seen.

Feed Additives

In 1992 the government began to investigate the price-fixing practices of the Archer Daniels Midland company (ADM). An informant told investigators that the company conspired with competitors in Japan to fix the prices of lysine, an amino acid added to animal feed (amino acids are building blocks of body proteins). Although such a common component of protein might not seem worthy of federal attention, lysine sales generated about $1 billion annually. The case drew particular attention because it involved the son of the company's chairman, Dwayne Andreas, a man known for his skill at courting politicians and for his generous contributions to both political parties. It also attracted attention when the chief informant was found to have stolen millions of dollars from the company (which he claimed represented bonuses) and lost his immunity from prosecution. Most remarkable was the central piece of evidence: a videotape of a 1993 meeting of ADM executives with those of the Ajinimoto company of Japan, in which they apparently haggled over prices. In a statement interpreted as expressing how *normal* such activities were, the videotape displayed an ADM official explaining that "We have a saying at this company . . . our competitors are our friends and our customers are our enemies."[24]

In 1998 a federal jury found the company guilty. As a result, Mr. Andreas resigned as chair, although he was expected to continue to exert influence over the company. Three ADM executives received prison sentences. During the course of the investigations, federal prosecutors discovered that the company also had discussed price fixing for citric acid—a feed additive manufactured by the Roche pharmaceutical company—with Cargill and other companies. Cargill denied the charge, but Roche paid a fine of $14 million to settle that particular case.[25] Roche also was involved in other questionable activities. Read on.

Wholesale Vitamins: Vitamins, Inc.

In late 1997 the vitamin industry was said to be "buzzing with speculation" over the names of companies that might be targets of a federal investigation into price fixing among sellers of wholesale vitamins. Companies in this $3 billion annual industry sold vitamins to makers of supplements, fortified foods, or animal feeds (the heaviest user). With sales of $1.4 billion per year, Roche was the largest supplier, but its prices did not seem to vary from those of its competitors. According to investigators, senior executives of the wholesalers—constituting what they called "Vitamin, Inc."—met in secret every fall for a decade to set production quotas, prices, and distribution for the global market. Antitrust officials of the Justice Department called these meetings "the most pervasive and harmful criminal antitrust conspiracy ever uncovered."[25] High officials of Roche, however, "pronounced themselves blameless and clueless" and attributed the illegal actions to lower-level staff: "You will understand that this was not part of our responsibility . . . [I]t is certainly not easy to understand the reasons for actions of employees who in secrecy organized a conspiracy of this kind."[26]

Eventually, the legal actions included a class-action suit by direct purchasers of wholesale vitamins such as Kellogg, Kraft, Coca-Cola, and companies making animal feed who complained that they had been cheated out of $5 billion or more. The investigations supported these allegations and led to dismissals of employees and to admission that the companies had participated in a global conspiracy to set prices and divide the world markets for vitamins. Early estimates were that the settlement would involve more than $1 billion, but three-quarters of the nearly 300 companies participating in the class-action suit (among them huge companies such as Tyson Foods and Quaker Oats) decided to seek settlements on their own. The remaining settlement amounted to just $255 million.[27]

Although it might seem self-evident that price fixing harms the public by making foods cost more, at least one business economist argues otherwise. According to his analysis, the prices of both vitamins and nonprescription drugs rose by about the same amount during the conspiracy period. In his view, "what sets the vitamin case apart is its international nature. Thanks to some recent treaties, the U.S. government can now prosecute foreign firms for violating American laws, and U.S. citizens can collect civil damages from those same firms. Thus, the vitamin case has had the remarkable effect of allowing Americans to walk away with more than $1.85 billion taken from European and Japanese firms without the slightest protest from any of their governments."[28]

What these three examples illustrate is the ability of companies to profit from price-fixing alliances. They are protected from price wars and can raise prices with impunity. Even a casual reading of these cases suggests that they are unlikely to be isolated instances. Indeed, by late 1999 at least 35 federal grand juries were investigating charges of price fixing in the food industry and the case of Archer Daniels Midland was considered just the tip of the iceberg.[25] According to a 1999 report, at least 22 food, agriculture, or food chemical firms ranked among the "top 100 corporate criminals of the decade" on the basis of the size of the fines they had paid for violating federal laws. Of these "leading" companies, 12 were convicted of price fixing; they paid a total of $994 million in fines ranging from a high of $500 million (Hoffman LaRoche for vitamins, ranked number 1) to a low of $400,000 (Cerestar Bioproducts for citric acid, tied for number 91). Other food companies on the top-100 list were convicted and fined for rigging bids, corrupting federal officials, concealing election campaign contributions, selling adulterated food, or contaminating the environment.[29] On the basis of such evidence, it is difficult to believe that such practices are uncommon in the food industry.

WORKING THE SYSTEM, SYSTEMATICALLY

As these last four chapters have indicated, lobbying is only one facet of a broad range of strategies used by food companies to maintain a favorable sales environment for their products. Because lobbyists must register, lobbying is just the best known of these strategies. A 1960s study of this practice viewed it as a *healthy* influence within the political system—one that keeps Congress informed about issues, stimulates public debate, and encourages participation in the political process. That study concluded that lobbying is unlikely to exert undue influence because "it is virtually impossible to steal or buy a public policy decision of any consequence in Washington."[30] Whether its author would reach such a comforting conclusion today is questionable. Not only are the financial stakes higher, but we now know much more about the relationship of money to congressional actions, particularly as taught to us by the makers of guns, drugs,[1] and, most notably, cigarettes.[31]

If the examples given here do not provide unequivocal proof that the ways in which food companies "work the system" to influence opinions, programs, and policies, they surely provide evidence for strong associations between funding sources and what Congress, agency officials, academic departments, researchers, and nutritionists say and do. For the most part, the strategies I have discussed here are legal. Furthermore, they are available to consumer groups as well as to food producers. Indeed, several examples in this book offer evidence that public action to oppose food companies and products on behalf of sound nutrition can be highly effective. It should be apparent, however, that food companies have vastly greater resources for pursuing these strategies than have consumer groups or, for that matter, responsible agencies of the federal government. The hundreds of millions of dollars available to the meat and dairy lobbies through check-off programs, and the billions of dollars that food companies spend on advertising and lawsuits, so far exceed both the amounts spent by the federal government on nutrition advice for the public and the annual budget of any consumer advocacy group that they cannot be considered in the same stratosphere.

As Michael Jacobson, the director of the Center for Science in the Public Interest observed in the mid-1970s, it is unfortunate that "good advice about nutrition conflicts with the interests of many big industries, each of which has more lobbying power than all the public-interest groups combined."[32] The controversies discussed in this book demonstrate that the connections between food lobbies and members of Congress, officials of federal agencies, and food and nutrition professionals raise unsettling questions about the independence of judgments and policy decisions. Such questions require even more public scrutiny than they have received to date.

The next section of the book begins our discussion of a different food industry strategy—a search for new marketing targets. In response to competition, food companies have expanded their efforts to find new consumers for their products and have initiated sales campaigns aimed at ethnic minorities, at international audiences, and (most egregiously, as discussed next) at young children.

PART THREE

EXPLOITING KIDS, CORRUPTING SCHOOLS

DURING THE TWENTIETH CENTURY, THE NUTRITIONAL HEALTH of American children improved dramatically in some ways—but not in others. Early in the century, many children died from the complications of infectious diseases made worse by diets limited in calories and nutrients. As scientists learned more about how diets could protect against disease, they introduced measures that virtually eliminated classic signs of severe undernutrition among American children. Fortification of foods with iron, for example, helped reduce rates of iron-deficiency anemia to their present low levels, and school lunch programs kept many children from going hungry. These accomplishments count among the greatest achievements of twentieth-century public health.

Today, the health consequences of undernutrition—illnesses due to deficiencies of vitamins, minerals, protein, or calories—are rarely observed except among children who are ill from other causes or those from households with the lowest income. Income is a major factor in children's nutrition. For example, the Public Health Service's 2000 review of national health data, *Healthy People 2010*, demonstrates that anemia due to iron deficiency is almost twice as common among 2-year-old children from families with incomes barely at the poverty level than it is among those from higher-income families (12% compared to 7%). Growth retardation (height-for-age below the 5th percentile for age and sex) affects 8% of low-income children under age 5. Thus poverty continues to be the single most important danger signal for nutritional deficiencies in American children.[1] Although nearly 90% of American households with children were "food secure" in 1999 (that is, they consistently obtained enough food for all members to maintain active, healthy lives), just 37% of households with below-poverty incomes are in this category—an improvement since 1900, but still well below what should be expected in such a wealthy country.[2]

Too little food, however, is only part of the problem. For all children, wealthy and poor alike, the principal nutritional concerns are eating too much of the wrong kinds of foods in particular, and consuming too many calories in general. Obesity, as we saw in the Introduction, is now the most serious dietary problem affecting the health of American children. Although many factors influence childhood obesity, the quality and quantity of the foods consumed are major contributors. Thus efforts to market food products directly to children deserve close scrutiny. As I explain in Chapter 8, food companies spend enormous creative energy and huge sums of money to entice children to buy their products or demand that their parents do so. Despite claims to the contrary, such efforts have little to do with good nutrition and everything to do with promoting food sales. The blatant exploitation by food companies of even the youngest children raises questions about the degree to which society at large needs to be responsible for protecting children's health in a free-market economy.

We shall see in these chapters that the creativity of food industry marketing extends beyond such standard channels of communication as television, magazines, billboards, store displays, and the Internet. It also targets schools. As described in Chapter 8, many American schools have been co-opted into a variety of partnerships that serve the interests of the food industry far more than they do children's health. Chapter 9 provides a detailed examination of a particularly disturbing example: "pouring rights" contract agreements between schools and soft drink companies.

CHAPTER 8

STARTING EARLY

UNDERAGE CONSUMERS

WHEREAS CONCERNS ABOUT CHILDREN'S NUTRITION ONCE focused on dietary insufficiency, the most serious dietary issue affecting today's American children is obesity—the result of eating more food than is needed, rather than too little. Obesity rates are rising rapidly among children and adolescents, especially those who are African-American or Hispanic. In the early 1990s, for example, 23% of white girls aged 6–11 were overweight, compared to 29% of Mexican-American girls and 31% of black girls.[1] Pediatricians report seeing children with high levels of serum cholesterol, high blood pressure, and "adult"-onset diabetes at earlier and earlier ages—all consequences of excessive caloric intake. Because obesity tends to persist into adulthood, this condition may well predispose overweight and obese children to cardiovascular and other chronic disease risks later in life.

The increasing prevalence of childhood obesity results from complex interactions of societal, economic, demographic, and environmental changes that not only encourage people to eat more food than needed to meet their energy requirements but also encourage people to make less healthful food choices and act as barriers to physical activity. In part as a result of the overabundance of food in the United States, and the consequences of overabundance for the food industry, the diets of most American children do not come close to meeting nutritional recommendations. In 1997 American children obtained a whopping 50% of their calories from added fat and sugar (35% and 15%, respectively), and only 1% of them regularly ate diets that resemble the proportions of the *Food Pyramid*. The diets of nearly half (45%) of all U.S. children failed to meet *any* of the serving numbers recommended in the *Pyramid*—not even one of them.[2] A survey the following year found that only 2% of teenagers in California met diet and activity recommendations.[3] As might be expected, children whose dietary patterns least resemble the *Pyramid* are most lacking in intake of essential nutrients, in part because they consume more soft drinks and other high-calorie, low-nutrient foods. Indeed, American children eat one out of every three meals outside the home, where foods are demonstrably higher in calories, fat, saturated fat, and salt as well as lower in more desirable nutrients.[4]

Such discouraging findings suggest the need for attention to the dietary habits of children and to the ways in which our society influences the quality and quantity of the foods they eat. Food marketing is only one of those influences, but it raises issues of special concern, especially when it is deliberately targeted to the youngest and most impressionable children. As this chapter explains, the marketing of foods to children is big business—in the home, in fast-food outlets, and in schools.

TARGETING CHILDREN

Marketers have long known that children make attractive customers, but attention to this group (and to younger and younger members within it) has increased sharply in recent years. The reasons are easy to understand: children control increasing amounts of money, and society has granted them increasing responsibility for purchasing decisions. It is difficult to know exactly how much money children now control as a result of allowances, gifts, and jobs, but even small amounts add up to very large numbers when computed across the entire population. Studies in the late 1980s reported that children spent an average of $4.42 per week each, for a combined total of more than $6 billion a year, and that they influenced annual family spending decisions involving another $132 billion. More recent studies have found that children as young as 3–5 years accounted for $1.5 billion in discretionary spending and influenced $15 billion more, that those aged 4–12 had a combined discretionary income greater than $27 billion, and that children in general influenced parental spending worth $188 billion.[5] The amounts controlled by children increase with age; children aged 7–12 have been reported to control $8.9 billion in spending money, and teenagers $119 billion, a figure that was expected to rise to $136 billion by 2001. Overall, children aged 6–19 years were thought to have influenced a staggering $485 billion in purchase decisions in 1999.[6]

The astonishing rise in children's purchasing power and influence can be attributed to a variety of societal trends. The decreasing size of families permits parents to devote more attention to individual children. Older parents are wealthier and can be more indulgent. Working and single parents delegate more responsibility to children by necessity. Putting these trends in old-fashioned terms, children these days appear more "spoiled." In other ways, however, they are *less* independent. Concerns about neighborhood safety mean that fewer children walk to school, play in parks, ride bicycles, or explore cities on their own. In the New York City of the 1940s and 1950s, my friends and I were permitted to take subways and explore the city from the time we were 8 years old—a freedom of action now utterly unthinkable for such young children. Changes in society discourage out-of-home activities and encourage television, video games, and Internet surfing. And, of course, these activities not only keep children sedentary but also expose them to countless advertisements for purchasable products.

Furthermore, increasing pressure from advertising messages reaches even the youngest children. At earlier and earlier ages, children are aware of advertised brands and establish firm preferences for them. Even very young children can identify stores that sell desired items, distinguish one product from another, and understand sales messages, the goals of retailers, and the purpose of money. By the age of 7 or 8, most children are *sophisticated* shoppers; they can shop independently, ask for information about what they want, and show off what they have bought to other children.[7]

Beyond the absolute amounts involved, discretionary spending by children establishes buying preferences and patterns that can be expected to last a lifetime. Given the importance of sound nutrition for good health, establishing appropriate preferences and patterns is especially important for foods. The development of lifetime loyalties to early purchases is well documented for foods and beverages,[1] and these products rank third in spending by teenagers, behind clothes and entertainment. In 1997 children spent nearly $8 billion of their own money on food and beverages, of which $1 billion each went for sweets and soft drinks. The amounts spent on food increase with age; in 1997, children aged 7–12 spent $2.3 billion of discretionary money on snacks and beverages, teenagers $58 billion.[5]

What do children choose to buy? Table 19 gives the percentages of children aged 7–9 and 10–12 who reported buying foods and beverages with their own money during the previous month. Half chose candy, more than one-third chose soft drinks and ice cream, and about one-fourth bought

TABLE 19. Percentages of children of ages 7–9 and 10–12 who reported purchasing foods with their own money during the past month

Product	Ages 7–9	Ages 10–12
Candy	55%	49%
Chewing gum	39	43
Soft drinks	34	46
Ice cream	33	39
Salty snacks	27	31
Fast food	16	25
Cookies	18	16

SOURCE: J. Pollack, *Advertising Age*, March 1, 1999:16.

fast food. Children also influence a substantial proportion of the total annual sales of certain foods: 25% of the total amount of salty snacks, 30% of soft drinks, 40% of frozen pizza, 50% of cold cereals, and 60% of canned pasta, for example.[5]

From such figures alone, it is easy to understand why children of any age present an irresistible marketing opportunity and why food companies spare no effort to reach them. Soft drink companies unapologetically name 8- to 12-year-olds as marketing targets. Advertisers encourage marketing directed to 9-year-olds as a logical consequence of the fact that children—and girls in particular—are maturing earlier. McDonald's produces commercials, advertisements, and a Web site aimed specifically at children aged 8–13. Other fast-food companies also are developing campaigns for preteens, and Campbell Soup views "appealing to children [as] one prong of a new effort to lift sales."[8] In January 2000 Quaker Oats began a $15 million, 5-month campaign devoted entirely to promoting sales of its heavily sugared Cap'n Crunch cereal to children. What is most remarkable about these practices is how *sensible* they appear to marketers: "Kids are a growing demographic and [the companies] are trying to get in on the ground floor."[9]

MARKETING TO YOUNG TASTES

To reach children of any age, food marketers employ a variety of methods, all highly successful. Advertising—on television and on the Internet—is only the most visible of these methods, for food companies also reach children by less obvious means, both in and out of school. The amount of money spent on marketing directed to children and their parents rose from $6.9 billion in 1992 to $12.7 billion in 1997.[10] Some of these funds pay for market research that is simply breathtaking in its comprehensiveness, level of detail, and undisguised cynicism. Anyone with access to a library can discover in a minute how best to exploit current trends and family dynamics to get children to buy or demand products.

Market researchers have defined the basic elements of advertising—package design, typefaces, pictures, content—most likely to get boys or girls of varying ages to want to purchase products. Most remarkable, they justify the results of this research as a *public service*: "Advertising to children . . . is nothing less than primary education in commercial life; the provision, in effect, of free and elementary instruction in social economics—a passport to street wisdom. Far from being further restricted, as many suggest, this education course should in fact be supported, encouraged, and enlarged."[11]

Food companies defend their targeting of children in a variety of ways, not all of them equally convincing. They rationalize their use of advertising to children as an expression of freedom of speech. They argue that advertised foods are not inherently unhealthful (recall the mantra "All foods can be part of healthful diets") and that advertising encourages children to eat breakfast or healthier food products. They maintain that no one food contributes to obesity more than any other and emphasize that exercise—not diet—is the key to weight control.

Paradoxically, despite their spending of billions of dollars on advertising directed at children, food marketers complain that this method isn't particularly effective: "In reality, there is no evidence that advertising is a major influence on children's food choices; at the same time, there is substantial evidence that it is not a major influence, and that other factors—notably inherent taste preferences and parents—are a much stronger influence."[12]

Given this alleged lack of influence, it is also paradoxical that food marketers claim that advertising *contributes* to nutrition education and argue that the primary responsibility for determining dietary intake rests with parents and caretakers who plan meals. Finally, food marketers propose that what's good for business is good for America: ". . . the idea that commercialism in general is evil is very misguided. It is the engine that drives our economy."[13]

What raises skepticism about these arguments, however, is the fact that food marketing to children is big business aimed at uncritical minds. Thus psychologists, among others, deplore this "unfair and conflict-ridden manipulation of the young" and urge restrictions on the use of psychological research by advertisers of foods and other products aimed at children.[14] But perhaps such critics are overreacting. Does advertising really sell *non-nutritious* food to children? Researchers who have examined this question answer it with a resounding "yes!"[15]

Indeed, it is so easy to demonstrate that advertising influences brand preferences that even children can prove it, as shown by two Oregon eighth-graders in a winning science fair project. The 13-year-old researchers asked their sixth- to eighth-grade classmates to state whether they preferred to drink Coca-Cola, Pepsi-Cola, or a nonadvertised store brand of cola. All respondents mentioned either Coke or Pepsi; none chose the store brand. The investigators then asked their classmates to rank the taste of coded samples of the three colas that could not be identified visually. The results: 73% of the respondents were not able to identify their preferred cola by taste, and 27% ranked the unpopular store brand as *best* in taste. They concluded, "Most of the people we tested said they liked Coke and Pepsi before the taste test because they're the original, popular cola brands. The reason they chose Coke or Pepsi had nothing to do with taste. . . . [We] think the advertising media targets their advertisements to appeal to teenagers because . . . [that's when you] develop buying habits and that's when you have more pressure to drink the brand that's cool."[16] One could hardly ask for better documentation of the reasons why businesses commit billions of dollars in efforts to reach underage consumers. Let us now take a look at how food companies marshal such efforts.

Television Advertising

The impact of television advertising on children's health, emotional state, and dietary habits has long been a cause of concern for at least three reasons: children watch television for so many hours, commercials are numerous and endlessly repeated, and children lack the critical facility to distinguish commercials from program content. In 1989 a Nielsen report found that the average child in the United States spent more time—at least 22 hours weekly—watching television than doing anything else except sleeping.[17] Today children are watching less television; in 1996, viewing among children 2–11 years old had declined 18% from a decade before. Children aged 2–7 now watch about 11 hours of television each week, but those aged 8–18 still watch about 22 hours. Unfortunately, the drop in television viewing does not mean that children have become more active and are expending more calories. On the contrary, they more than compensate by using computers to surf the Internet or play video games. Together, these sedentary visual activities amount to an average of 38 hours per week for the average child aged 2–18.[18]

One recent trend is an increase in viewing of programs designed especially for the youngest children. Because no child is too young to be targeted by television food marketers, many of these programs are linked directly to commercial products. Teletubbies, the public television program for toddlers, for example, was sponsored first by Burger King and later by McDonald's; McDonald's distributed toys representing the four characters. In the late 1990s, the Nickolodeon channel, designed for somewhat older children, was in 63 million homes, accounted for more than half of children's viewing time, and was one of the three most profitable networks in television. The children's television-advertising market, once considered "soft" because it accounted for just $750 million in 1998, quickly hardened: it accounted for about $1 billion just a year later.[19]

Not surprisingly, these expenditures of money on television advertising are richly rewarded. Research indicates that children respond best to commercials designed to appeal to desires for sensual gratification—play, fun, friends, and nurturance (in that order)—and, to a lesser extent, to concerns about achievement, overcoming opposition, and resisting undue influence. Moreover, prior to the age of 9 or 10, children do not readily understand the difference between commercials and programs. After that age, most children grasp the purpose of commercials, but there is still substantial blurring of the distinction. Even high school students have difficulty distinguishing between commercials and programming when confronted with sales messages cloaked as entertainment, information, or public service announcements. Apparently, many children do not see commercials as fundamentally different from any other form of television program content.[7]

The rising frequency of commercials is alone sufficient to raise questions about impact, especially those aired on Saturday mornings during prime-time children's programming. Despite differences in the ways that studies have been conducted over the years, they demonstrate a sharp increase in commercial bombardment. In 1987 researchers counted 225 commercials on major network channels during Saturday morning hours; the number increased to 433 in 1992 and to 997 in 1994. Of these commercials, 160 (71%), 264 (61%), and 564 (57%), respectively, advertised foods and beverages of dubious nutritional value: presweetened breakfast cereals, candy, fast food, sodas, cookies, chips. Researchers counted not a single commercial for fruits, vegetables, bread, or fish.[20] The percentage of commercials for foods may have declined, but the absolute number more than tripled, which means that children are subjected to far more frequent advertising of foods of low nutritional quality.[19]

That televised commercials influence the food choices, preferences, and demands of children—particularly younger children—has been well understood since the early 1970s. Researchers consistently have linked snack choices and food requests to televised commercials, especially to those repeated frequently. The conclusion from such studies seems inescapable: television advertising works well and is especially effective for the most frequently aired commercials such as those for sugared cereals, candy bars, and soft drinks.[21]

Many studies also have described how television viewing affects the caloric intake, health, fitness, and social outlook of American children. Children who watch the most commercials tend to consume more calories, a finding consistent with the well-documented connection between hours spent watching television and obesity.[22] Researchers, impressed by the strong correlation between television watching and blood cholesterol levels, have concluded that questions about viewing habits convey more precise information about early risk for heart disease than conventional questions about family history. Given such observations, it is not surprising that at least one study has found turning off the television set to be a promising approach to prevention of childhood obesity.[23]

Particularly distressing are reports that food commercials stimulate "antisocial" behavior in children, not just inappropriate demands for advertised products. Beer commercials, for example, influence fifth- and sixth-graders to have more favorable beliefs about drinking, greater knowledge of beer brands and slogans, and more strongly stated intentions to drink beer as adults.[24] Most troubling, researchers classify food commercials aimed at children as "high emotional/low analytic" and as overly dependent on "socially negative" material: violence (observed in 62% of the commercials), conflict (41%), trickery (20%), or some combination of these three features (64%):

> Upon reflection, it may not be a mystery that advertisers relied so heavily on these individual or combined themes, because conflict and violence are central to so much of children's TV programming. . . . The violence and conflict seen in food ad stories may simply present children with familiar themes. . . . [F]orms of deception are practiced by children as young as 2 and 3 years of age . . . so they might have little trouble appreciating its implications in food ad stories.[25]

Such disturbing findings, among others, have prompted organizations such as the American Academy of Pediatrics to recommend limits on television viewing, promotion of critical viewing skills, and controls over the content of programs and commercials directed toward children.[17] The academy recognized that the ultimate control of children's television viewing rests with parents and caretakers, but it also called on industry and government to take responsibility for what gets aired. In 1999 the American Public Health Association joined other health groups to sponsor "Healthy Kids: Campaign for Less TV" and National TV-Turnoff Weeks to encourage children and adults to replace television viewing with other activities likely to be more constructive, rewarding, and conducive to health. Such campaigns, useful as they are, assign responsibility for controlling television viewing to individual consumers, parents, and caretakers and do not necessarily target food companies, television stations, or government regulators.

Beyond Television

The advantage of television as a marketing device is its wide reach, but today's children have replaced at least some commercial programming with videos and video games. For younger children, another source of the decline in television watching turns out to be day care. Day care centers tend to keep televisions turned off during the day except to show selected videos. Thus marketers realize that "to reach kids, you have to be in a lot of different places. . . . [N]ew technologies and other activities are beginning to take them away."[26] One such place is the Internet; by the late 1990s, one-third of American households had personal computers, a development that has created a huge market for online advertising to children as well as adults. About 12 million children aged 2–12 (25%) were online in 2000, and their numbers were expected to grow to 32 million just within the next few years.[27]

Places to advertise to children are limited only by the marketer's imagination. Food companies put their logos on toys, games, clothing, and school supplies. They produce magazines, sponsor clubs, distribute coupons, buy product placements in movies, obtain celebrity endorsements, and even add their logos to baby bottles and Macy's Thanksgiving Day balloons. The M&M candy company, for example, offers an entire catalog of logo items (such as toys, caps, jackets, watches, key chains, magnets, playing cards, and cups) and has opened stores all over the world to sell them. McDonald's offers cups, toys, placemats, movie coupons,

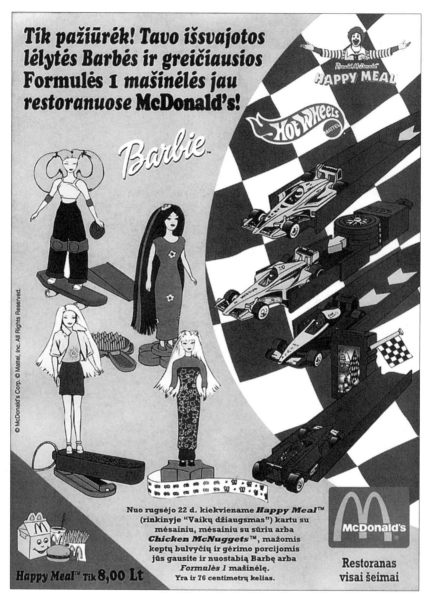

FIGURE 18. This flier for McDonald's "Happy Meals" came from one of its outlets in Vilnius, Lithuania. The meal-plus-toy cost the equivalent of about $2 in October 2000.

special toys and mugs, and logo-labeled items for holidays, birthdays, and celebrations, and it does so in its outlets throughout the world, as shown in Figure 18.

Several companies license counting books for young children that require the purchase and use of brand-name candies, cookies, and sugar-sweetened cereals. These books thoroughly undermine any instruction not to play with food. They teach children to count by using candy, cereal, or cookies as tokens and placing the foods on designated parts of the pages or in cutout spaces. They also teach children to "need" those foods. The books come with a convenient discount coupon, and the product is pictured on every page. Despite their obvious commercial purpose, the books sell well; more than 1.2 million copies of the Cheerios version were purchased just from 1998 to 2000. The books are popular with teachers and parents, even those who are uncomfortable about promoting top-of-the-*Pyramid* foods in this way. Listen to this teacher's explanation: "You hate to always use food, but it is such a hit with the kids because they can count them and then it is so rewarding for them to eat them."[28] No food marketer could possibly ask for more. Figure 19 shows two such books—one for Kellogg's Froot Loops and the other for Oreo Cookies. The Oreo book requires children to count (and, presumably, eat) their way through ten cookies before reaching "and now there are none."[29]

Soft drink companies are especially comprehensive in their approach to young consumers, as illustrated by the list in Table 20. Coca-Cola puts its logo on so many items that it runs a chain of stores to sell them; it even has stores at international airports. At least 15 books catalog the company's toy delivery trucks, Olympic pins, and other such collectibles. Figure 20 shows several such toys for people of all ages: a Coca-Cola "Picnic" Barbie doll, Volkswagen Beetle, and stapler, and one of the infamous (as explained in the next chapter) baby bottles imprinted with soft drink logos, in this case, Diet Pepsi's. For all such items, the customer pays for the advertising. A teenager wearing a tee shirt with a company logo is a walking advertisement for its products, as are adults who collect food logo items.

The attention to detail involved in marketing soft drinks to teenagers is especially impressive. The Coca-Cola company, for example, sends multiple copies of "Coke cards" to "teen influentials"—school officers, cheerleaders, and sports participants—expecting that they will pass the extras along to their network of friends. And they do; one of the Portland science fair winners told me that she had received six Coke cards and shared five with friends, precisely as the company intended. In exchange

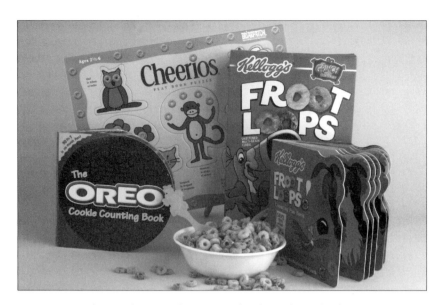

FIGURE 19. These "educational" counting books and puzzles for young children require the use of cereals or cookies as tokens, provide discount coupons to encourage adults to purchase these products, and advertise the food throughout. (Photo by Enrique Caballo, 2001)

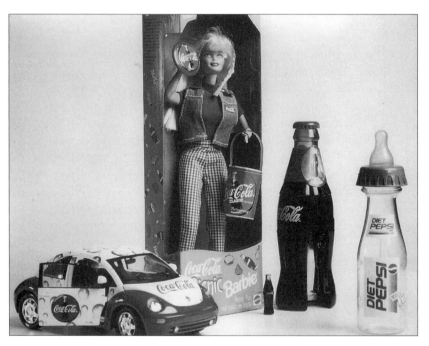

FIGURE 20. Toys like these convert children into advertisers as well as consumers of soft drinks. (Photo by Shimon and Tammar Rothstein, 2000)

TABLE 20. Examples of methods used by soft drink companies to market their products to children outside of school and at school

---

Marketing methods that target children outside of school
  Television advertising
  Internet advertising
  Magazine advertising
  Internet interactive computer games
  Toys, clothing, and other items with logos
  Discount cards, coupons
  Telephone cards
  Celebrity endorsements of products
  Product placements in movies
  Supermarket placements
  Fast-food chain tie-ins
  Prizes

Marketing methods that target children at school
  Channel One (required television watching, with commercials)
  Soft drink "pouring-rights" agreements
  Logos on vending machines, supplies, and sports facilities
  Hallway advertising
  Advertisements on free book covers
  Advertisements on school buses
  Sports uniforms, scoreboards
  Contests
  Free samples
  Coupons for fast food
  Club and activity sponsorship
  Product placements in teaching materials

---

for soda purchases, the cards provide discounts for such activities as sports, video rentals, fast food, candy, haircuts, and voice-mail. The cards are specific to geographic location; the company issues more than 300 different versions for teenagers all over the country. Coke's main competitor, Pepsi-Cola, has organized grassroots marketing programs, an entertainment Web site, and a national promotion through MTV, the music cable-television channel, to convince elementary school children that its soft drinks are "cool."

Do prizes, premiums, games, and Coke cards induce children to request the products? Of course they do. Children love such items, and food marketers explicitly reinforce such desires. Because "kids and families will be the next source for new and future customers," Nabisco publishes a guide to restaurant owners to explain how to use its Oreo cookies as a marketing tool. This book explains the fundamental elements of successful marketing to young children: entertainment, fast and friendly service, immediate gratification, familiar brand names, fun-to-eat desserts, and an environment that gives "mom and dad" comfort, reasonable prices, value, and quality time. Its suggestions are specific: keep the kids busy with crayons and placemats, provide premiums, and give kids cups to take home—all with Oreo logos. It also encourages businesses to use public service as a marketing tool by dispensing Oreo premiums to reward Little League teams or as prizes for school or community events.[30] No marketer could afford to pass up such opportunities.

FOCUSING ON SCHOOLS

Not all families own television sets or computers, but most American children attend school. Given their purchasing power, numbers, potential as future customers, and captive status, it is no wonder that food companies view schoolchildren as an unparalleled marketing opportunity. A General Accounting Office investigation found it difficult to distinguish commercial from noncommercial activities in schools because such intrusion into everyday life is so intrinsic to U.S. society. The study noted that many commercial activities, such as those listed in Table 20, produced no tangible benefits for the schools, although the benefits to advertisers were quite evident.[31]

It may well be true that corporations have genuine concerns about the state of education in this country. It is also the case that in exchange for advertising, corporations contribute resources desperately needed by financially strapped school systems. But in this exchange, the line between philanthropy and exploitation is very fine indeed. Marketing executives are well aware of the line they are crossing: "In the past, there was maybe more of a feeling that shameless promotion in school wasn't right. . . . I think in today's business climate, that's definitely beginning to change."[32]

Although, as discussed in the next chapter, many school districts actively seek industry partnerships, some school officials remain unconvinced that advertising in schools is good for either children or society:

> It must be the dream of marketing executives. The law requires your future customers to come to a place 180 days a year where they must watch and listen to your advertising messages exclusively. Your competitors are not allowed access to the market. The most important public institution in the lives of children and families gives its implied endorsement to your products. The police and schools enforce the requirement that the customers show up and stay for the show. The disturbing implications . . . are numerous and profound.[33]

Channel One and More

The most prominent, most scrutinized, and most vilified intrusion of commercialism into school life surely is Channel One, the 12-minute television program beamed into 12,000 schools throughout the United States and viewed daily by 8.3 million students. Two minutes out of every program are devoted to commercials. The private company responsible for Channel One provides, for the entire school, television sets and installation hardware estimated to be worth about $17,000. In exchange, the company *requires* students in 80% of the classrooms to watch the program on 90% of school days. The commercials pay for the programming; in the mid-1990s, a 30-second commercial cost $200,000, thus enabling the company to earn an annual profit of $30 million. The cost of advertising on Channel One and other school venues must be worth the investment, because about 12,000 companies do so.[34] Food companies are particularly prominent among school advertisers, and it is difficult to imagine a food or beverage that is *not* marketed in schools. Table 21 gives selected examples of food companies that advertised in schools in the early 1990s.

Channel One elicits particularly pointed criticism, not only of its commercial intrusion, but also of the mind-numbing "stupidity" of its news programming and the hidden costs of the time it wastes, which are estimated at $1.8 billion a year.[35] The *New York Times* quoted one critic explaining that "there's no money passing hands, but to give up that hour a week of school time makes these the most expensive TV sets you ever laid eyes on. . . . That school time was purchased by taxpayers. If you watch Channel One for 90 percent of the school days, it adds up to 31

TABLE 21. Selected list of food companies advertising in schools or in television programs or magazines that specifically target children in schools

American Home	Beatrice Foods	Bird's Eye
Campbell Soup	Carnation	Coca-Cola
ConAgra	Dannon	Del Monte
Domino's	Frito-Lay	General Foods
Gerber's	Hershey	Kellogg's
KFC	Kraft	Lawry's
McDonald's	Nabisco	Nestlé
Oscar Mayer	Pepsico	Planters
Procter & Gamble	Quaker Oats	Seven-Up

SOURCE: Consumers Union, Mount Vernon, NY, 1990.

hours a year. . . . This is required commercial television. We have an obesity crisis with adolescents in this country, and here we have government schools telling children to eat Snickers and drink Pepsi."[36] Critics also are troubled by studies showing that children do not readily distinguish Channel One's commercials from its entertainment, news, and public service programs and that they are confused about such distinctions. Children say, for example, that they believe Channel One advertisers such as Pepsi-Cola are "deeply committed to helping them cope with their emotional and psychological problems."[15]

Channel One's privileged position in schools has been reported to be the result of an intense and expensive lobbying effort in Washington and even more so in states like New York that bar the company from public schools. Given this effort, it is difficult to imagine that this statement from a Channel One executive could be anything but disingenuous: "The reality is the sponsors of Channel One News are playing a tremendous, important role in getting this free and independent journalism to the kids. . . . The same people who have gripes about Channel One point an identical finger at 'Sesame Street' and the Girl Scouts for commercializing kids. We're perfectly happy to be in that company."[36]

Beyond Channel One, at least 13 firms are devoted specifically to helping companies market products to children in schools. They help food advertisers place logos or samples on book covers, videos and curriculum guides, guides to nutrition, mathematics educational materials, and reading software. No fewer that 75 food-related corporations or groups offer teaching materials to schools.[37] Such materials are remarkable for their attitude, as Consumers Union terms it, of "NIMF—Not In My Food."[38] Thus Kellogg's materials emphasize fat (not sugar) as a concern, the Egg Board's materials minimize cholesterol, and Nabisco's materials emphasize concerns about saturated (but not total) fat. Among the more widely used materials are those produced by the National Dairy Council; as noted in Chapter 3, its nutrition guides display the dairy food group first, recommend more daily servings than the *Pyramid*'s, and do not necessarily promote low-fat products.

Corporate-sponsored teaching materials invariably give prominence to their own products in pictures, if not in words. A Consumers Union review of such materials—many of them prepared in collaboration with academic-sounding organizations—concluded that most were commercial, incomplete, biased, and oversimplified. For example, mathematics educational materials sponsored by Mars, Inc., and developed by Scholastic, Inc., were judged "incomplete, biased, and commercial." The reviewers were concerned that the materials listed candy only as an energy-producing food, made such statements as "Eating SNICKERS is a good way to get quick energy that will keep you kicking all day long," and contained the Team SNICKERS logo on every page.[38]

These kinds of partnerships enable food companies to advertise in schools under the guise of education. Since 1973, for example, Campbell Soups has offered a program called "Labels for Education" that has encouraged 50 million children in thousands of schools to redeem soup labels for basketballs, computers, and minivans. Because food products—no matter how sweet, salty, or high in calories—are claimed by their makers to be benign, school boards readily permit companies to promote them without giving the arrangements anywhere near the degree of scrutiny that would be applied to similar proposals from a cigarette company, for example.

Opposition to school commercialism is unlikely to come from financially strapped school officials grateful for whatever help they can get, from parent–teacher associations, or, regrettably, from nutritionists. A recent survey reported 70–80% of nutritionists to believe that school-based marketing programs are beneficial and that food companies should be permitted to offer teaching materials to children; just 40% thought that food companies were inappropriate sponsors of teaching materials.[39]

Other groups, however, do recognize the problem. Industry publications and those of advocates feature nearly identical articles—"Schools for Sale" and "Students for Sale"—arguing that school commercialism has gone too far.[40] Filling the gap are organizations such as the Center for Commercial-Free Public Education (Oakland, California) and the Center for Analysis of Commercialism in Education (University of Wisconsin, Milwaukee). These groups publicize the most blatant conflicts of interest in books and articles, file petitions with state legislatures, encourage lawmakers to ask for investigations and to introduce bills restricting commercial activities in schools, and demand that marketers stop advertising on Channel One. By 2001, their efforts were gaining increasing publicity and support.

Corporate Takeovers

A somewhat different form of commercialism is the relatively recent corporate takeover of school food service operations. Understanding why this particular aspect of commercial intrusion deserves attention requires a brief review of the history of school breakfast and lunch programs.

School meal programs began during the Great Depression of the 1930s. From the outset, they had two purposes: to help dispose of surplus agricultural commodities owned by the government as a result of price-support agreements with farmers, and to help prevent nutritional deficiencies among low-income schoolchildren.[41] Because chronic disease risk factors were not an issue at that time, the rules specified meals that used surplus commodities and were higher in fat, saturated fat, sugar, and salt—and lower in fiber—than recommended in later years.

Since 1946, the government has supported a program, administered by the USDA, to provide free or reduced-price breakfasts and lunches to schoolchildren from low-income families. The USDA reimburses schools at a fixed rate for the cost of the meals and for administrative and technical support; it also gives schools more than a billion pounds of surplus agricultural commodities annually. In 1999 federally supported meal programs served nearly 27 million children in 97,000 schools at a cost to taxpayers of $7.3 billion.[42]

The school meal programs have long been caught in a no-win situation. On the one hand, advocates argue that all children—regardless of family income—should have access to "universal" free meals. On the other, reformers object to the notoriously poor taste, appearance, and nutritional quality of the meals served in many schools and to the waste and low participation rates (58% of eligible children) that occur as a consequence. Over time, with increasing recognition of the need to promote diets that would reduce the risk of chronic diseases as well as nutrient deficiencies, advocates have increasingly demanded improvements in the nutritional quality of school meals.[43]

In 1994 Congress required the USDA to bring school meals into compliance with the *Dietary Guidelines*, which meant that the agency would need to propose new rules to reduce the amounts of fat and sugar in school meals—and therefore in the use of foods that contain them. Table 22 lists the amounts of some food commodities used in school lunches in 1993 and indicates the anticipated effect of the proposals on food purchases and, by implication, on revenues to producers. Although the USDA tried to show that the changes would have minimal impact on commodity purchases (except butter, which, in any case, was supplied through government surpluses), the new rules meant that schools were likely to buy smaller amounts of meat, cheese, and frying potatoes, but larger amounts of poultry, fruit, vegetables, and nuts. Indeed, USDA economists estimated that the proposed changes would "displace" as

TABLE 22. Food commodities in the National School Lunch Program and the effects of converting menus to meet the *Dietary Guidelines*[47]

Commodity	Pounds Used, millions	Effect on purchases[a]
Butter	55	Eliminate; use surpluses
Cheese	135	Decrease
Chicken	245	Decrease, or increase low-fat[b]
Turkey	105	Decrease, or increase low-fat[b]
Beef	485	Decrease
Pork	280	Slight increase or no change
Potatoes	674	Decrease[c]
Vegetables	1,218	Increase
Fruits and juices	1,097	Increase
Peanuts	44	Increase

[a]These estimates assumed only minimal changes in existing menus or the use of less fat in food preparation. An alternative "scenario" required no changes in commodity purchases but called for foods lower in fat, sugar, and salt.

[b]Higher-fat preparations would decrease use of the commodity; lower-fat preparations would increase its use.

[c]Most potatoes are served fried; this proposal would decrease fat content.

much as 55 million pounds of butter, 90 million pounds of cheese, and 126 million pounds of beef annually.[44]

As might be expected, commodity groups likely to lose market share opposed the proposals, but so did school food service groups who thought them too difficult to achieve without increased funding. Advocacy groups also complained that the resulting meals were not nutritionally adequate for low-income children. The proposals were enacted over such protests but quickly amended to grant significant concessions to the food industry. For example, although federal surveys indicated that 50% of children's fat intake comes from whole milk,[2] the former rules required school lunches to offer it and the dairy industry was able to block any change in that rule. Soft drink producers also blocked proposed restrictions on sales from vending machines, and fast-food companies won the right to continue selling items that had to meet nutritional standards only if they were sold as part of reimbursable school meals.[45]

Legal loopholes permitting the sale of high-profit items encouraged large food service corporations to move into the school meal business. In 1994–1995, about 8% of schools participating in federal meal programs had contracted with companies such as Marriott, Aramark, and Daka to run their food service operations, a doubling since 1987–1988. By 1996 about 1,000 of the 15,000 school districts in the United States had arrangements with such companies. Marriott, for example, ran food service operations in 3,500 schools in 350 districts, and Aramark was in 330 districts with 2,300 schools. Districts favoring such contracts tend to be those with lower participation rates in the federal programs (and, therefore, lower reimbursements). They move their programs to management companies in the hope that costs will decline and revenues increase. Indeed, the companies have improved student satisfaction, reduced food waste, and saved money in some—but not all—schools.[46]

Management companies are required to serve meals that meet all federal nutrition standards, but their need to profit from the enterprise makes critics wonder whether nutritional quality is sacrificed to cost considerations, especially when the companies introduce food courts. Food courts are popular because they sell the heavily advertised fast foods that students consider "cool." The increasing use of brand-name fast foods by school meal programs adds to concerns about nutritional quality. In 1990–1991 only 2% of schools offered brand-name food items, but 13% did so in 1995–1996. In 1995 Pizza Hut sold products in about 5,000 schools, a 20% increase in four years, and Taco Bell served about 2,000 schools in 1995 (both companies are PepsiCo subsidiaries).[47] In 1997, 30% of public high schools sold fast foods from one or another of nine chains. At least one high school is actually licensed as a fast-food franchise; it pays royalties to the parent company and keeps the profits, which are said to be $100,000 annually. The philosophy of this type of franchising is quite straightforward: "You get the customers what they want, where they want it, and when they want it."[48] For the companies, meal programs offer an additional advantage beyond income: "We want to get the brand out in front of kids. . . . [I]f they have a good experience in the cafeteria, we hope they'll buy it on weekends."[49] Even schools that keep fast foods to a minimum occasionally hold "brand days" when they offer well-advertised foods in rotation with regular offerings, despite concerns about nutritional quality.

It is easy to understand why schools might welcome corporate takeovers. With a big company in charge, they no longer have to deal with the consequences of serving foods that kids don't like or with any other aspect of the complicated, messy, and expensive food service business. When management companies take over, the students return to the cafeteria, the operation stops losing money, and the workers keep their jobs and enjoy them more. Schools pay more for fast foods, but they also can add a higher markup and clear a larger profit. In the late 1990s, students might be charged 40 cents for a reduced-cost federal meal, but a fast-food meal could be sold for $2 to $3. The nutritional issues and the fact that only a few fast-food items meet the USDA's nutritional guidelines (and are not, therefore, eligible for federal reimbursement) were of little concern to some school food managers. As one manager explained, "I'm not here to address all the ills of society in our cafeteria."[49]

Because the higher costs of fast-food lunches put them out of the reach of low-income children, some schools do not permit them. The rare administrators of such schools are concerned about financial issues but even more concerned about social implications: "We'll try to keep the kids from buying your sodas, your chips, your candy and your shoes and jackets that can cause conflicts among children. We'll stand up for the children. They're not for sale."[33] Participating schools, however, deny that they are selling out to corporate interests and contributing to children's obsessions with brand names. "The kids need something to eat . . . and we want to make it as pleasant for them as we can."[49] In such discussions, nutrition hardly ever emerges as an issue.

MARKETING TO CHILDREN: IMPLICATIONS

Among the many disturbing aspects of food marketing to children is its barely disguised cynicism. Marketers will do whatever they can to encourage even the youngest children to ask for advertised products in the hope of enticing young people to become lifetime consumers. In doing so, food companies have enormously increased the burden on caretakers to control television viewing, resist requests for food purchases, and teach critical thinking to children whose analytical abilities are not yet developed. Most parents of my acquaintance tell me that they are constantly arguing with their children over food choices. Parents vary in the ways they deal with children's demands for advertised foods, but many prefer to reserve family arguments about setting limits for dealing with aspects of behavior that they consider more important. Food marketers depend on caretakers to be too busy to want to deny requests for fast-food meals or snack foods, whether or not consuming such foods inappropriately raises caloric intake.

Schools constitute a logical extension of this cynicism in action. The simplicity of contracting out food service, the potential financial rewards, and the ease of getting children to eat fast foods constitute much of the rationale for schools' having given up responsibility for what kids eat, whether or not they teach nutrition in the classroom. Thus the quality of school meals cuts to the heart of issues of social responsibility in our society.

Even when parents promote good dietary practices at home, they may be too busy to pay attention to what their children eat at school. Whether school officials like it or not, they have been delegated the responsibility for teaching children about appropriate food choices and setting an example in practice.

What is especially disturbing about the commercial takeover of school meals is that it is so unnecessary. For many years, it has been evident that schools are perfectly capable of producing nutritionally sound lunches that taste just fine and are enthusiastically consumed by students as well as teachers.[50] From my own observations, a healthy (in every sense of the word) school meals program requires just three elements: a committed food service director, a supportive principal, and interested parents. Children deserve a learning environment in which each of these elements is firmly in place. Once school meals get taken over by companies concerned about market share, profit, and stockholders, nutritional considerations inevitably are assigned a lower priority.

Nowhere are these kinds of issues brought into sharper focus than in the debates about the snacks and soft drinks served outside the school meal programs and, therefore, in competition with them. Of particular concern are exclusive contracts between companies that produce soft drinks—forbidden in school lunch programs—and school districts. Because so much money is involved, and because the nutritional implications are so profound, the next chapter focuses on the development and significance of soft drink "pouring rights" contracts.

CHAPTER 9

PUSHING SOFT DRINKS

"POURING RIGHTS"

I HAD NEVER HEARD OF "POURING RIGHTS" UNTIL LATE IN 1998 when I received a telephone call from a representative of the New York State School Food Service Association, inviting me to comment on that topic at its next meeting. She explained that the term referred to a recent development in food marketing: large payments from soft drink companies to school districts in return for the right to sell that company's products—and only those products—in every one of the district's schools. I was aware that colleges and universities had negotiated vending contracts with soft drink companies, and I knew that nutritionists and school food service directors had long been concerned that soft drinks and other top-of-the-*Pyramid* foods were sold in competition with the more nutritious foods provided by federally supported school meal programs. Although these contracts seemed to raise special concerns about their effects on children's diets, I had not heard debates about their health implications at professional meetings, nor had I heard discussions of their potential for fostering an environment that might actively promote soft drink consumption at the expense of more appropriate food choices. As I soon learned, the loudest protests against these contracts were coming instead from competing soft drink companies. These companies objected to restraints on *their* trade and on consumers' "freedom of choice" in the marketplace. As this chapter explains, soft drinks raise nutritional issues that place them at the forefront of present-day dietary concerns. For this reason, pouring-rights contracts illustrate some of the more disturbing consequences of "eat more" marketing imperatives.

WHY CARE ABOUT SOFT DRINKS?

For the purposes of this discussion, a soft drink is a soda made from car-bonated water, added sugar, and flavors. Diet sodas substitute artificial sweeteners for the sugar but are not consumed by children to any great extent. By this definition, a soft drink is the quintessential "junk food"—high in calories but low in nutrients. A 12-ounce can contains about 1.5 ounces of sugar and 160 calories, but so little else of nutritional value that the Center for Science in the Public Interest rightfully refers to soft drinks as "liquid candy."[1] From a nutritional standpoint, water or almost any other beverage is a better option. As shown in Table 23, a 12-ounce glass of orange juice—even that reconstituted from cans—provides substantial amounts of vitamin A, folic acid, potassium, and other vita-mins and minerals along with its sugar and calories, as does an equivalent amount of 1% low-fat milk. Worse, soft drinks are the single greatest source of caffeine in children's diets; a 12-ounce can of cola contains about 45 milligrams but the amounts in more potent soft drinks can exceed 100 milligrams—a level approaching that found in coffee.[2]

If soft drinks were occasional treats, no nutritionist would be the slightest bit concerned about them. But they are produced and con-sumed in vast quantities. As shown in Table 24, soft drinks have replaced milk in the diets of many American children as well as adults. School purchases reflect such trends. From 1985 to 1997, school districts decreased the amounts of milk they bought by nearly 30% and increased

TABLE 23. The nutrient composition of soft drinks, per 12-ounce serving, in comparison to orange juice and low-fat milk

	Coca-Cola	Pepsi	Orange Juice[a]	Low-Fat 1% Milk
Calories	154	160	168	153
Sugar, g	40	40	40	18
Vitamin A, IU	0	0	291	750
Vitamin C, mg	0	0	146	3
Folic acid, µg	0	0	164	18
Calcium, mg	0	0	33	450
Potassium, mg	0	0	711	352
Magnesium, mg	0	0	36	51
Phosphate, mg	54	55	60	353

SOURCE: J.A.T. Pennington, *Bowes & Church's Food Values of Portions Commonly Used*, 16th ed. (Philadelphia: J.B. Lippincott Co, 1994) IU = international units, g = grams, mg = milligrams, and µg = micrograms.

[a]Made from frozen concentrate.

TABLE 24. Beverages available, gallons per person per year,[a] in the U.S. food supply, 1970-1997

	Soft Drinks		Juice	Milk
	Diet	Regular		
1970	2.1	22.2	5.7	31.3
1975	3.2	25.0	6.9	29.5
1980	5.1	29.9	7.4	27.6
1985	7.1	28.7	8.3	26.7
1990	10.7	35.6	7.9	25.7
1995	11.8	39.8	8.7	24.3
1997	11.6	41.4	9.2	24.0

SOURCE: J. J. Putnam and J. E. Allshouse. *Food Consumption, Prices, and Expenditures*, 1970–1997. (Washington, DC: USDA, 1999).
[a]One gallon = 128 ounces. The annual supply of 12-ounce soft drinks in the United States in 1997 is equivalent to 442 regular drinks and 124 diet drinks per capita.

their purchases of carbonated sodas by an impressive 1,100%.[3] From 1970 to 1997, the production of sugar-sweetened sodas increased from 22 to 41 gallons per person per year. These volumes require translation; they mean that the yearly *per person* supply of 12-ounce soft drinks in the United States is equivalent to 442 regular and 124 diet drinks (total 556). On average, enough regular soda is produced to supply every American adult, child, and infant with 1.2 daily 12-ounce drinks, or nearly 200 calories per day from this source alone. The production of diet sodas also rose during this period, from 2 to nearly 12 gallons per person per year.

I must emphasize that these are *production* figures that for the most part overestimate consumption; they do not necessarily reflect the amounts people actually drink. Surveys of actual dietary intake, on the other hand, tend to underestimate consumption, but they too indicate increasing intake of soft drinks by children, and especially by teenagers. As shown in Table 25, children begin drinking these beverages very early in life and steadily increase the amounts they consume through adolescence and young adulthood. One national survey reported that children aged 2–17 increased their average daily intake of sugar-sweetened soft drinks from just under 7 ounces to nearly 10 ounces just from the early to mid-1990s.[4] USDA data from 1994–1995 indicated that girls aged 12–19 drank 12 ounces of regular soda (160 calories) on average, and boys drank 21 ounces (280 calories). Diet sodas barely enter into this picture; on an average day, girls were drinking an additional 2 ounces per day of diet soda, and boys 1 additional ounce.[5] For children at the higher levels

TABLE 25. Reported daily consumption of carbonated soft drinks, in ounces, and percent consumed as regular soda rather then diet soda, by age and sex, 1994–1995[5]

Age	Total	Males	Females
All ages	12 (75%)		
1–2	1.5 (100%)		
3–5	4 (88%)		
6–11		8 (88%)	7 (86%)
12–19		22 (95%)	14 (86%
20–29		29 (69%)	16 (75%)
30–39		18 (78%)	13 (62%)
40–49		14 (71%)	12 (50%)
50–59		11 (64%	9 (44%)
60–69		6 (67%)	5 (60%)
70 and older		4 (50%)	3 (67%)

of intake, soft drinks can contribute hundreds of empty calories. One analysis suggests that one-fourth of adolescents drink 26 or more ounces of soft drinks per day (a minimum of 325 calories); these heavy users take in 600 daily calories more from all sources than nonusers, and they drink much less milk and fruit juice.[6]

The extra calories from soft drinks replace calories from more nutritious foods and are more than sufficient to account for rising rates of obesity and related risk factors among American schoolchildren. Indeed, the relationship between soft drink consumption and body weight is so strong that researchers calculate that for *each* additional soda consumed, the risk of obesity increases 1.6 times.[7] Consumption of soft drinks is well known to contribute to tooth decay especially when it is sipped throughout the day, and adolescents who consume soft drinks display a risk of bone fractures three- to four-fold higher than those who do not.[8] Parents of teenagers tell me that their children deliberately use caffeine-containing soft drinks to stay awake in school. These parents are concerned about the effects of caffeine on their children's behavior and about the potential for "addiction," especially because companies deliberately market caffeinated sodas to children as young as age 9.[2]

MARKETING SOFT DRINKS TO KIDS

Carbonated soft drinks are big business in the United States; they generated more than $50 billion in annual sales just in this country in the late

1990s. Sales are dominated by two companies, Coca-Cola and PepsiCo, whose relentless competition for market share is known as the "Cola Wars." In 1999 Coca-Cola sold 160 brands of soft drinks in 200 countries for worldwide sales of nearly $19.8 billion, on which it earned $2.4 billion in profit, less than in previous years. In the United States alone, Coca-Cola held a 44% market share worth $7.5 billion in 1999 sales.[9] PepsiCo is distinctly number 2, holding a roughly 30% share of the U.S. market. Both companies were doing well, but the market for soft drinks grew so rapidly in the late 1990s—four times as fast as that for any other food or beverage—that all companies were seeking to expand.[10]

To expand its sales base, Coca-Cola's explicit strategy is to put a can of Coke within arm's reach of as many people in the world as possible. The company's most evident marketing strategy is advertising. Coca-Cola's global advertising budget exceeded $1.6 billion in the late 1990s. In 1999 the company spent $867 million for advertising in the United States alone—$174.4 million for Coca-Cola beverages, $68.4 million for Sprite, $41.4 million for Minute Maid, and $17.6 million for Powerade.[9] In addition, Coca-Cola places its logo where it is most likely to be seen by large numbers of people. The company has supported the Olympic games since 1928 and sponsors numerous local sporting events. Its foundation gives away more than $12 million annually for scholarships and educational programs particularly aimed at helping minorities and women.[11] Over the years, these combinations of activities have firmly established Coca-Cola as an American icon.

Because it is difficult to compete with icons, PepsiCo spends even more on advertising. Its total *domestic* advertising budget was $1.31 *billion* in 1999—$165 million for Pepsi beverages, $37.7 million for Mountain Dew, and most of the remainder for Doritos, Tostitos, Cheetos, and FritoLay snack foods. The huge costs of the Cola Wars, and increasing competition from sweetened juice drinks, have forced soft drink companies to seek new markets. Both companies, for example, aggressively target African-American and Hispanic consumers with "guerrilla-marketing tactics" to distribute products in urban neighborhoods.[9]

As part of this effort, soft drink companies seek consumers among younger and younger children. They approach this task quite systematically through the methods described in Chapter 8. Because the overall strategy is to establish brand loyalty as early in a consumer's life as possible, marketing efforts begin with the parents of young infants. Some soft drink companies go so far as to license their logos to makers of infant-feeding bottles. The manufacturer of the bottle shown in Figure 19

(Chapter 8) justifies its use in historical terms; he recalls that soft drink bottles were routinely used to feed milk or formula during the Depression. The company's public relations materials explain that the logo-labeled bottles are "designed to be fun and enjoyable . . . [such that] the positive effects of the bonding experience will be increased for both parent and child."[12] It may indeed seem like fun to feed infant formula to a baby in a Pepsi or other soft drink bottle, but studies show that parents who buy such bottles are much more likely to feed soft drinks to their children than those who do not buy them.[13] Moving up in age targets, PepsiCo states explicitly that its strategy is to expand soft drink consumption among children aged 6–11.[14]

POURING-RIGHTS CONTRACTS: THE LOGICAL NEXT STEP

An obvious way to reach this younger age group is through schools. In the early 1990s, having sold their products for many years through vending machines on school and college campuses, soft drink companies increased their efforts to reach the student market, at first focusing on colleges and universities but later turning to elementary, middle, and high schools. Pouring-rights contracts emerged as a particularly effective marketing strategy. These contracts usually involve large lump-sum payments to school districts and additional payments over 5 to 10 years in return for exclusive sales of one company's products in vending machines and at all school events. According to the General Accounting Office, about 200 school districts in the United States were participating in such agreements by 2000.[15]

For soft drink companies, a stable base of sales in schools is only the most evident benefit of pouring-rights contracts; the agreements also result in constant advertising through display of company logos on vending machines, cups, sportswear, brochures, and school buildings. In this manner, *all* students in the school, even those too young or too difficult to reach by conventional advertising methods, receive constant exposure to the logos and products. The use of a single brand is designed to create loyalty among young people who have a lifetime of soft drink purchases ahead of them.

Furthermore, the financial advantages to soft drink companies are substantial. For one thing, sugar and water are inexpensive ingredients. For another, the earlier contracts typically called for a charge of $1.00 for a drink purchased from vending machines, or $24 for a case of 12-ounce cans. In 1999, for example, the wholesale cost of a case was $4.99—half the retail price charged by my local Manhattan convenience store, but still leaving $19.01 to cover supply, labor, overhead, and funds donated to the school district. Even taking the large initial lump-sum payments and sales taxes into consideration, soft drink companies were unlikely to lose money on those deals.

I could not obtain reliable sales figures, but school food service directors laughed at the suggestion that students might consume an average of one case (24 12-ounce sodas) per year; they thought one soda *per day* was more realistic, at least for high school students. The quoted comments of a marketing consultant hired by 63 school systems to negotiate such contracts support this higher estimate.[16] An official of a school district in New York state told me that his students drink so many sodas that the biggest problem is keeping the vending machines stocked, and teachers of my acquaintance give similar accounts. If just *half* the students in a district of 10,000 students consumed one soda per day, gross sales should have been more than $25,000 per week. To such figures must be added sales of drinks at sports and community events. Yet in one New York state contract, the amount that Coca-Cola guaranteed to the district over the *entire* 10-year period came to a total of just $15 for each student. These comparative figures explain why a PepsiCo official described such contracts in 1998 as "a pretty high stakes business development," and a Coca-Cola official said that his company would "continue to be very aggressive and proactive in getting our share of the school business."[17]

It must be noted that more recent contracts deal with larger amounts of soda. By 2001, soft drink companies were routinely placing 20-ounce sodas in vending machines, and pricing them at $1.00–1.50. The larger sodas clearly encourage "eat more." They provide 250 calories each and are a better value (5.0–7.5 cents per ounce compared to 8.3 cents per ounce for the 12-ounce can). In addition, they are vended in portable screw-top plastic bottles that permit sipping throughout the day rather than downing in one gulp. This last feature particularly distresses dental groups alarmed about how the sugar and acid in soft drinks so easily dissolve tooth enamel.[8]

Nevertheless, it is not difficult to understand why administrators of financially strapped school districts would find these contracts irresistible. As the American population has aged, as the gap between rich and poor has widened, and as the proportion of low-income school children has increased, the tax base for public schools has consistently eroded. Schools barely manage to provide for basic educational needs, let alone activities that might appear as frills. It is easy to understand why school districts in Colorado, Ohio, and Texas would contract with Coca-Cola, Pepsi, or Dr Pepper for pouring rights worth millions of dollars, why larger school districts would auction their rights to the highest bidder, and why school districts would hire consultants to help them negotiate the best possible deals. The Center for Commercial-Free Public Education, an advocacy organization in Oakland, California, announced that nearly 200 school districts in 33 states had entered into such contracts by early 2000, a four-fold increase in just 2 years.[18] In the contract that set the standard, a 53-school Colorado district relinquished its Pepsi vending machines when it signed an $8 million, 10-year agreement with Coca-Cola that included cash bonuses for exceeding sales targets and incentives such as a new car for a senior with perfect attendance and high grades.[19]

Even smaller contracts might provide sports, arts, or computer facilities not otherwise available from state or local resources. The 1998 contract between the North Syracuse Central School District in New York state and Coca-Cola, for example, is a 10-year agreement that requires all 10 of the district's schools and preschool programs—with a combined population of 10,100 students—to use Coca-Cola products exclusively in all vending machines, and at all athletic contests, booster club activities, and school-sponsored community events. The contract calls for the company to install, maintain, and stock at least 135 vending machines in schools throughout the district, for which it guarantees a payment of $1.53 million—$900,000 upon signing and the rest distributed in annual installments of $70,000. The contract stipulates that the company is to pay additional commissions on purchases that exceed target amounts and is to donate 150 free cases of Fruitopia drinks, provide drinks to fund-raising groups for resale, and also include software, coupons, or other premiums for each vending machine placed.[20] With the assistance of a powerful state legislator, the district was able to leverage this contract to obtain state aid for a $6.5 million sports facility for the high school. These terms were considered so favorable that the New York State Education Department used them to develop a prototype contract. In 1999, the 18-school district in Albany, the state capital, negotiated a contract with Coca-Cola worth just $667,000 but only for five years, because the school board wanted to retain some flexibility in the marketplace.[21]

The most questionable aspect of these contracts is that they link returns to the companies and to the schools to amounts that students drink. At first glance, the financial advantages to the schools may seem impressive, especially because a significant part of the funding comes in an immediate lump sum that is not tied to sales. Most schools use the funds for sports facilities—scoreboards seem to be a particular favorite—but some buy furniture, sound systems, or computers; support student employment; and occasionally pay for scholarships. But because the contracts provide additional benefits for consumption levels that surpass quotas, school administrators are placed in the position of pushing soft drinks to faculty, staff, and students. Not that they necessarily mind doing so. In a letter widely circulated on the Internet and reprinted in a national magazine, a Colorado district administrator who signed himself "The Coke Dude" announced payments of $3,000, $15,000, and $25,000, respectively, to his elementary, middle, and high school principals—along with some ground rules:

> We must sell 70,000 cases of product . . . at least once during the first three years of the contract. If we reach this goal, your school allotments will be guaranteed for the next seven years. . . . If 35,439 staff and students buy one Coke product every other day for a school year, we will double the required quota. Here is how we can do it. . . . Allow students to purchase and consume vended products throughout the day. . . . I know this is "just one more thing from downtown," but the long-term benefits are worth it.[22]

Given the financial benefits of such contracts, it is understandable why many school administrators might resist thinking about, let alone dealing with, the agreements' ethical implications or health consequences. School officials justify the contracts as breaking no new ground: soft drink vending machines already exist in schools, soft drinks already pervade American culture, children are not forced to drink sodas, and contracts can be written to safeguard students' rights to drink other brands. From this standpoint, the benefits of soft drink contracts appear to outweigh any nutritional or other concerns they might raise. On this precise issue, the administrator of an Ohio school district with a new PepsiCo contract wrote,

> We have worried about whether we're forcing students to pay for their education through the purchase of soft drinks. In the end, though, we have decided that is not the case, because each student has the option to buy or not to buy. . . . Americans drink 13.15 billion gallons of carbonated drinks every year—which means somebody is making a lot of money. Why shouldn't schools get their share? In the end, everyone wins: the students, the schools, the community. And for once, even taxpayers get a break.[23]

Early in 1999, at the New York State conference I attended, the participating school food service directors expressed strong disagreement with such views. They were deeply troubled by a broad range of issues related to the length, exclusivity, and financial terms of the contracts, to the lack of adequate federal oversight of foods sold in competition with school meals, and to the widespread failure of schools to enforce even the weak rules that do exist. In particular, they worried about the consequences of pouring-rights contracts for the economic viability of school food service operations and the integrity of the schools' educational mission—all for good reason.

The typical pouring-rights contract period greatly exceeds the tenure of most school boards; boards cannot be held accountable when schools are locked into contracts that may prove unfavorable—financially or otherwise—in later years. Not surprisingly, the exclusivity feature frustrates competing soft drink companies that would like to sell *their* products to school children. A representative of one such company told conference participants that publicly supported schools have no right to dictate what students eat, when parents and children might want something else. Only in prisons, he said, are brands forced upon populations in this manner.

Indeed, the exclusivity of the contracts leads to situations so patently absurd as to elicit nationwide media attention. In one incident, a high school in Georgia suspended a senior student because he wore a shirt sporting a Pepsi logo to a "Coke Day" rally sponsored by the student government. To avoid such embarrassing attention, New York State Education Department contracts include a noteworthy clause that explicitly permits students, employees, and guests to drink and wear products that bear competing logos on school grounds.[20]

A critical question is whether the contracts encourage greater consumption of soft drinks. People who track trends in pouring-rights contracts think that is exactly what they do: "What we have seen in just about every exclusive contract around the country is a resulting increase in the amount of soda consumed by students. . . . There's almost always an increase in the number of vending machines, and they're put into schools that previously didn't have them. . . . They're also putting machines in schools with younger children."[24] If children are drinking soft drinks, they are less likely to be eating more nutritious foods, especially those offered in school meal programs. This brings us to the issue of competition with school meals. As we shall see, pouring-rights contracts affect federal regulations for competitive foods, and we must now turn to a discussion of this otherwise obscure area of federal policy.

COMPETING FOR STUDENTS' COINS AND APPETITES

Soft drinks have long concerned federal regulators. In 1914, for example, Harvey Wiley, then head of the forerunner of today's Food and Drug Administration, said of such products, "While the miscellaneous bottled soft drinks on the market with the exception of those bearing habit-forming drugs, such as Coca-Cola (caffeine), cannot be said to be absolutely injurious, they represent to my mind second grade products of miscellaneous composition which does not recommend them for consumption by the young. . . . Why give your child [these] . . . when you can always obtain . . . pure fruit juices obtained direct from the lime, the berry, the orange or lemon?"[25]

Sales of soft drinks in schools, however, are permitted as a result of amendments to the Child Nutrition Act of 1966, which in turn amended provisions of the National School Lunch Act of 1946. As outlined in Table 26, the history of regulations dealing with sales of soft drinks and other "junk foods" (graciously defined by Congress as "foods of minimal nutritional value") is part of a 50-year saga of nearly annual tinkering with the rules that govern the school lunch and school breakfast programs. The regulations for sales of soft drinks and other "competitive" foods—foods that children might buy instead of federally supported meals in the school cafeteria—constitute a minuscule part of the saga, but they illustrate the way commercial interests dominate congressional decisions about matters that affect the health of children.

For more than 30 years, in efforts to protect the nutritional and economic integrity of federally subsidized school meal programs, groups such as school food service officials, nutritionists, and advocates for children's health sought regulations to restrict sales of competitive foods in public schools. For decades, soft drink companies—often joined by principals, school boards, and state education departments—opposed any "time-and-place" restrictions on when or where soft drinks and other competitive foods might be sold. The results of this historical conflict readily reveal why advocates view the current regulations as promoting the commercial interests of soft drink companies far more than they do children's health.

By the late 1960s, coin-operated vending machines selling soft drinks and snacks were already well established in schools. Parents, school officials, health authorities, and even Congress could recognize as "an obvious fact of life" that sales of such foods directly competed with federally supported meal programs "for the children's coins and appetites."[26]

TABLE 26. Selected events in the history of regulations governing sales of soft drinks and other competitive foods of "minimal nutritional value" in elementary and secondary schools

1946	National School Lunch Act passed to promote use of surplus agricultural commodities in school meals as a way to improve the nutritional status of low-income children.
1966	Child Nutrition Act requires USDA to develop regulations governing nutritional aspects of school meal programs.
1970	Amendments to 1966 act ban sales of competitive foods in or near school cafeterias during mealtimes but allow individual foods served in school meals to be sold competitively at other times and places, in effect restricting only soft drinks and candies.
1972	Amendments permit sales of competitive foods during mealtimes if proceeds benefit schools or school groups, and transfer authority to regulate competitive foods from USDA to state and local boards of education.
1977	Amendments restore USDA's authority to regulate competitive foods.
1978	USDA proposes rules restricting sales of foods of "minimal nutritional value"—soft drinks, water ices, chewing gum, certain candies—from the beginning of the school day until after the last lunch period; withdraws proposal in response to comments.
1979	USDA again proposes rules; PepsiCo organizes letter-writing campaign opposing USDA authority.
1980	USDA issues final rules similar to those proposed in 1978. National Soft Drink Association sues to overturn regulations; loses, appeals, and wins in 1983.

Congress, therefore, asked the USDA secretary "to take a hard look at some of the competition to the balanced meal offered within schools . . . [at] the availability of candy bars, soft drinks and a snack line in the school cafeterias."[27] In 1970 Congress passed amendments that allowed the USDA to block sales of competitive foods at the same time and place as school meals were offered (that is, in the school cafeteria during lunch periods) but permitted any food *ever* served as part of a school lunch to be sold at *other* times and places. This arcane distinction meant, for example, that cake could be sold but soft drinks could not.[28]

As a result of these rules, soft drink companies lost revenue, but so did the schools. To protect the ongoing income they derived from sales of snack foods, school officials joined soft drink companies in pressuring Congress to allow competitive foods to be sold at *any* time and place (again, this meant in the cafeteria during lunch periods), provided that the proceeds went to the schools or to approved student organizations. They also induced Congress to remove the USDA's authority to regulate

TABLE 26. *(continued)*

1983	U.S. Appeals Court rules that USDA cannot impose "time-and-place" restrictions on sales of competitive foods.
1985	USDA revises rules; prohibits sales of competitive foods of minimal nutritional value only during lunch periods in cafeterias; permits such sales at all other times and places, with no restrictions on allocation of revenues.
1990	Citizens Commission on School Nutrition recommends restrictions on availability of non-nutritious foods in schools.
1991	American Dietetic Association and American School Food Service Association recommend restricting or banning sales of competitive foods in schools.
1994	Senate introduces bill to restrict or ban school sales of soft drinks and other foods of minimal nutritional value. Congress reaffirms 1985 rules but permits USDA to propose "model language" recommending time-and-place restrictions on sales in elementary schools.
1995	Center for Science in the Public Interest (CSPI) petitions USDA to require competitive foods to meet standards for good nutrition.
1998	CSPI publishes *Liquid Candy: How Soft Drinks Are Harming Americans' Health*; urges schools to stop selling soft drinks.
1999	USDA places soft drinks at the "eat less" tip of its *Food Guide Pyramid* for children aged 2–6.
2000	Public Health Service calls for an improvement in the dietary quality of meals and snacks served in schools. Text of *Dietary Guidelines* suggests reducing intake of added sugars by limiting use of soft drinks. General Accounting Office issues report on school commercialism.

sales of competitive foods and, instead, to delegate decisions about such sales to state and local boards of education. These decisions effectively deregulated competitive foods, leading critics to charge that "profit had triumphed over nutrition."[26] After 1972, sales from vending machines and other competing venues increased in many schools. In 1977, during the more liberal Carter administration, Congress viewed sales of competitive foods as an abuse of the school meal programs and restored the USDA's regulatory authority. Yet in doing so, Congress demanded and received assurances from the USDA that the agency would not actually *ban* competitive foods but would only restrict sales of soft drinks and other foods of minimal nutritional value that "did not make a positive contribution to children's diets."[29]

With its newly regained authority, the USDA then attempted to ban sales of foods of minimal nutritional value just until after the end of the last lunch period. Because this plan provoked a deluge of angry public comments, the USDA withdrew it and solicited additional input. Some

4,200 comments were submitted in response, filling a 15,000-page record. In 1979 the USDA again proposed this idea, this time defining foods of minimal nutritional value as those containing less than 5% of the Recommended Dietary Allowances for eight nutrients (protein, vitamin A, ascorbic acid, niacin, riboflavin, thiamin, calcium, and iron) per 100 calories or per serving. This definition meant that the restrictions would apply only to carbonated soft drinks, water ices, certain candies, and chewing gum. Even this revised proposal elicited more than 3,000 comments, of which 562 could be traced to a PepsiCo directive to its employees suggesting that they tell the USDA that its health objectives would be better achieved through nutrition education. Despite these pressures, the USDA held firm; its 1980 final rules continued to ban vending of soft drinks until the end of the school lunch period.[30]

In the early 1980s, encouraged by the election of a more conservative administration, soft drink producers tried a more aggressive tactic. They took the USDA to court, charging that its regulations were "arbitrary, capricious, and an abuse of discretion . . . and in excess of statutory jurisdiction." The District Court dismissed the complaint, stating that "it is an obvious fact of life that a . . . vending machine, no matter where located, can act as a magnet for any child who inclines to the non-nutritious."[26] Soft drink producers appealed the decision and won. The Appeals Court ruled that the intent of Congress was simply to control sales of "junk foods" during meal service and that the USDA had no right to otherwise restrict the time and place of sales of competitive foods—even those of minimal nutritional value. The court did allow one exception: Competitive foods other than those of minimal nutritional value could be sold in the cafeteria during meal service if the proceeds went to approved student groups. In practice, this decision meant that the USDA could prohibit the selling of soft drinks only in the cafeteria during meal service periods and had to allow sales of sodas at any other time or place.[31]

As might be expected, this ruling stimulated sales of competitive foods (with the equally predictable result that school food service operations lost revenue) leading advocacy groups to renew their efforts to restrict such sales. They encouraged Senator Patrick Leahy (Dem-VT), then chair of the Senate Agriculture Committee, to introduce a bill to reinstate a complete ban on sales of soft drinks and other competitive foods of minimal nutritional value until the end of the last lunch period. Predictably, Coca-Cola opposed the bill and organized a letter-writing campaign among school principals, superintendents, and coaches who feared losing revenues generated by vending machines. The *New York Times* quoted

Senator Leahy as complaining that "the company puts profit ahead of children's health. . . . [K]ids have no money, no political clout, no political action committees. . . . If Coke wins, children lose."[32] In hearings on his bill, the senator charged that "some local officials were being misled by Coca-Cola or other bottlers into believing that they had to allow soda machines in their schools." Congress, he said, should put the health of children above corporate profits.[33]

According to the *New York Times*, a spokesman for Coca-Cola argued that his company makes "no nutritional claims for soft drinks . . . but they can be part of a balanced diet. Our strategy is ubiquity. We want to put soft drinks within arm's reach of desire . . . [and] schools are one channel we want to make them available in." A lobbyist for the soft drink industry explained to a reporter, "You have no evidence that the consumption of soft drinks is in any way harmful."[34] This same lobbyist told a Senate committee, "We question whether there is a need for 'Big Brother' in the form of USDA injecting itself into . . . decisions when it comes to refreshment choices."[33] School principals also opposed the bill on the grounds that it would interfere with their ability to bring in revenue for discretionary activities.

Such objections convinced Congress to retain the permissive regulations. In discussions of amendments to the School Lunch Act passed in 1994, a Senate committee suggested that the USDA should instead develop "model language" to restrict sales of soft drinks and other such foods in *elementary* schools before the end of the last lunch period, but it left the decision about whether to adopt that language to the discretion of state and local school authorities. Congress advised the USDA to send a letter to secondary schools reminding them that federal laws restricted profit-making sales of soft drinks in food service areas during lunch periods.[35] When advocacy groups called on the USDA to impose tighter controls on vended and competitive foods, officials explained that Congress had given the agency no authority to regulate the sale of foods *outside* the food service area.[36]

As had been the case since 1972, the 1994 amendments explicitly invited state and local school authorities to impose more stringent restrictions on sales of competitive foods, and several have done so. New York State regulations enacted in 1987, for example, follow the earlier, more restrictive USDA proposals: "From the beginning of the school day until the end of the last scheduled meal period, no sweetened soda water, no chewing gum, no candy including hard candy, jellies, gums, marshmallow candies, fondant, licorice, spun candy and candy coated popcorn, and no water ices except those which contain fruit or fruit juices, shall be sold in any public school within the state."[37]

Although reliable data on compliance are difficult to obtain, advocates, teachers, and school officials tell me that state and federal rules are routinely ignored. To begin with, soft drink companies circumvent the rules by donating sodas to schools for free distribution during school meal periods, a development that prompted Senator Leahy to introduce additional legislation to stop such practices: "Nutrition doesn't go better with Coke or Pepsi at lunchtime . . . [T]his is a loophole—big enough to drive a truck through—that hurts our children . . . not unlike the old days when the tobacco companies would hand out free cigarettes to kids."[38] Furthermore, the companies developed sweetened fruit "drinks" that can be sold on lunch lines; these contain just barely enough juice (5%) to get around being defined as a food of minimal nutritional value.

Some evidence, limited though it may be, suggests the ubiquity of rule breaking. A survey of 55 Minnesota high schools found that 95% of the schools that had vending machines left them unlocked and thus accessible during some school hours, 29% left them unlocked all day, and 15% left them open during the lunch period—despite state regulations that discourage sales of soft drinks during lunch periods. The same survey also found that 60% of the vending machines were located in cafeterias and that another 33% were near the cafeterias.[39] A nationwide survey by the General Accounting Office found that 20% of U.S. schools gave students access to vended snacks and drinks during lunch periods and that two-thirds allowed other competitive foods to be sold during lunchtimes.[40] A more recent USDA survey reported that about one-fourth of all schools had vending machines located in or near the cafeteria.[41] If nothing else, these studies prove that opportunities for violating regulations are readily available.

On this basis, advocates in New York City organized a class-action suit against the board of education, the chancellor of education, and five school principals to enforce a universally ignored city regulation that flatly prohibits "the sale of non-nutritious food, either directly or through vending machines" in public schools. Noting that the money for competitive junk foods in schools "comes from the poorest section of New York City—public school parents—who can least afford it," the suit argued that officials are obligated to comply with existing laws.[42] After a two-year delay, the court ruled that the Board of Education must comply with the law and stop selling foods of minimal nutritional value until after the last lunch period. If schools wanted to sell foods such as sweetened soft drinks during lunch periods, they would have to ask the head of the city's school food service operations for permission. Whether schools will comply with these directives, which carry no penalties, remains to be seen.

UNDERMINING NUTRITIONAL GOALS

Advocates maintain that if schools are doing their job properly, school meals should contribute to healthful eating habits, should be fully integrated into educational activities, and should receive adequate financial support. They believe such purposes would be best served if food service departments managed sales of all food in schools, rather than administrators or sports officials for whom nutrition and health are not necessarily high priorities. Advocates especially fear that competitive foods jeopardize the economic viability of school meal programs, because these programs are expected to be self-supporting with federal reimbursements and must have adequate sales volume to survive. The short time devoted to lunch periods in many schools also discourages students from eating full meals and encourages the purchase of competitive foods that can be eaten on the run.

This combination of circumstances has forced school food service departments to put substantial effort into recruiting participants through development of in-house food brands, restaurant-type menus, food courts, food carts, and new food items that can be purchased separately from meals. They also are forced to seek ways to improve the image of school meals, stimulate demand for more healthful food choices, and involve students in decisions about how to make school meals more appealing. All of these actions make excellent sense from a business standpoint, but only some of them reinforce the schools' educational mission.[43] The dilemma is best illustrated by beverage purchases. In the 1990s, milk and other dairy products accounted for nearly one-fourth of the food costs incurred by schools. Perhaps to reduce such costs, school purchases of sweetened fruit drinks increased by 180%. Fruit drinks cost less than milk, and although they are only marginally more nutritious than sodas, they may be served on lunch lines under the regulations. Using them saves money for the schools.[3]

That soft drink companies deliberately compete with school meals seems quite evident from testimony at congressional hearings. During hearings for the 1994 School Lunch amendments, for example, a high school food service director testified that when Coca-Cola distributed free 20-ounce bottles of soda, participation in the lunch program declined by half; children drank soda instead. She reported that Coca-Cola had provided her school with cash incentives, bicycles, computers, and catered events and that it would be difficult for her principal to give up such perquisites. She concluded, "Without government regulations, Coca-Cola will always win."[33] Soft drink industry lobbyists, however, consistently argue that no evidence links the sale of their products to poor nutrition, to any other health problems, or to low participation rates in school lunch programs. Others, however, state frankly that the preferred placement for vending machines is near the cafeteria, just where the Minnesota survey found them to be.

As a side issue, it should be noted that pouring-rights contracts have economic implications beyond school meal service. Because they affect the sales of milk, the contracts also affect the livelihood of community dairy farmers. Milk used to be the only beverage provided to school-children. Once sodas were permitted, milk sales declined. As shown in Table 24, this change has contributed to the overall decline in the annual production of milk in the United States from 31 gallons per capita in 1970 to 24 gallons in 1997.

From its inception, the purpose of the school lunch program was to improve the nutritional status of children, while providing an outlet for surplus agricultural commodities. Figuring out how to use school meals to promote nutritional goals has not been easy, however, and has occupied Congress since 1966. In implementing the provisions of the 1994 School Lunch amendments, the USDA accepted improved nutrition as a goal when it recognized that school meals could establish "childhood eating patterns that influence lifelong habits" and specified reductions in the fat, sugar, and salt content of the lunches to bring them into compliance with federal *Dietary Guidelines*.[44]

In doing so, the school meal programs also were brought into compliance with Public Health Service 10-year plans to improve the health of Americans. Since 1980, the plans have called for information about healthful dietary patterns to be included as part of comprehensive health education curricula in elementary, junior high, and senior high schools. Part of the reason for paying attention to school nutrition education is that it has been demonstrably effective, especially when supported by meals served in school cafeterias. Participants in school meal programs have been shown to consume better diets than nonparticipants. If students replace school meals with competitive foods of minimal nutritional value, the quality of their diets can be expected to deteriorate.[45]

One goal of the 10-year plan released in 2000 is to increase the percentage of children and adolescents aged 6 to 19 years whose intake of meals and snacks at schools contributes appropriate proportions of nutrients and calories. The plan specifically recognizes that students today have "increased food options" at school. Thus, creating an environment supportive of healthful diets would help schools promote health as well as learning readiness.[46] Because this goal applies to foods served in snack bars, school stores, and vending machines, improving the nutritional quality of competitive foods has now been incorporated as a formal component of national nutrition policy. It is as yet uncertain whether and how government agencies will implement this policy.

PRESERVING "THAT BRIEF SHINING OASIS"

The attention that soft drink companies have recently focused on children in grades K–12 can be seen as part of the increasing intrusiveness of commercial interests into American schools. Companies routinely market food products to children in and out of school; these activities are now so common as to be taken for granted and accepted with minimal debate. The companies—and the school officials who contract with them—implicitly assume that soft drinks are appropriate fare for school-age children, rather than milk, juice, or water, any of which would be a better nutritional choice.

Here too, the level of cynicism is especially disturbing. What are we to make of the comments of a PepsiCo official who casually mentions that "marketing to the 8- to 12-year-old set is a priority," as though it were unquestionably appropriate for a soft drink company to direct sales efforts to such young children? [14] And how are we to take the following comment attributed to a consultant who helps schools obtain contracts? He says that pouring-rights contracts make schools more realistic for children: "If you have no advertising in schools at all, it doesn't give our young people an accurate picture of our society."[16]

Pouring-rights agreements clearly teach students that school officials are willing to compromise nutritional principles for financial reasons, even when the linking of payments to higher-consumption goals puts them in the position of advocates for soft drink consumption. When a school administrator tells a reporter that "the nutrition aspect is important, but I'm ambivalent about it," he reveals his priorities; such ambivalence contributes to student attitudes that nutrition and health are not important concerns.[47] All too rare is the school administrator who is brave enough to say, "Matters involving money properly stop at the schoolhouse door" or to insist that "education and marketing are like oil and water."[48] All too few newspapers are willing to admit discomfort with the deals schools make with soda companies, and to argue that "the more things in a school that are for sale . . . the less the school can claim to offer that brief shining oasis" from the rampant commercialism aimed at children everywhere else.[49]

The well-financed promotion in schools of soft drinks and other foods of poor nutritional quality directly undermines federal efforts to improve the dietary intake of children and to reduce rates of childhood obesity. Even though colleges (and now entire cities, such as Huntington Beach, California) have become advertising vehicles for soft drink companies, elementary and secondary school students surely deserve some protection against commercial interests that contribute to poor nutrition outside of school, as well as within.

Soft drinks, of course, constitute just one example of industry marketing to children, but the health effects of this product are becoming increasingly well documented. Thus a good starting place for nutrition advocacy for children is to encourage consumption of water, juices, and low-fat milk but to discourage consumption of sodas and sweetened fruit drinks, except as occasional desserts. In what must be considered a courageous move in this direction, the USDA braved the wrath of the soft drink industry when it pictured "soda pop" at the tip of its 1999 *Food Guide Pyramid* for children aged 2–6.[50]

Anticommercialism advocates urge students to identify and resist school marketing, communities and states to require firm adherence to existing regulations, and school boards to disallow exclusivity agreements and pouring-rights contracts altogether. By the end of 2000, more than 30 school districts in California, Tennessee, and Wisconsin, for example, had refused such deals after protests by parents, students, and school officials. Philadelphia refused an offer from Coca-Cola for $43 million over a 10-year period, and Michigan turned down a contract that would have covered 110 school districts encompassing nearly half a million students.[18] At the national level, advocates are lobbying for federal regulations to restrict sales of competitive foods in general, and those of minimal nutritional value in particular, and to expand the definition of such foods to include the new "juice" products and other such foods. Others are considering a range of pricing, tax, and other "environmental" strategies to improve the diets of schoolchildren, similar to those that I and others have proposed to address current trends in obesity.[51]

By 2001, such advocacy was beginning to have an effect. Days before the inauguration of President George W. Bush, the USDA asked Congress to "strengthen the statutory language to ensure that all foods sold or served anywhere in the school during the school day meet nutrition standards."[52] Soon after, Senator Leahy introduced a new bill to require the USDA to ban or limit the sale of soft drinks and other competitive "junk foods" before the end of the lunch period on the basis that "schoolchildren are a captive market for soda vendors . . . [and] our kids pay the price when we give soft drink companies free reign to market their products in school."[53] In Minnesota, a state senator introduced a bill to ban sales of soda pop while school is in session, but it "failed in the committee BIG TIME" under pressure from lobbyists for soft drink companies and school boards.[54]

Despite such victories, but surely in response to the threat of legal intervention, Coca-Cola announced that it would no longer require exclusivity in school contracts. Advocates, however, viewed this "retreat" as a corporate decision that would enable the company to remain in schools, and business analysts thought it would have little financial effect on the company, since school beverage sales "only" accounted for 1% of its $20 billion in annual revenue.[55]

Although pouring-rights contracts are only one component of an arsenal of food company marketing techniques, issues related to societal inequities are central to the significance of these contracts as a public health concern. Congressional reluctance to favor children's health above the rights of soft drink producers is a direct result of election laws that require legislators to obtain corporate funding for their campaigns. Like most corporations, soft drink companies donate funds to local and national candidates. More rational campaign financing laws might permit Congress to take positions based on public good rather than private greed.

Similarly, if American public schools were funded adequately, the blatant commercialism inherent in pouring-rights contracts and other marketing efforts in schools would almost certainly be subjected to debate, and departments of education, school boards, principals, and coaches would be less likely to enter into such agreements without far more public discussion than now occurs. As one San Francisco school board official explained, "Education cannot be funded by potato chip contracts. . . . [C]ome back and talk to me about nothing being wrong with these contracts when there are Coca-Cola banners in the House of Representatives and members of the U.S. Senate can only have a TV set if they watch Channel One for 15 minutes a day."[56] Pouring-rights contracts may solve immediate problems of school funding, but their social cost is high, not least because they erode efforts to establish adequate federal, state, and local funding for public education. These contracts, therefore, point to the need for much greater public attention to overall commercial pressures on children and for a much greater level of critical scrutiny of such pressures by school officials, legislators, health professionals, and the public.

In these chapters, I have focused on the ways in which food companies use advertising and marketing methods to expand their base of consumers by targeting young people. In the next section, we move on to an even more powerful strategy: resistance to regulation. Part IV examines the ways in which food companies—in this case, those that sell dietary supplements—were able to obtain almost complete deregulation of their products and, in the process, weaken the ability of the Food and Drug Administration to regulate foods, as well.

PART FOUR

DEREGULATING DIETARY SUPPLEMENTS

WE NOW TURN TO A NEW TOPIC: HOW A RELATIVELY MINOR segment of the food industry—the makers and sellers of dietary supplements—convinced the public and Congress that its products did not need to be regulated according to the strict standards applied to conventional foods or to drugs. Supplement makers do not need to demonstrate that their products are safe and effective before selling them. What is left of supplement regulation is based on the assumption that supplements are safe until proved otherwise, and Congress places the burden of responsibility on the beleaguered Food and Drug Administration (FDA) to do such proving. The industry also achieved a regulatory system that holds claims for the efficacy of supplements—their ability to perform as advertised on the label—to a remarkably low standard.

The industry-driven deregulation of supplements would not concern us so much if its consequences were less profound. Most supplements, after all, do appear safe. Their cost is low compared to that of medications, and most people who take supplements can afford to buy them.[1] What *is* of concern is how little we know about the thousands of products available. Research on supplements other than vitamins and minerals is in its infancy, and few products have been tested adequately for safety or health benefits. While investigations are in progress, the supplement industry "jumps the data," makes extravagant claims for the ability of its products to prevent or treat disease, demands less and less federal control over its practices, and goes to court to enforce those demands. The makers of conventional foods, watching sales of supplements increase at a greater rate than they themselves can achieve, also are demanding—and getting—the same kinds of loose regulations for foods. It is difficult to believe that this situation is in the best interest of public health.

Although the supplement industry has always couched its political efforts in terms of health benefits or "freedom to choose," its more immediate rationale was and is economic. Supplement makers do not want to have to conduct lengthy, expensive clinical trials to prove that their products are safe or useful. They would like blanket permission to market supplements as promoting whatever health benefits seem convenient. Given a choice between following rules that apply to foods and following rules that apply to drugs, they prefer the more favorable. They like regulations that assume supplements are safe. They want to be able to make the kinds of health claims permitted for prescription drugs without having to conduct clinical trials to prove that supplements actually meet those claims. Before the mid-1990s, however, the laws required the FDA to make supplements follow the rules either for foods or for drugs. As we shall see, in pressing Congress to exempt supplements from either set of rules, the industry undermined the FDA's regulatory authority over foods and drugs as well as over supplements, to the great detriment of the public.

In the context of this discussion, supplements are products taken in addition to food, and for some health purpose, in the form of pills or potions. They include the common nutritional supplements—vitamins, minerals, and other essential nutrients—as well as herbs and diet supplements. Although more than 15,000 such products are sold in the United States, the supplement industry makes up only a small fraction of the food industry as a whole; it accounts for no more than 3% of total U.S. food sales. The use of supplements is growing rapidly, however, and at least half of the adult population take one or more on a regular basis in the belief that the products will improve health, well-being, strength, or endurance, will compensate for poor dietary habits, or will prevent or treat one or another kind of illness.[2] Because so many people take supplements, and because people who take supplements tend to be better educated and better off economically then non-takers, they constitute a powerful political force in support of the industry. In these chapters, we will see how supplement makers used this force in their own self-interest.

It seems reasonable to expect that everyone would be concerned about whether supplements are safe, whether they do what they claim to do, and whether the benefit of taking them outweighs any financial or health risks they might induce. When it comes to supplements, however, the world is divided into two broad and sometimes overlapping categories: people who believe that supplements are useless unless demonstrated to be effective through standard methods of scientific proof ("science-based") and those who believe that supplements are beneficial whether or not their benefits can be scientifically proved ("belief-based," for want of a better term). We shall see in these chapters how the supplement industry exploited this dichotomy to escape testing requirements and to gain the ability to suggest claims for benefits, whether or not such claims could be substantiated according to accepted standards of scientific proof.

Today, marketers of supplements are permitted to make practically any claim they want for the health benefits of their products, they may vary the ingredient contents of their products with impunity. They do not have to remove potentially harmful products from the market unless taken to court by the FDA, and they do not have to prove that their products bestow the benefits claimed for them. This remarkable situation is the result of the industry's persistence and skill in generating public pressure on Congress to restrict the FDA's regulatory mission. These chapters explain how such a small segment of the food industry was able to achieve this political coup. Chapter 10 lays the groundwork by explaining how federal food and drug regulations applied to dietary supplements and how the food industry as a whole worked to undermine regulations that restricted the ability of companies to claim health benefits for their products. Chapter 11 describes how Congress came to require the FDA to approve health claims for conventional foods and supplements and then increasingly passed laws relaxing restrictions on those claims. Chapter 12 discusses the implications of supplement deregulation for the food industry and for public health.

CHAPTER 10

SCIENCE VERSUS SUPPLEMENTS

"A GULF OF MUTUAL INCOMPREHENSION"

EARLY IN 1999 I TOOK A EUROPEAN VISITOR, NEWLY APPOINTED as director of his country's equivalent to our Food and Drug Administration (FDA), on a field trip to my local health food store. I thought that he might be interested in the vast array of dietary supplements and the benefits claimed for them, as indeed he was. His home agency demanded proof that supplements were safe and effective before permitting them to be sold as health remedies, and his country (like others in Europe) does not permit misleading health claims on product labels or in advertisements.[1]

Like most health food stores, the ones in my neighborhood offer thousands of products. Many of them are the familiar nutritional supplements—vitamins and minerals—that have been studied for years and produce effects on health that are well documented by research published in respected scientific journals. But most of the products are herbs, botanicals, food extracts, enzymes, and diet or fitness formulas that have barely been investigated, if at all. Some may have been used as traditional remedies for millennia, but almost none has been studied with anything like the scientific precision needed to define active ingredients, biological effects, safe levels of intake, or the ability to alleviate symptoms of illness.

Despite the paucity of research, health food stores routinely shelve supplements as remedies for specific conditions: allergies, bone health, colds, toxins, fatigue, heart health, immune function, women's health, or just the generic "feel good." Even a casual glance explains why the products might trouble a government official responsible for food safety and consumer protection. Their names alone—Blood Builders, Brute

Strength, CholesAid, Estra-Prime, Herbal Laxative, Joint Fuel, Liver Support, Neuro-Mind, Osteo-Cal, Prosta-Care, RxMemory, Sound Asleep, Stress Formula—imply function. The label of a product that we picked at random from the "immune support" shelf stated that it contained black elderberry extract, echinacea, zinc, propolis, and vitamin C. The brochure for the product explained that these ingredients are all "well documented" for their health-promoting benefits, a statement guaranteed to raise questions in the mind of even a moderately skeptical health official.

Of course, the nutrients in this product (zinc and vitamin C) should promote immune function; *all* essential vitamins and minerals are required for a healthy immune system, and these two have received more attention than most. But what about black elderberry, echinacea, and propolis? To help answer this question, the store conveniently provides a desk copy of *Prescription for Nutritional Healing*, a book that matches hundreds of supplements with the conditions they are supposed to alleviate.[2] The book describes echinacea as "anti-inflammatory and antiviral" but provides no citations to research studies that might support that role. A somewhat better-researched work, the *Physicians' Desk Reference for Herbal Medicines*, explains that black elder is a folk medicine used for colds, coughs, and fevers but warns that "proof of efficacy is not available."[3]

On balance, the ingredients in this particular immune supplement seemed unlikely to be harmful, but beyond the sources of information available in the store, there is no way to know whether the product truly contains the ingredients listed on its label, whether the ingredients are active or safe, or whether the product performs as advertised. No government agency has approved or evaluated the contents, let alone determined that they will work. As explained in the brochure that accompanied the product, the claim for health benefit "has not been evaluated by the FDA, and the product is not intended to diagnose, treat, cure, or prevent any disease."

In contrast to the protection afforded European consumers, Americans get little or no help from government in evaluating dietary supplements. The present anarchy in the dietary supplement marketplace is the result of decades of political action by the makers of these products, culminating in the industry's crowning achievement—the Dietary Supplement Health and Education Act of 1994, an act invariably referred to as DSHEA (pronounced "D'Shay"). As we shall see, DSHEA gave the industry everything it wanted and then some; it deregulated dietary supplements and undermined the FDA's regulatory authority over supplements and conventional foods as well. After DSHEA, the FDA could no longer take the kind of responsibility for ensuring the accuracy of information on product labels that consumers had come to expect.

DSHEA, in turn, must be understood as an attempt by Congress to balance two sets of competing priorities: on the one hand, the rights of consumers to buy products perceived as harmless (whether or not they actually do good) and, on the other hand, the responsibilities of federal regulatory agencies and the concerns of scientists and consumer advocates about the physical and economic harm that supplements might cause. This balancing act has a long and complicated history involving multiple agencies and organizations. Running through this history is a conflict between two modes of judgment about supplements and about more general health issues—one based on personal belief systems and one based on scientific belief systems. Between these viewpoints lies the great "gulf of mutual incomprehension" that the writer and scientist C. P. Snow described decades ago in his classic lecture on *Two Cultures*.[4] For consumers, the result is confusion, misinformation, and lack of protection against health claims that at best are unwarranted and at worst are false.

This chapter begins with an introduction to DSHEA as a major departure from the way the FDA has regulated foods, drugs, and supplements. It next explores differences in the ways in which scientists and nonscientists decide whether a supplement is worth taking, to illustrate how the gap between the two kinds of belief systems is expressed. It then explains how the supplement industry was able to exploit the differences between these belief systems to achieve its marketing objectives—and to do so under the guise of promoting health and basic democratic values.

CONGRESS VERSUS FDA: DSHEA, 1994

In enacting DSHEA, Congress was responding to an industry-led campaign framed as giving Americans the "freedom to choose" dietary supplements. Although the industry earned annual revenues of just $4 billion in 1994, its constituency included at least half of the adult population. Congress, therefore, recognized that "the nutritional supplement industry is an integral part of the economy of the United States" and prohibited the Food and Drug Administration (FDA) from enforcing any "unreasonable regulatory barriers" that might deter anyone from buying the products.[5]

DSHEA's Key Provisions

DSHEA contained four provisions designed expressly to prevent federal interference with the interests of the supplement industry. First, it expanded the legal definition of dietary supplements beyond the familiar vitamins and minerals to include the less-well-researched herbal, botanical, and diet products. Second, DSHEA specified that manufacturers did not need to demonstrate that their products were safe before selling them. Instead, Congress required the FDA to prove that products were unsafe before the agency could order them removed from the market. Furthermore, DSHEA eliminated the FDA's independent authority to take products off the market. Instead, the FDA would now have to obtain approvals of such action at four bureaucratic levels: two at FDA itself (its legal counsel and commissioner) and two at the FDA's parent agency, the Department of Health and Human Services (DHHS)—its general counsel and the DHHS secretary. Once all of these people had approved the proposed action, DSHEA required the FDA to give the manufacturer a 10-day warning notice. Only then could FDA initiate a lawsuit to have the product withdrawn. While these cumbersome steps were proceeding, manufacturers could continue to sell their products.

It should be evident from these rules that Congress was making one blanket assumption—that the supplements then on the market were safe. Indeed, DSHEA "grandfathered" the safety of supplements that were on the market prior to October 15, 1994. After that date, Congress required makers of new supplement products merely to think ahead. Just 75 days before putting a product on the market, its manufacturer must send the FDA some evidence (unspecified) of a history of use or benefit. If the FDA has reason to believe that a product is so unsafe that it should not be marketed, the agency must obtain the required approvals, warn the manufacturer, and demonstrate in court within that 75-day period that the supplement poses a public health risk.

Finally, DSHEA granted a concession long sought by the supplement industry. Marketers would now be able to label their products with "statements of nutritional support" proclaiming how ingredients might alleviate a nutrient deficiency, improve the structure or function of a part of the human body (a "structure/function" claim), or promote general well-being. To use such claims (which are now collectively referred to as structure/function statements), a supplement maker need only notify the FDA 30 days after marketing the product, have on hand some substantiation (also unspecified) for the statement, and include on the label the

DSHEA disclaimer: "This statement has not been evaluated by the Food and Drug Administration. This product is not intended to diagnose, treat, cure, or prevent any disease."[5]

DSHEA's provisions marked a sharp departure from previous regulatory policies. For most of the twentieth century, the FDA prohibited supplement makers from claiming that their products could be used to treat one or another condition. From the FDA's standpoint, if manufacturers claimed that their food or supplement was good for a disease, they were claiming drug-like benefits for their products, and the agency should regulate the products as it did for drugs.[6] Drug regulations require manufacturers to demonstrate through controlled scientific and clinical studies that the products not only are safe for human consumption but also are more effective as remedies than placebos or comparable drugs. (See the Appendix for a discussion of placebo effects and other related research issues.) Given the time and expense involved in research needed to demonstrate such benefits, manufacturers would do practically anything to avoid having their products considered drugs. They wanted to be able to use claims about health benefits to market their products, but FDA policies prevented them from doing so.

Some Fine Distinctions

In passing DSHEA, Congress let stand a distinction it had made in 1990 between a *disease claim* that would render a supplement a drug and a *health claim*—by definition, a statement preauthorized by the FDA about the relationship between a dietary factor and a medical condition or risk factor. DSHEA specified, however, that the FDA was not to demand scientific proof of statements of nutritional support (structure/function statements) as long as they were "truthful and not misleading" and did not use such words as *diagnose, treat, prevent, cure,* or *mitigate.* In setting these rules, Congress intended the FDA to bring its regulatory policies in line with the far more lenient policies of the Federal Trade Commission (FTC), the federal agency responsible for regulating statements in product *advertisements* as opposed to labels.

It should be obvious by now that understanding DSHEA's provisions demands close attention to several mind-numbing distinctions:

- FDA (foods, drugs, supplements: safety and labels) versus FTC (advertising)
- Conventional foods versus dietary supplements versus drugs

- Nutritional versus herbal and other types of dietary supplements
- Food labels versus advertisements
- Disease claims versus health claims versus statements of nutritional support (structure/function claims)

Such distinctions are invisible in supermarkets and health food stores and cannot possibly matter to the average consumer, but they thoroughly preoccupy supplement marketers, lawyers, and federal regulators. This chapter explains the terms as they occur and sometimes repeats the definitions for clarity.

FDA versus FTC

Let us begin with the critical differences between the missions and philosophies of the two federal agencies involved in regulating dietary supplements, the Food and Drug Administration (FDA) and the Federal Trade Commission (FTC). The FDA's mandate is to promote *safety:* its job is to ensure that conventional foods, dietary supplements, and drugs are safe and labeled accurately, and that drugs do something useful according to "science-based" standards—in other words, as verified by clinical trials. The FTC has a decidedly different mission: to promote *business competition.* One way it does so is by preventing unfair commercial practices such as false advertising. Thus both agencies are involved in regulating certain actions of supplement companies. In a 1954 agreement, the FDA retained regulatory authority over statements on food *labels* and associated handouts, but the FTC assumed responsibility for ensuring the fairness of food *advertisements.* Because advertisements and labels are subject to different rules issued by different agencies, the regulation of health claims for supplements and foods becomes exceptionally messy. Naturally, the supplement industry finds the FTC's regulatory philosophy far more favorable to its interests than that of the FDA.

Table 27 summarizes the peculiar results of this division of responsibility. Unlike those of the FDA, FTC policies do not carry the force of regulations. The FTC does not distinguish between health claims and statements of nutritional support, does not require marketers to obtain approval of health claims before using them in advertisements, and demands less substantiation of such claims. The FTC simply requires advertising statements to be truthful and not misleading and to be substantiated with "competent and reliable scientific evidence," taking into consideration what a product is, how likely it is to be beneficial, and what

TABLE 27. Comparison of Federal Trade Commission (FTC) and Food and Drug Administration (FDA) policies on health claims for dietary supplements

Policies	FTC[a]	FDA[b]
Regulate	Food advertising	Food labels
Constitute	Policy statements	Regulations
Distinguish claim types	Treats all claims equally, but defers to FDA	Has different rules for health and nutrient-content claims versus structure/function (s/f) statements.[c]
Scientific support	"Truthful, not misleading, substantiated." Qualifying information disclosed.	"Truthful, not misleading, substantiated" for s/f statements. For nutrient-content and health claims: "authoritative statements published by federal agencies or the National Academy of Sciences, based on consensus and deliberate review of the evidence."
Scientific standard	"Competent and reliable scientific evidence," considering type of product, benefits, consequences, costs, feasibility, expert opinion	For s/f statements: "scientifically valid evidence." For health claims: "significant scientific agreement."
Notification	Not required	Required
Health claims		120 days before marketing
Structure/function claims		Within 30 days of marketing
Prior approval	Not required	Required for health claims, not required for structure/function claims
DSHEA disclaimer for structure/function claims[d]	Not required, but sometimes desirable	Required

[a]FTC policies refer specifically to supplements but also apply to conventional foods.

[b]FDA regulations for nutrient-content (such as "good source") and structure/function claims for conventional foods also apply to dietary supplements; FDA intends to extend these rules to health claims for supplements.

[c]*Health claims* are FDA-approved statements about the relationship between a food or supplement and a disease or health condition. *Nutrient-content claims* refer to levels of nutrients in products compared to standards (such as "good source"). *Structure/function (s/f) statements* refer to benefits for correcting nutrient deficiencies, improving a bodily structure or function, or promoting well-being.

[d]The Dietary Supplement Health and Education Act of 1994 (DSHEA) requires structure/function statements on supplement labels to be accompanied by the following disclaimer: "This statement has not been evaluated by the Food and Drug Administration. This product is not intended to diagnose, treat, cure, or prevent any disease."

TABLE 28. Acceptable structure/function statements authorized by the Dietary Supplement Health and Education Act of 1994 (DSHEA) compared to unauthorized health claims that cause dietary supplements to be regulated as drugs

Acceptable Structure/Function Statement[a]	Unauthorized Health (Drug) Claims[b]
Helps maintain cardiovascular function.	Protects against heart disease.
Promotes healthy cholesterol level.	Lowers cholesterol.
Promotes healthy joints.	Reduces pain of arthritis.
Supports regularity, healthy intestinal flora.	Alleviates constipation; laxative.
Promotes urinary tract health.	Prevents urinary tract infections; improves urine flow in men over age 50; diuretic.
Supports the immune system.	Helps patients with reduced or compromised immune function.
Improves absentmindedness.	Improves cognitive functioning in the elderly.
Reduces stress and frustration.	Herbal Prozac.

[a]DSHEA permits manufacturers to make structure/function statements if they can demonstrate (by unspecified criteria) that the statements are truthful and not misleading. Such statements require no prior authorization by the FDA for use on labels but must be accompanied by the DSHEA disclaimer.

[b]Claims that products diagnose, mitigate, treat, prevent, or cure disease will cause FDA to regulate them as drugs unless manufacturers obtain prior FDA authorization for a health claim.

experts say about it.[7] The net result of these differences is that the FTC permits in advertisements statements about health benefits that the FDA does not permit on product labels.

Because these differences are sufficiently ambiguous to be easily misunderstood by anyone other than a lawyer who specializes in such things, the FTC has produced an *Advertising Guide for Industry* to explain how supplement marketers should interpret the effects of DSHEA. The FDA has issued an analogous guide concerning the use of health claims on the labels of conventional foods and dietary supplements. The FDA also has proposed rules to explain the difference between acceptable *structure/function* statements and unapproved *disease claims* that would cause products to be regulated as drugs.[8]

Despite these efforts, there is little doubt that DSHEA succeeded in blurring the distinctions among the various categories of claims. The comparative statements in Table 28 illustrate this problem. With DSHEA, the supplement industry won the right to state that an untested product promotes healthful cholesterol levels, but not that it lowers cholesterol; that it supports regularity, but not that it relieves constipation; that it maintains healthy joints, but not that it reduces symptoms of arthritis. The label of the black elderberry product that I mentioned at the beginning of the chapter may—and does—state that the product promotes immune function, but not that it prevents or cures colds, infections, or AIDS (acquired immunodeficiency syndrome). In advertisements, however, marketers are permitted to make much more blatant statements about health benefits, just as long as they can produce a supporting study if anyone asks for it. The books in health food stores are protected by First Amendment rights to free speech, and DSHEA explicitly prohibits the FDA from considering books, pamphlets, and fliers distributed at the point of sale as "labeling." Note, however, that no matter what the manufacturer claims for the black elderberry or any other product, neither the FDA nor the FTC would be likely to pay much attention unless someone filed a complaint of an adverse effect. Both agencies deal with dietary supplements on a case-by-case basis *after* people start reporting problems with their use.

THE "TWO-CULTURE" PROBLEM

In deregulating dietary supplements, Congress effectively shifted safety responsibility from industry to the government. The government, therefore, effectively shifted this responsibility to the public. In demanding only semantic restrictions on what marketers can claim about health benefits, Congress weakened not only the FDA's ability to protect the public from supplements that are in fact hazardous but also its ability to control the inappropriate marketing of foods, food additives, and even drugs. This achievement was hailed as a tremendous victory by the supplement industry. As one of its lobbyists gloated, "DSHEA stands for the unusual precedent that the FDA was wrong. . . . [T]his is one of the first times where an agency got not just publicly slapped on the wrist, but, in a congressional setting, they lost power. The agency lost big for the first time."[9]

To explain how this "victory" was accomplished, this chapter and the next review the contentious history of dietary supplement deregulation. As we shall see, the driving force in these events was—and continues to be—pressure from the dietary supplement industry to promote its marketing interests. The events, however, also reflect the expression of two conflicting views of the role of science in public policy. In theory, the FDA's policies are supposed to be science-based, which means that the agency requires products to be proved safe and effective according to commonly accepted ("mainstream") standards of scientific evidence. In contrast, the industry takes what I call a "belief-based" approach to dietary supplements; supplement makers argue that adults have the right to decide for themselves, on the basis of their own personal beliefs and experience, whether a product is worth taking and is effective.

The profound differences between these two approaches are summarized in Table 29. People who hold belief-based attitudes tend to view supplements as natural products that (1) promote health, (2) correct dietary deficiencies due, for example, to poor eating habits, depletion of nutrients from soil, pollution, stress, or aging, and (3) are far less likely than FDA-approved drugs to be harmful. In contrast, people who adopt science-based approaches tend to believe that most dietary supplements are of questionable content and safety and that any health benefits claimed are largely unproven. For the most part, the rationale for both sets of views is demonstrably factual; it is only the *interpretation* that differs. For example, none of the statements listed under belief-based approaches in Table 29 demonstrates that taking a particular supplement will make someone healthier. Similarly, the statements in support of a science-based approach do not prove that a particular supplement is unsafe or ineffective. From a scientific perspective, the preponderance of available evidence suggests that if they were tested, the great majority of supplements now on the market would prove to be no more effective than placebos and that a few would be demonstrably harmful. Science-based regulators would prefer to see the results of research studies demonstrating a supplement's safety *and* effectiveness before approving it for marketing.

The conflict between science-based and belief-based views of dietary supplements perfectly illustrates the "gulf of mutual incomprehension" that C. P. Snow saw to lie between scientists and nonscientists.[4] I first experienced this gulf when teaching nutrition to medical students, who might be expected to hold science-based approaches to dietary supplements. I described a clinical trial that had demonstrated beyond question that improvements in symptoms of the common cold reported by participants had been due to placebo effects, *not* to the vitamin C tablets they mistakenly thought they were taking (see the Appendix). After the lecture, the students surrounded me seeking advice about how much vitamin C they should take or recommend to patients. Even people trained in science take supplements and believe they are useful, either for "nutritional insurance" or for other belief-based reasons used by nonscientists—reasons connected only marginally to convincing scientific evidence of benefit.

TABLE 29. Two cultures: comparison of belief-based and science-based approaches to deciding whether dietary supplements are needed, effective, or safe

Belief-based approach

Need

Diets do not always follow dietary recommendations.
Foods grown on depleted soils lack essential nutrients.
Pollution and stressful living conditions increase nutrient requirements.
Cooking destroys essential nutrients.
Nutrient-related physiological functions decline with age.

Efficacy

People who take supplements are healthier.
People feel better when they take supplements.
Studies demonstrate the health benefits of supplements.
Benefits are sometimes greater at amounts higher than can be obtained from food.

Safety

Supplements are safe within a broad range of intake; safety problems are rare.
Herbal products have been used for thousands of years.
Supplements cause less harm than many prescription drugs.

Science-based approach

Need

Food is sufficient to meet nutrient needs.
Foods provide nutrients and other valuable substances not present in supplements.
People who take supplements are better educated and wealthier; they are healthier whether or not they take supplements.

Efficacy

Research demonstrates health benefits of diets and foods, not of single nutrients.
Higher-than-recommended doses of few single nutrients improve health.
Health claims for many supplements often address issues (such as "stress") that are difficult to evaluate scientifically.
The health benefits of most supplements are unproven.
Many "benefits" of supplements can be explained as placebo or other self-healing effects.

Safety

Excessive doses of many nutrients are demonstrably toxic.
High levels of single nutrients interfere with the functions of other nutrients.
The safety of many herbal products is untested and, therefore, unknown.
Herbal supplements vary in composition, potency, and quality.

As this chapter illustrates, the FDA's attempts to impose science-based regulatory standards on an industry with wide appeal to a public that subscribes to belief-based views of dietary supplements caused the agency no end of woe—astonishing amounts of work followed by increasing isolation from the public, from the courts, and eventually from Congress, which voted for personal beliefs over science when it passed DSHEA.

FROM "BRAZEN QUACKERY" TO REGULATION—AND BACK AGAIN

In a sense, DSHEA marked a return to the days of "flagrant and brazen" quackery that first induced the federal government to become involved in regulating over-the-counter health remedies.[10] Prior to the Food and Drug Act of 1906, nostrums, panaceas, and patent medicines promised cures for every conceivable health problem. Many products contained alcohol or opiates that (not surprisingly) made people feel better, if only for a few hours. In addition to their addictive properties, such remedies appealed to the public's disenchantment with the ability of doctors to relieve illness and pain. Because many symptoms of illness resolve on their own, it was easy enough to find products that "worked," and to identify people who could give testimonials of cures. Manufacturers could include whatever ingredients they liked and advertise the health benefits of products without interference; indeed, patent medicines accounted for the largest category of advertising expenditures in the United States in 1900. Then, as now, reformers argued that education alone could never be sufficient to protect the public against widespread and uncontrolled hucksterism.

In the wake of public concerns about food safety elicited by publication of *The Jungle*, Upton Sinclair's muckraking report on the meat industry, Congress passed the Food and Drug Act of 1906. This act permitted the Bureau of Chemistry, the forerunner of FDA, to regulate nostrums and to ensure that their labels did not contain false and misleading statements about ingredients. In 1911 the bureau proposed that the false-and-misleading criterion should also apply to claims for therapeutic benefits (that is, to disease claims) made on product labels. Because the 1906 act did not actually state that "false and misleading" applied to such claims, manufacturers sued for the right to continue marketing their products, and they won initial court decisions as well as appeals to the Supreme Court. Congress amended the act in 1912 to permit the bureau to take action against products making disease claims, but only if the claims were both false *and* fraudulent, a requirement that the bureau found difficult to meet.

Thus in the early years of the twentieth century, the interactions among the industry, regulatory agencies, the public, the courts, and Congress established a cyclical pattern that continues to the present day. With respect to dietary supplements, the cycles follow a pattern that goes like this:

- Manufacturers market products using implausible and unprovable health claims.
- The FDA responds by proposing regulations that require consistent ingredients and scientific substantiation for the claims.
- Marketers file objections, organize massive letter-writing campaigns, lobby Congress, and file lawsuits.
- The courts rule in favor of the industry and force the FDA to revise the proposed regulations.
- Supplement companies object to the new rules, renew their lobbying efforts, file new lawsuits, and organize more letter-writing campaigns.
- In response to the "will of the people," Congress passes laws limiting FDA authority.
- Marketers take advantage of the greater leniency afforded by the new law.
- The cycle continues.[11]

Table 30 summarizes the various laws Congress has enacted since the mid-1970s that increasingly have supported nonscientific, belief-based approaches and weakened the FDA's regulatory authority over dietary supplements.

FDA VERSUS NUTRITIONAL SUPPLEMENTS

Although most supplements on today's market are herbals and botanicals, the ability of manufacturers to make claims for their health benefits derives from application of the FDA's science-based view of nutritional supplements—vitamins and minerals. The FDA's position on nutritional supplements dates from the early years of the twentieth century. As soon as vitamins were discovered and their nutritional functions identified, manufacturers began using them in supplements and advertising them as

TABLE 30. Congressional acts that have weakened the FDA's authority to restrict the contents of dietary supplements or of label statements about health benefits

1976   Proxmire Amendment (Public Law 94-278), says the FDA may *not*:
- Set limits on the amount of a vitamin or mineral allowed in a supplement.
- Classify a supplement as a drug if its dose exceeds a level that FDA considers nutritionally rational.
- Restrict the combination of vitamins or minerals in supplements.

1990   Nutrition Labeling and Education Act (NLEA) (Public Law 101-535), directs the FDA to:
- Authorize health claims on foods and supplements when they are substantiated by "significant scientific agreement among qualified experts."
- Decide whether to authorize ten specific claims for foods and supplements.
- Develop a separate authorization process for supplement health claims.

1992   Dietary Supplement Act (Public Law 102-571):
- Prevents the FDA from applying its restrictions on health claims for conventional foods to dietary supplements for one year.
- Requires the FDA to repropose rules for supplements.
- Orders an investigation of the FDA's management activities related to supplement regulation.

1994   Dietary Supplement Health and Education Act (DSHEA) (Public Law 103-417):
- Defines supplements as amino acids, herbs, botanicals, metabolites, and diet products as well as vitamins and minerals.
- Makes the FDA responsible for proving that a supplement is harmful, rather than making the manufacturer prove that it is not harmful.
- Ends the FDA's independent authority to remove harmful products from the market.
- Makes the Secretary of Health and Human Services responsible for initiating court proceedings against harmful products.
- Permits products to remain on the market while obtaining approvals and while court proceedings are underway.
- Prohibits the FDA from considering brochures provided at the point of sale as part of a package label.
- Authorizes "structure/function" statements when they are accompanied by the following disclaimer: "This statement has not been evaluated by the Food and Drug Administration. This product is not intended to diagnose, treat, cure, or prevent any disease."

1997   Food and Drug Administration Modernization Act (FDAMA) (Public Law 105-115):
- Requires the FDA to permit nutrient-content and health claims for *conventional foods* when these claims are substantiated by published, authoritative statements of federal public health agencies or the National Academy of Sciences.
- Permits the FDA to apply these criteria to supplements.

a necessary means to overcome weaknesses in the food supply or daily diet. Right from the start, the prime targets of supplement marketing were middle-class women—the group least likely to have nutrient deficiencies (except, perhaps, iron-deficiency anemia) but most likely to be concerned about family health. This strategy helped the industry to grow rapidly. By 1935, vitamins accounted for as much as one-fourth of the total sales of leading drug companies and one-third of sales in the average drugstore. Retail vitamin sales rose from $32.2 million in 1935 to $82.7 million in 1939—during the Great Depression.[12] Although concerned about such trends, the FDA could do little about the labeling or advertising of questionable products until Congress, in 1938, passed amendments that eliminated the need for the FDA to prove claims "fraudulent."

In the 1950s, the regulatory cycles became increasingly contentious when the FDA took a much more aggressive and confrontational stance against the makers of nutritional supplements. In 1954, a year in which an estimated half-billion dollars was spent on "nutritional quackery," the FDA proposed to establish "standards of identity"—precise formulas used for ingredients in foods such as ketchup and ice cream—that would enable the agency to regulate supplements as an entity rather than case by case. This proposal resulted from concerns about the unrealistic claims made for nutritional supplements and fears of toxicity from high doses of certain vitamins. Thus the FDA proposed to require all vitamin and mineral supplements to contain a defined set of nutrients at defined levels; otherwise, the products would be considered drugs.

This proposal constituted only the first of the many steps needed in the unbelievably tedious process of issuing food or supplement regulations. Like other federal agencies, the FDA is required to open all proposed rules for public comment and to consider all comments in developing its final regulations. Typically, the FDA announces proposed rules, calls for comments, considers the comments, proposes revised rules, opens the revisions to comments, considers these comments, proposes final rules for comment, and, only after considering these *further* comments, issues final rules. At best, this process takes years and involves a succession of interminably lengthy notices—in very fine print—in the *Federal Register*.

In this early case, industry and other groups argued that the FDA's proposed standards of identity were totally unnecessary for vitamin and mineral supplements of such evident safety and physiological function. A citizens' advisory committee agreed and urged the FDA to increase its *educational* efforts, rather than engaging in litigation against potential quackery, and to put greater effort into helping the industry deal with the

FDA's scientific concerns. The standards-of-identity threat encouraged supplement makers to join together to form an association, the National Health Federation (NHF), which soon began lobbying congressional representatives and informing consumers about the need to protect their freedom to choose supplements. In 1961 and 1962, the FDA and the American Medical Association (AMA) held joint national conferences on quackery that suggested to the industry that the FDA was colluding with mainstream medicine to require a doctor's prescription for anyone who wanted to take a vitamin or mineral supplement.

Despite warnings of the near-hysterical level of industry concern about its proposals, the FDA continued to pursue science-based standards. Because research did not show much benefit from nutritional supplements in healthy people, the agency not only continued to advocate the unpopular standards of identity but also proposed that supplement labels include a disclaimer: "Deficiency symptoms have been induced only under experimental conditions, and there is no convincing evidence that the ordinary diet requires supplementation with these nutrients."[13] As might be expected, this proposal elicited an outpouring of industry opposition; the National Health Federation generated 40,000 of 54,000 letters sent to the FDA on this issue.[10]

Nevertheless, the FDA persisted in maintaining a strict, science-based approach. In 1966 it again proposed standards of identity, this time specifying an even more restrictive disclaimer to be displayed "in prominent type": "Vitamins and minerals are supplied in abundant amounts by the foods we eat. The Food and Nutrition Board of the National Research Council recommends that dietary needs be satisfied by foods. Except for persons with special medical needs, there is no scientific basis for recommending routine use of dietary supplements."[14]

Again led by the National Health Federation, supplement companies and their supporters deluged Congress with more than two million letters—more mail than was later generated by Watergate—protesting the proposed rules and demanding that Congress intervene. A lobbying organization of the pharmaceutical industry, joined by 12 drug companies producing vitamin supplements, took the FDA to court on a technicality: The group argued that the FDA could not implement its proposals because it had never held hearings on this issue. Even critics concerned about "FDA's failure to serve as an effective counterweight against the 'corporate greed and irresponsibility' of the $125-billion food industry" complained bitterly about the agency's narrow interpretation of the scientific evidence related to nutritional supplements.[15]

During the next few years, the FDA held the required hearings; these were said to have generated 32,000 pages of testimony and more than 20,000 letters arguing against every possible aspect of the proposals. One of the FDA's most controversial proposals was to classify as a drug any supplement of vitamin D or vitamin A—which can induce toxic symptoms in adults at doses 5 to 15 times higher than recommended levels—if its dose just *slightly* exceeded those levels. This proposal alone elicited 2,500 comments and 1,000 signatures on petitions, nearly all of them unfavorable.

Holding fast to the view that supplements are "nutritionally irrational," the FDA eventually published final regulations in 1973; these specified the upper and lower limits of supplement potency, and retained the classification of vitamin A and D as drugs but dropped the requirement for the unpopular disclaimer noted above. The industry sued. In response, the courts intervened, struck down the standards of identity, and prohibited the FDA from classifying high-potency supplements as drugs for reasons such as lack of nutritional need or toxicity—reasons that the court considered "irrelevant."[16]

CONGRESS INTERVENES:
THE PROXMIRE AMENDMENT, 1976

At about this time during the early 1970s, under pressure from the industry and the public, Congress introduced several bills to prevent the FDA from regulating the dosages of nutritional supplements. In 1976 these attempts succeeded when Congress passed an amendment to the Food, Drug, and Cosmetic Act—the Proxmire Amendment—as a rider to a health bill that was certain to pass.[17] The Proxmire Amendment firmly disallowed standards of identity, and it said that the FDA absolutely must not set limits on the amounts of vitamins and minerals in supplements, classify supplements as drugs, demand that supplements contain only useful ingredients, or bar supplements from including useless ingredients.

From the standpoint of supplement marketers, "Proxmire meant the survival of our industry. . . . [W]ithout that, the FDA . . . could have crippled us"[18] To science-oriented commentators who believed that supplements should be proved useful before their manufacturers were permitted to make health claims for them, the Proxmire Amendment was "the first retrogressive step in federal legislation . . . since 1906,"[10] or, as expressed by the then FDA commissioner, "a charlatan's dream."[18]

Subsequent court actions further diminished the FDA's authority to apply drug laws to supplements. Then in 1979, after 25 years of futile effort to regulate the supplement industry as a whole, the agency gave up, withdrew its proposals, and returned to enforcement on a case-by-case basis. Later that year, the FDA made one last attempt to classify nutritional supplements as over-the-counter drugs. It recruited a panel of nutrition scientists to produce a monograph on vitamin and mineral supplements and used the monograph in a way that could not have been better designed to provoke opposition: It defined vitamin and mineral supplements as drugs that would be "labeled for use in the prevention or treatment of a deficiency *when the need for such therapy has been determined by a physician* (emphasis added)." This meant, for example, that the label of a supplement of vitamin C (ascorbic acid), a vitamin safe except at extraordinarily high doses, would have to say, "for use in the prevention of vitamin C deficiency when the need for such therapy has been determined by a physician" *and* would need to include this warning: "Patients with gout and/or a tendency to form kidney stones may be at increased risk when taking more than the recommended dose. Diabetics taking more than 500 milligrams vitamin C daily may obtain false readings in their urinary glucose test." And as though *that* were not enough, if the vitamin C occurred in the form of sodium ascorbate and contained more than 125 milligrams of sodium per dose, the label must add: "Do not take this product if you are on a sodium-restricted diet except under the advice and supervision of a physician."[19]

With this level of overkill, it is not difficult to understand how industry groups could convince Congress to intervene by introducing a bill to prohibit the FDA from defining nutritional supplements as drugs. Although the bill did not pass, the FDA wisely withdrew the controversial monograph. At that point, manufacturers could market vitamins or minerals in any dose, but if labels claimed that the pills mitigated, treated, cured, or prevented diseases or symptoms, the FDA would consider the products to be drugs and insist that they be regulated as such.

BREACHING THE HEALTH-CLAIMS BARRIER: KELLOGG'S ALL-BRAN, 1984

If the FDA was adamant about health claims for supplements, it was even more insistent about health claims for foods. It applied the same logic: if food labels claimed benefits for disease prevention, manufacturers were marketing the foods as drugs. Events in 1984, however, forced the FDA to retreat from this position, this time as a result of pressures from *food* companies urging the agency to develop a more liberal policy on health claims. As the chair of the National Food Processors Association explained, the no-claims policies badly hurt sales: "Many food processors have experienced stabilized or reduced sales of traditional processed foods because they have been unable to inform consumers about the current state of knowledge linking these products and cancer and heart disease."[20]

The initial break in the FDA policy came as a result of an unexpected maneuver from a surprising source, the Kellogg cereal company. Kellogg had created a new marketing campaign for its line of All-Bran cereals. As shown in Figure 21, the cereal boxes said, "The National Cancer Institute believes eating the right foods may reduce your risk of cancer. Here are their recommendations: Eat high fiber foods. A growing body of evidence says high fiber foods are important to good health. That's why a healthy diet includes high fiber foods like bran cereals."

Kellogg had developed this text by "working closely" with the National Cancer Institute (NCI), a sister agency to the FDA within its parent agency, the Department of Health and Human Services (DHHS). According to reports at the time, the institute's scientific staff and legal advisors had reviewed the material to check the accuracy of the statements and to make sure that they did not imply that the NCI endorsed the product. From the standpoint of the NCI and political appointees in DHHS, the Kellogg campaign would "infuse millions of dollars of private sector funds into the promotion of cancer prevention messages."[21]

Kellogg's alliance with the NCI largely excluded the FDA and caught the agency by surprise.[22] According to an FDA staff member who was present at meetings at the time, "FDA was never consulted, nor . . . did Kellogg ever suggest to NCI that there might be any FDA concern about the matter. . . . [I]ncredible as it may be . . . it never occurred to [NCI] that there were any regulatory implications of putting what they considered to be a perfectly reasonable public health education message on cereal boxes."[23]

FDA staff realized immediately that the Kellogg campaign seriously threatened the agency's regulatory authority over label statements. They understood that if the campaign was not stopped, health claims might "become commonplace and beyond the reach of the agency."[24] A reporter quoted Dr. Sanford Miller, then the head of FDA's Center for Food Safety and Applied Nutrition, as expressing skepticism about the scientific basis of the Kellogg statements: "This ad is incorrect because

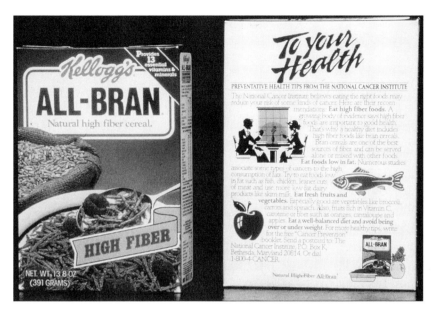

FIGURE 21. Kellogg evaded FDA restrictions on health claims in 1984 when its cereal box displayed a recommendation from the National Cancer Institute to "eat high-fiber foods," implying that eating this cereal might help prevent cancer. (Courtesy National Cancer Institute)

there's no evidence that this kind of fiber can help. It's a scientific issue. . . . How far can you simplify? . . . [T]he agency simply hasn't figured out a way it can protect its very powerful tool in regulating claims on food, and, at the same time, allow [claims] to go on."[25]

The FDA's attempt to block the Kellogg campaign failed, however. It was overruled at higher levels within DHHS, not least because the FDA position was inconsistent with the deregulatory ideology of the administration of President Ronald Reagan. Political appointees in DHHS and the FDA did everything but outright endorse the Kellogg advertisements. As the commissioner of the FDA explained to the National Food Processors Association, "The profit motive alone does not account for your . . . serious consideration of innovative approaches to food labeling. I think we'd both agree that an informed public can make better decisions about the products that it buys and consumes. . . . FDA's job is to encourage this trend . . . by cooperating with industry to make healthful products available."[22]

The FTC also enthusiastically endorsed the Kellogg advertisements and recommended that other companies follow suit. According to the

FTC's director of consumer protection, Kellogg's claims "appear to be exactly the kind of adequately substantiated and responsible vehicles for providing beneficial information to the public that we believe it is important for regulatory programs to encourage, not discourage."[24]

Kellogg, although conceding that the fundamental purpose of its campaign had been to sell All-Bran, asserted that its actions were a *public service* and that the company would be irresponsible if it sold health-promoting products and did not tell people about them.[26] Researchers at the FTC confirmed that the campaign indeed had informed consumers about the value of fiber to health and that it also had caused a shift from low-fiber to high-fiber cereals. When an FDA analysis revealed an astonishing 47% increase in the market share of All-Bran within the first six months of the campaign, the message to the food industry was clear: Health claims sold products.[27]

Opposed by the NCI and the FTC, and bereft of support from the upper echelons of their own agency and department, FDA professional staff could do little beyond expressing unhappiness that Kellogg had failed to consult them in advance. Instead, an associate FDA commissioner (politically appointed) announced the agency's new position: The FDA would give food advertisers a "cautious green light . . . to use health claims in promotions."[28] The agency would begin developing regulations for claims that companies could use on food labels to explain how their products might reduce the risk of heart disease, cancer, and other diseases, but without "opening the door to outright fraudulent ones."[29]

Supplements, however, would not be able to take advantage of this new marketing opportunity. An NCI official viewed the evidence for "the associations between cancer and foods . . . [as] for food only, not supplements," a statement interpreted as indicating that the FDA also would refuse to "extend to food-supplement marketers the same liberalized labeling and advertising freedoms that food marketers appear to have won."[28] The Council for Responsible Nutrition (CRN), a trade organization representing manufacturers and marketers of dietary supplements, immediately charged that regulatory agencies were demonstrating a "not-for-supplements" bias, and they threatened lawsuits.[30]

In June 1985, the CRN sent a letter to the FDA commissioner suggesting that his agency allow supplement labels to include "statements of nutritional support" that were substantiated by research acceptable to federal or private agencies: "Statements that speak in terms of modifying the diet so as to enhance the body's ability to resist disease, or to reduce the long-term risks of developing disease, would be classified as nutritional, rather than therapeutic. Such claims would be permitted in food labeling and advertising so long as not false or misleading."[31]

The CRN and three other organizations—Kellogg, the National Food Processors Association, and, oddly enough, the consumer advocacy organization Center for Science in the Public Interest—filed petitions asking the FDA to develop a uniform policy on health claims to establish a level playing field for both conventional foods and supplements. In 1987 the FDA issued "cautious and deliberate" proposals to permit health claims on the labels of foods and nutritional supplements. These were to be "truthful and not misleading" and "supported by [1] valid, [2] reliable, [3] publicly available scientific evidence derived from [4] well-designed and conducted studies [5] consistent with generally accepted scientific procedures and principles [6] performed and evaluated by persons qualified by expertise and training in the appropriate disciplines" [numbers added for emphasis].[32] Each of these six elements of substantiation constituted a standard that companies would have to meet.

Such heavily science-based proposals satisfied neither consumer nor industry groups. Several consumer organizations opposed the entire concept of health claims, which they believed were likely to confuse the public, to reduce the credibility of information on food labels, and to be unenforceable by an agency already strapped for resources.[33] A committee of the New York Academy of Medicine, opposed to the very idea that a health benefit might relate to any single type of product in a food package, argued that nutrition research is so indefinite that the biomedical community could hardly be expected to reach consensus on "whether a given class of foods, food supplements, or a specific nutrient is beneficial."[34] Food companies, on the other hand, considered the requirements for scientific substantiation to be far too stringent, knowing that the FDA would require them to produce documentation to support every single one of the six substantiation elements. Instead, the industry much preferred the FTC approach, which encouraged advertising statements that would "make an important contribution to public welfare."[35]

Industry complaints about the FDA's proposed substantiation criteria led President Reagan's Office of Management and Budget (OMB) to delay publication of the final rules for one year, then for two more. This interference resulted from a White House executive order to OMB to review the fiscal effects—meaning any negative impact on industry—of regulations that were currently under review by federal agencies. With such impact in mind, the OMB view of the FDA proposal was "We don't like it, it's too restrictive."[36] Some members of Congress recognized that

OMB interference would weaken the FDA. They held hearings to demonstrate that "the intervention of OMB ideologues who seek unregulated market entry of food products bearing disease-specific health claims" meant that the FDA was "telegraphing to industry that it is becoming a 'paper tiger.'"[33]

The supplement industry also opposed the FDA proposals, particularly because one feature seemed especially alarming. The proposals said,

> Individual diets are not composed of isolated substances or even isolated foods; rather, they contain thousands of combinations of nutrients and other compounds. From the standpoint of general public health education, it has generally been found more practical and effective to emphasize overall dietary patterns that enhance good health than to attempt to identify individual compounds. For these reasons, although the agency will apply the same criteria to the labeling of dietary supplements, it may be more difficult for dietary supplements to meet the criteria.[32]

The Council for Responsible Nutrition continued to argue that the FDA's differing approaches to foods and supplements reflected a pervasive antisupplement bias, were illegal under the Proxmire Amendment, and would be challenged in court. Further, the CRN complained about the restrictive substantiation criteria: "Consensus should not be viewed as some kind of holy grail. . . . [R]ather . . . consensus is more like the Cheshire cat, appearing and disappearing unpredictably."[18] The CRN again petitioned the FDA to consider the supplement industry's alternative proposals:

> CRN suggests that those statements that discuss the relationship between diet and disease . . . in terms of the effect of the food on the *structure or function* of the body—be distinguished from those that discuss the prevention of disease in a therapeutic or pharmacological context. . . . CRN proposes that nutritional statements . . . be substantiated by "peer-reviewed published studies or other well-controlled studies of the type that scientists qualified in the relevant field would consider reliable for such purposes." . . . [A] statement would not be inadequately substantiated solely because it did not reflect a consensus of scientific or medical opinion [emphasis added].[32]

It is a tribute to the effectiveness of supplement industry lobbying efforts that suggestions made by its leaders in 1985 and again in 1987 were eventually incorporated as elements of the 1994 DSHEA. In 1987, however, the CRN proposals merely encouraged the White House to continue to delay publication of regulations until the FDA could guarantee that they "would not be too restrictive on industry."[37]

HEALTH CLAIMS PROLIFERATE

With so much opposition to restrictions on health claims coming from so many sources, federal agencies were unenthusiastic about pursuing misleading claims. When the FDA did take action against one small company that was marketing a putative "cholesterol-lowering" supplement that could not possibly do so, the courts ruled that it was unfair of the government to pick on that company rather than a larger corporation such as Kellogg or RJR Nabisco. Food companies took advantage of this period of "free-for-all" regulatory inaction to label or advertise more and more products with health claims based on the FTC's less stringent requirements for scientific substantiation. Appearances of nutrient-content claims (such as those proclaiming that products were low in fat or cholesterol or high in fiber) increased from 25% of the food advertisements in women's magazines in 1975 to more than 50% of those advertisements in 1990. Claims were especially prevalent in advertisements for meat and high-fat products, apparently to counteract any idea that such foods might be unhealthful.[38] Some consumer groups and their sympathizers in Congress wanted to end the regulatory impasse and force the FTC to use the FDA's more stringent substantiation standards, but their initiatives did not get very far. Food and supplement industries were lobbying for precisely the opposite goal—to compel the FDA to follow the more relaxed approach of the FTC.

By 1989 40% of all new food products—and nearly $4 billion in food advertising—contained a health message of one kind or another.[39] With the federal government immobilized on this issue, states took over regulatory enforcement against companies making deceptive claims for juices that were mostly sugar and water, for vitamins advertised as giving energy, and for high-fat foods said to lower blood cholesterol levels. The state cases often were settled when companies stopped making the claims and paid court costs. Kellogg, however, retaliated by suing a Texas legal official for slander after he was quoted as characterizing some of the company's health claims as lies.[40]

This chaotic legal situation finally ended when Congress passed the Nutrition Labeling and Education Act of 1990, which, as discussed in the next chapter, forced the FDA to begin authorizing health claims for foods and supplements. Until Kellogg broke the health-claims barrier, the FDA had managed to keep the labels of foods and supplements relatively free of statements implying that consuming them would prevent or treat disease. Even in the face of overwhelming political opposition, FDA staff maintained that the agency's role was to hold foods and supplements to the same level of scientific substantiation of benefit that it required for drugs. If supplement makers could not prove that their products enhanced immune function, for example, the labels should not be allowed to say that they could. To makers and takers of supplements and to their supporters in Congress and federal agencies, this science-based standard seemed unnecessary as well as bad for business. The division between the "two cultures" became even more pronounced in the years just prior to the passage of DSHEA, as discussed in the next chapter.

CHAPTER 11

MAKING HEALTH CLAIMS LEGAL

THE SUPPLEMENT INDUSTRY'S WAR WITH THE FDA

NO PERSON MAKING A FIRST VISIT TO A HEALTH FOOD STORE today, perhaps bewildered by the vast array of supplements and the statements made about their purported purposes, could possibly imagine that as recently as 1990, claims about health benefits were strictly prohibited. Until then, if the labels suggested that supplements might be useful for preventing or treating a specific condition, the FDA considered them drugs and demanded evidence that they were beneficial as well as safe. To the supplement industry and to supplement users, the FDA's science-based regulation seemed inappropriate, if not downright obstructive. Makers and sellers of supplements banded together to oppose the FDA's policies. In doing so, they appealed to the huge proportion of American adults who take supplements. They based these appeals on the beliefs listed in Table 29 (Chapter 10), but also on the right of adults to exercise freedom of choice in the marketplace. Their highly successful organizing of grass roots support induced Congress to pass the Dietary Supplement Health and Education Act of 1994 (DSHEA), which forced the FDA to permit a wide range of claims for which scientific support was limited, weak, or nonexistent. This chapter explains how the supplement industry achieved this "victory."

The previous chapter described how Kellogg's All-Bran campaign produced two results: It convinced the food industry—and makers of dietary supplements—that claims about health benefits could help sell products, and it forced the FDA to begin writing regulations in the late 1980s that would, for the first time, permit such claims to be made. Because the FDA insisted that manufacturers submit scientific evidence to support their claims, the White House blocked the FDA from releasing its initial proposals. In 1990, in what appeared to be a policy reversal, the White House finally permitted the FDA to repropose its science-based rules for health claims on food and supplement labels. This time, the FDA proposed to approve only those health claims substantiated by the (1) totality of (2) published evidence, from (3) well-designed studies, (4) conducted in a manner consistent with standard methods, about which (5) significant scientific agreement must exist (6) among qualified experts.[1]

The FDA identified six possible claims for relationships of dietary factors to disease risk that were least likely to run afoul of the "significant scientific agreement" standard. Each suggested a *reduction* in risk: high calcium and reduced risk of osteoporosis, low salt and high blood pressure, low fat and heart disease, low fat and cancer, high fiber and heart disease, and high fiber and cancer. Even though the FDA seemed willing to concede these six claims, its proposals elicited the usual furor. To the industry, the six distinct substantiation elements were too restrictive. The president of the Council for Responsible Nutrition, J. B. Cordaro, viewed the FDA proposal as "the most retrogressive, anti-consumer rule put out by the Government in years. . . . [I]t will discourage companies from putting out information on health and from modifying their products to be more healthy." But Congressman Henry Waxman (Dem-CA) said that the FDA should be doing *more*, not less, to regulate health claims: "In today's market, the industry has an incentive to make exaggerated and inaccurate health claims on foods. I hope the FDA will finally begin prohibiting health claims unless the agency first finds they have a sound scientific basis."[2]

Late in 1990, a House committee investigated the circumstances that had caused the FDA to take so long to reissue its proposals. The committee concluded that White House interference had held up the rules for three years and that the FDA's political leaders had "kowtowed" to the Office of Management and Budget (OMB) at virtually every step in the process, with the result that the agency's "regulatory powers [had] been neutered." The committee termed as "at best, disingenuous" the assertion by OMB that it merely was giving advice that the FDA was free to ignore. This committee's assessment, however, was not unanimous; one dissenting member characterized the House report as "another ideologically motivated subcommittee assault on American capitalism and Republican Administrations who support creating wealth through capitalism instead of imposing poverty through bureaucracy."[3]

During this contentious period, the FDA was collecting comments on its health-claims proposals and simultaneously working on rules for the design and content of labels on food packages. As we shall see, three separate lines of regulatory proposals—for food labeling, health claims on food labels, and health claims for dietary supplements—became thoroughly entangled with each other and with a host of political issues as broad as environmental protection and states' rights. Throughout, the FDA continued to execute its mission as a science-based regulatory agency and to apply science-based standards to all aspects of consumer protection, including health claims on food package labels.

In writing rules for labeling, however, the FDA had to deal with a regulatory quagmire. By the late 1980s, only about 30% of food package labels were required to list nutrient contents (because they contained added nutrients or made statements about them), another third was labeled voluntarily, and the rest were not labeled at all. A later FDA Commissioner, Dr. David Kessler, viewed the food-labeling rules of that era as the result of a 50-year-old patchwork rather than a coherent policy for informing the public about the nutritional content of foods. Food package labels, said Dr. Kessler, were the result of politics, not science, and had become "so opaque or confusing that only consumers with the hermeneutic abilities of a Talmudic scholar can peel back the encoded layers of meaning. That is because labels spring not from disinterested scientific reasoning but from lobbying, negotiation, and compromise."[4]

In March 1990, the secretary of the Department of Health and Human Services (DHHS), Dr. Louis W. Sullivan, finally announced FDA proposals for "sweeping changes" in food labels: "The grocery store has become a Tower of Babel, and consumers need to be linguists, scientists and mind readers to understand the many labels they see. Vital information is missing, and frankly some unfounded health claims are being made."[5]

Consumer organizations generally viewed the labeling proposals as a forward step, as did food industry groups hoping for an end to confusion in the marketplace. In his remarks, however, Dr. Sullivan suggested that some states might want to "add to the information required." The food industry viewed this idea as an open invitation to states to enact more stringent food-labeling laws than those proposed by the FDA and as a politically motivated effort of a Republican administration to strengthen states' rights during an election year. Food industry protests were especially pointed because some trade associations already had agreed in principle to mandatory nutrition labeling. They had done so, however, only with the understanding that federal regulations would prevent states from enacting more restrictive laws governing the amounts of *pesticides* that would be permitted in foods.[6]

Just three months later, Dr. Sullivan announced that his department had reversed its position and now favored uniform federal standards for food labels that would totally override state and local laws. This announcement was considered premature, however, because the White House again had stopped the FDA from releasing the revised labeling rules, this time because the OMB director reportedly favored the rights of states to make their own food-labeling laws.[7] Therefore, efforts to permit health claims for dietary supplements were inextricably enmeshed in the politics of even more complex issues: labeling on food packages, food safety, electoral politics, and states' rights.

CONGRESS INTERVENES AGAIN: FOOD-LABELING RULES, 1990

Dr. Sullivan may have had another reason for announcing FDA's blocked food-labeling rules. He may have wanted to discourage Congress from passing laws that might embarrass the FDA by ordering it "to do what it proposes to do, and more."[8] Congress, however, did precisely that when it preempted the FDA's years of work on food labeling by passing the Nutrition Labeling and Education Act (NLEA) of 1990 (see Table 30 (Chapter 10). The NLEA, widely viewed as "a win–win for consumers and the food industry," applied nationally and did not allow states to make their own food-labeling rules. Although its major purpose was to specify the content and format of labels on foods, the NLEA also addressed health claims. It directed the FDA to consider authorizing health claims for foods as well as dietary supplements so long as the claims could be substantiated by "significant scientific agreement" among "qualified experts." Furthermore, it required the FDA to consider ten specific claims. In doing so, it specified substantiation requirements less stringent than those proposed by the FDA but more restrictive than the FTC's.

The FDA, however, had just found compelling evidence to justify stricter standards for dietary supplements. In 1989 at least 1,500 people who took supplements of tryptophan (an amino acid present in all food proteins and human proteins) became seriously ill—and nearly 40 of them died—from the effects of a rare blood and neurological syndrome. Although the precise cause of the syndrome has never been determined, its symptoms were clearly related to use of the supplement.[9] As a result of this tragedy, the FDA appointed an internal task force to recommend ways in which it could "improve" (translation: strengthen) its regulatory methods for supplements. While the committee review was under way, the FDA was dealing with the 6,000 or so comments that had been filed on its 1990 proposals for health claims—many of which argued for *less* restrictive scientific standards.[10]

FDA staff must have been especially busy at that time, because the agency also was working on labeling rules for conventional foods, rules that critics feared would be used as a "holy war against misleading claims."[11] In November 1991—in what was widely regarded as an all-time "first"—the FDA and the USDA jointly released a gigantic (nearly 600-page) *Federal Register* notice proposing definitions, portion sizes, and health claims for labels for packaged foods as well as on meat and poultry products over which, in the peculiar division of federal responsibility for food labeling, the USDA holds jurisdiction. This level of collaboration between the two agencies was unprecedented.[12]

The release of these regulations came after yet another delay, this one because the White House Office of Management and Budget wanted the USDA to "think twice" before letting meat products be labeled in a way that might reveal their high content of fat and cholesterol. President George Bush called for a moratorium on all pending regulations that might adversely affect industry, including the joint labeling rules proposed by the FDA and the USDA. By that point, virtually all of the major food lobbying groups had filed complaints about one or another of the rules on the basis that labels might make some foods appear healthier than others: "Should government be allowed through the food label, to tell each consumer to eat less of this or more of that?"[13] The Grocery Manufacturers of America, for example, argued that labeling represented "regulatory excess, and appears to be designed to protect consumers against themselves. . . . [F]oods do not, *per se*, possess nutrition characteristics such as being "low" or "high" in a nutrient. Virtually all "low" nutrient foods can be said to lose their low characteristic if eaten in sufficient quantity."[14]

Early in 1992, reportedly at the request of OMB, the FDA suggested some revisions that might make the food-labeling rules more acceptable to industry. These proposals, visibly a retreat from the original plan, now allowed nutrient-content claims that a food could be labeled "reduced" in an undesirable nutrient when its manufacturer removed just 3 grams of fat, 40 calories, or 140 milligrams of sodium. The FDA's initial proposal had been to demand reductions of 50%, 33%, and 50%, respectively.

This change meant that a package of macaroni and cheese containing 20 grams of fat, for example, could be labeled as having "less fat" if it contained 17 grams of fat, in contrast to the reduction to 10 grams that would have been required by the previous proposals. With this contentious political climate for food labeling now well established, we can return to the FDA's actions on supplements.

FDA ENFORCES RULES, EVOKES INDUSTRY BACKLASH

In the spring of 1992, the FDA task force committee released its report on dietary supplement regulation. Noting that 30 years had elapsed since the FDA had first proposed rules for supplements, the committee recognized "that the regulated industry believes that FDA has historically been biased against the use of dietary supplements. Although these beliefs are unfounded, the Task Force is aware that its recommendations will be closely scrutinized . . . [and] has, therefore, conducted an objective and unbiased examination of all issues."[15]

Unbiased or not, the task force concluded that safety must be the primary regulatory consideration and that the industry should take responsibility for ensuring the safety of its products. Its report recommended that the FDA strictly enforce rules for supplements, establish purity and identity standards and safe levels of intake for vitamins and minerals, regulate amino acid supplements as drugs, and regulate all other supplements as "food additives" (which meant that safety would have to be demonstrated for new products)—just what the FDA had wanted all along. The FDA now had to deal with these recommendations as well as the public comments on the food-labeling proposals before it could issue final rules for health claims.

While the rule-writing staff of the FDA was hard at work, other FDA units were stepping up enforcement activities. In the late summer of 1992, a front-page story in the *New York Times* told a shocking tale: Armed FDA agents in Washington state had stormed an alternative-medicine clinic that treated patients with injected vitamins and minerals. The *Times* said that the raid included "F.D.A. agents, dressed in bullet-proof vests, bursting into the clinic and commanding clinic employees to freeze." The *Times* interpreted this action as "part of the agency's increased efforts to stop manufacturers of nutritional supplements from making unproven claims for their products, to bar their use by doctors unless first approved by the agency, and to halt their sale as medicines."[16]

The *Times* characterized the FDA as opposed to the idea that supplements "can be effective, whether or not they are backed by science." It reported protests to the FDA action, among them a press conference at which celebrities urged the public to "start screaming at Congress and the White House not to let the F.D.A. take our vitamins away" and editorials demanding that "if there is any plausible excuse for the Gestapo-like tactics . . . it had better be forthcoming and fast."

Just one week later, however, the *Times* published a carefully worded retraction of many of the statements in its article ("The article erred in saying that the proposed regulations would classify vitamins and minerals as drugs . . . and would restrict or prevent the sale of most medicinal herbs"), but the damage had been done. "I am one of the millions of Americans outraged by the Food and Drug Administration's unwarranted efforts to keep me from purchasing the nutritional supplements I desire," wrote one *Times* reader. Another complained that the FDA "is overreaching its authority to a frightening degree and extending into areas that consumers are far better able to deal with themselves individually. "The FDA," wrote a third, is trying "to gull the public into not fighting to have the proposed rules changed."[17]

At this point, nothing the FDA could do or say would dispel such fears, nor could it convince anyone that restricting supplement sales was forbidden under the provisions of the Proxmire Amendment. The *Times* story only confirmed public suspicions that the FDA planned to regulate supplements as drugs, and it gave the supplement industry just the incident it needed to exploit such concerns. Reportedly, more than a dozen groups formed to ask the White House and Congress to intervene on behalf of the industry.

One such group was the Nutritional Health Alliance (NHA). Led by the owner of a dietary supplement company, the NHA conducted an opinion poll demonstrating that more than "two-thirds of all Americans do not believe that the FDA should be able to classify vitamins, minerals, and herbs as drugs solely because the product makes a truthful health claim. . . . [S]ome 82% of the country feel that . . . [they] should not have to obtain a doctor's prescription to purchase those products."[18] The alliance placed magazine advertisements announcing a "coordinated effort [that] promises to be the most effective grass-roots lobbying campaign in history." If the current FDA proposals were enforced, the advertisements warned, "50% of all nutritional supplements will no longer be available to Americans within the next 12 to 18 months." Figure 22 shows one such advertisement.

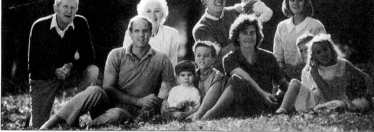

Fight for your family's rights

The FDA Is Once Again Attempting To Take Away Your Family's Right To Choose Safe And Beneficial Nutritional Supplements

Almost from its inception, the FDA has voiced AMA policy in attacking preventative health care and in particular, nutritional supplementation.

The results are 2 billion dollars a day in health care costs and millions of concerned Americans who cannot afford health insurance.

The American family with its back to the wall, is struggling to pay sky-rocketing health care costs. How anguished will they be when they discover that most of the pain, suffering and dollars spent might well have been avoided.

How is the FDA attempting to take away your family's nutritional rights?

§ If the current FDA and Congressional actions are passed and enforced, 50% of all nutritional supplements will no longer be available to Americans within the next 12 to 18 months. Indeed, your family's right to choose safe and beneficial nutritional supplements may cease to exist.

§ The FDA Task Force Report released in April may undermine the existing Proxmire Law, which protects nutritional supplements from overregulation by the FDA.

§ If HR 3642/S. 2135 are passed, the FDA will be empowered with police powers and the ability to levy heavy civil penalties that will be used indiscriminately against dietary supplements and force most health food stores out of business.

§ The new NLEA regulations give each of the 50 states the same enforcement powers as the FDA to also indiscriminately impose and enforce severe penalties against honest suppliers of quality nutritional supplements.

§ In preparation for increased enforcement activities, the FDA has hired 100 criminal investigators led by a 20-year veteran of the U.S. Secret Service. These new G-men will be unleashed on the supplement industry to enforce unwarranted restrictions designed to limit your access to preventative health care.

Protecting your health care rights

The Nutritional Health Alliance (NHA) is an organized coalition of manufacturers, retailers, health care professionals and concerned consumers who are committed to protecting your nutritional right to choose wellness over illness.

What the NHA is doing to protect your family's nutritional rights

▸ Preventing the FDA Task Force from undermining the Proxmire Law and attacking nutritional supplements such as herbs, amino acids and trace minerals.

▸ Lobbying against HR 3642/S. 2135 to prevent oppressive FDA police powers from destroying our country's nutritional supplement industry.

▸ Clarifying the NLEA regulations to guarantee your right to receive valid health claims and beneficial dosages of nutritional supplements.

▸ By supporting legislation to enhance the Proxmire Bill which will eliminate all present and future attacks on nutritional supplements.

▸ With your help, the NHA will organize the largest Congressional letter writing campaign in history. The FDA and Congress will see that the people's right to choose dietary supplements will once again continue to survive.

This coordinated effort promises to be the most effective grass-roots lobbying campaign in history, surpassing even the battles of the 70s which led to the passage of the Proxmire Law by a unanimous vote. The Proxmire Law is intended to prohibit the FDA from overregulating nutritional supplements.

• Tel: 516 249 7070 •

Nutritional Health Alliance

NHA

Protecting Your Right to Choose

What you can do to protect your family's nutritional right to choose wellness over illness!

Send your donations to the NHA to protect your family's nutritional rights. The NHA will send you information on key issues, a list of the key legislators who are against your nutritional rights and sample letters to help you influence these Congressmen to protect your rights.

❑ $20   ❑ $30   ❑ $40   ❑ $50   ❑ $100

Send your donations to:
Nutritional Health Alliance
P.O. Box 267, Farmingdale, NY 11735
THE NUTRITIONAL HEALTH ALLIANCE is a non-profit organization
Contributions may not be tax deductible.

FIGURE 22. Supplement manufacturers joined together to elicit popular support for industry opposition to the FDA's regulatory proposals. This advertisement from the now defunct Nutritional Health Alliance appeared in *Longevity* magazine in August 1992.

Although such information was misleading if not downright false, it helped to convince Senator Orrin Hatch (Rep-Utah) to introduce the Health Freedom Act of 1992, which would have blocked the FDA from using health claims as an excuse to regulate supplements as drugs. The senator was reported to have "entered the controversy after hearing from constituents in his home state, including both consumers and makers of dietary supplements" and to have concluded that the FDA "can put anybody out of business if they want to."[19] Although his bill did not get very far, it encouraged Congress to pass the Dietary Supplement Act of 1992; this act blocked the FDA from applying its forthcoming labeling rules for conventional foods to dietary supplements for another year—until the end of 1993. If, however, the final FDA rules allowed some health claims, supplement makers could use them immediately.

The Nutritional Health Alliance claimed credit for getting the bill passed and for giving the industry some additional time to organize opposition: "Working with Senator Orrin Hatch and Congressman Bill Richardson, we obtained a stay of execution from the FDA's efforts to overregulate, restrict and eliminate the dietary supplement industry. Congress was persuaded to extend the deadline for regulation for only one year, and that's all the time we are likely to get."[20]

In the midst of this furor over supplements, the FDA was contending with more than 47,000 comments filed on its proposed rules for food labeling. Because those proposals included rules for health claims that might apply to supplements as well as to foods, we need to turn now to the ways in which producers of conventional foods were putting their own kinds of pressures on the FDA.

WHITE HOUSE BLOCKS LABELING RULES, THEN RELENTS

The FDA intended to release revised final rules for food labeling by November 8, 1992, the deadline established by Congress when it passed the Nutrition Labeling and Education Act of 1990 (NLEA). In the byzantine way in which Congress does such things, the NLEA specified that if the FDA failed to meet that deadline, its proposed rules (the ones issued in conjunction with USDA) would go into effect unrevised.

Once again, political forces intervened, this time pressures from the USDA, which had not yet agreed to make its final rules for meat labels consistent with those of the FDA. Although USDA officials knew that meat and dairy foods were major sources of fat in American diets, they did not want package labels to suggest that consumers should eat less of those foods. An editorial in the *New York Times* said bluntly, "By blocking an overhaul of food labeling rules . . . Agriculture Secretary Edward Madigan put the interests of the meat industry ahead of the health of Americans."[21] Furthermore, the Philip Morris company wanted to be able to label its subsidiary Kraft cheese products as low in fat and asked the White House to prevent the FDA from doing anything that would block such claims.

Although the administration of President George Bush at first had been siding with the USDA, all parties concerned agreed that some compromise was in order. The food industry pressured the White House to concede so the rules would "get published once and for all." Bill Clinton had just won the presidential election, and if the rules did not get published before his administration took office, "months and months of litigation and uncertainty for food companies and consumers" were likely to ensue.[22] Once the FDA agreed to raise the limit on the amount of fat allowed in "low-fat" products, the Bush administration finally accepted the rules.

The final labeling rules appeared for public comment as an 875-page *Federal Register* notice on January 6, 1993. The criteria for scientific substantiation of health claims continued to be highly restrictive. The FDA would authorize only health claims supported by (1) published scientific evidence from (2) well-designed studies (3) conducted according to standard scientific procedures, evaluated with (4) significant agreement among (5) qualified experts.[23] On the basis of these criteria, the FDA proposed to authorize seven of the health claims mentioned in the NLEA regarding links between food components and specific diseases. Table 31 summarizes these initial NLEA claims and also lists subsequent claims authorized by the FDA through mid-2001.

One especially interesting feature of the food-labeling rules involved a loophole: the regulations allowed food companies to use the word "healthy" with few restrictions. Manufacturers could claim that jelly beans, for example, were healthy because they are low in fat and salt. FDA plugged that loophole by promulgating the so-called "jelly bean rule" to restrict use of the term *healthy* to foods low in fat and saturated fat, limited in sodium and cholesterol, and containing at least 10% of the recommended amount of at least one key nutrient: vitamin A, vitamin C, iron, calcium, protein, or fiber. Recognizing that this rule would encourage manufacturers to fortify foods to levels that would meet this definition of *healthy*, the FDA also developed a policy to prevent manufacturers from fortifying foods for the sole purpose of making that claim.[24] As

TABLE 31. Health claims authorized by the FDA for conventional foods and, in some cases, dietary supplements (*indicated in italics*)

NLEA health claims: authorized in 1993 in response to requirements of the Nutrition Labeling and Education Act of 1990

Food or *Supplement*	Health Claim Authorized
Fiber-containing fruits, vegetables, and grain products	Reduced risk of coronary heart disease
Fiber-containing grain products, fruits, and vegetables	Reduced risk of cancer
Fruits and vegetables	Reduced risk of cancer
Dietary saturated fat and cholesterol	Increased risk of coronary heart disease
Dietary fat	Increased risk of cancer
Calcium	Reduced risk of osteoporosis
Salt	Increased risk of hypertension
Folic Acid[a]	Reduced risk of neural tube birth defects

Health claims authorized subsequently in response to industry petitions or lawsuits

Date	Petitioner	Food or *Supplement*	Claim: Reduced Risk
1996	National Association of Chewing Gum Manufacturers	Dietary sugar alcohols	Tooth decay
1997	Quaker Oats Company	Dietary soluble fiber from whole oats	Coronary heart disease
1998	Kellogg	Dietary soluble fiber from psyllium seed husks	Coronary heart disease
1999	General Mills	Whole-grain foods[b]	Coronary heart disease and certain cancers
1999	Protein Technologies International (DuPont)	Soy protein	Coronary heart disease
2000	Lipton (Unilever): Take Control margarine	Plant sterol	Coronary heart disease
	McNeil Consumer Healthcare: Benecol margarine	Plant stanol esters	Coronary heart disease
	Tropicana	Potassium-containing foods[b]	High blood pressure and stroke
	Plaintiffs in *Pearson* v. *Shalala*	*Omega-3 fatty acid supplements*[c]	Coronary heart disease
2001	Plaintiffs in *Whitaker* v. *Thompson*	*Folic acid, vitamin B$_6$ and vitamin B$_{12}$ supplements*	Vascular disease
	Plaintiffs in *Pearson* v. *Thompson*	*Folic acid supplements (0.8 milligrams)*	Neural tube defects (more effective than lower amounts in food)

SOURCE: FDA. Online: http://vm.cfsan.fda.gov/. Accessed August 9, 2001.
[a]Approved for supplements later in 1993 and for foods in 1996.
[b]The FDA took no action on the petition within 120 days, thereby approving it by default as a claim based on authoritative statements.
[c]Approved as a "qualified" claim that must be accompanied by a detailed explanation.

we will see in the next section, the agency could not easily enforce this policy when manufacturers began adding herbal supplements to foods. In any case, the jelly bean rule prompted further objections. Even though the FDA had exempted fresh fruits and vegetables from the regulation, the National Food Processors Association objected that the rule would exclude foods such as green beans, raisins, and apple juice from being designated as healthy because their content of certain vitamins and minerals was not high enough.[25] The rule stuck, but the complaints continued.

As shown in Table 31, the food-labeling rules also affected dietary supplements. They permitted just one claim—that calcium supplements could reduce the risk of osteoporosis. Although the FDA had approved the other claims for foods, it refused to apply them to supplements. It also denied the remaining three claims specified in the NLEA: that antioxidant vitamins could reduce the risk of cancer, that zinc could improve immune function in the elderly, and that omega-3 fatty acids could reduce the risk of coronary heart disease. These claims, the agency said, failed to meet one or more of the five criteria for scientific substantiation noted above. These refusals sent a signal to the industry that the FDA would not easily authorize claims for supplements.

FDA ISSUES RULES, ELICITS BACKLASH: THE INDUSTRY MOBILIZES

With rules for food labels out of the way, the FDA turned its attention to supplements. In June 1993, it expanded its definition of supplements to include not just vitamins and minerals but also herbals, botanicals, and other such products. It continued to say that its rules for conventional foods also applied to supplements. It firmly disagreed with industry that this policy "would deny millions of Americans dietary information that they need to improve their health and thereby cost the nation millions of dollars in health care expenditures that could have been avoided."[26] In announcing the supplement-labeling proposals, FDA Commissioner David Kessler told a reporter that the industry was pushing hard for deregulation of its products but had not given "assurances that the products are appropriately manufactured, that what's on the label is actually in the bottle, that they bear adequate directions for use to insure safety or that basic safety data has been collected and reviewed."[27]

The Council for Responsible Nutrition immediately charged that the FDA's substantiation requirements were "biased, unnecessarily restrictive and would limit dissemination of scientific information."[28] The council demanded that the FDA create a new unit that would regulate these products separately, permit use of individual scientific articles as substantiation (rather than the totality of evidence evaluated by experts), and broaden the definition of nutritive value to include the role of supplements in protection against chronic as well as deficiency diseases. A lawyer for the supplement industry said that if the FDA proposals went into effect, its products would have to be taken off the market because health claims are "the lifeblood of the industry."[27]

Letters from supplement users—by the hundreds of thousands—poured into Congress and the FDA in what appeared to be a large and spontaneous consumer movement, which it most certainly was not. Instead, the protests had been orchestrated by supplement trade organizations, using "scare tactics to give cover to lobbyists and lawmakers in Congress trying to free the industry of government controls."[29] The Nutritional Health Alliance directed much of this campaign. The Alliance's "Campaign '93," for example, advertised, "Write to Congress today or kiss your vitamins goodbye! Can we stop the FDA this year? It's now or never. 1993—the year for nutritional freedom."[30]

The group took credit for the letters arriving on Capitol Hill and used them as evidence for the effectiveness of its efforts to educate consumers about "threats to the continued availability of dietary supplements." And well it might; its campaign set a new standard in grassroots organizing. The alliance sent displays about how to write to Congress to 1,500 General Nutrition Center stores, planned "blackout" days (during which stores shrouded supplements in black crepe and refused to sell them), mailed information packets to every member of Congress, provided retailers with personalized letters to sign and mail, printed 500,000 fliers to put in shopping bags, produced window banners, elicited letters from 50,000 mail-order customers, distributed videos to 400 television stations and audiotapes to 10,000 radio stations, and topped all this off by intensifying "its aggressive direct lobbying campaign on Capitol Hill."[31] Figure 23 shows one of the posters that was so effective in advertising this campaign.

As part of these efforts, the alliance had recruited a "team of lobbyists with ties to key lawmakers" and raised at least $80,000 in election funds for Senator Hatch, who continued to propose legislation drafted by the supplement industry. The senator was reported to have close ties of his own to supplement companies in his home state of Utah, to hold a small financial interest ($50,000 or less) in one firm, to have employed three aides who later took jobs as supplement industry lobbyists, to have raised

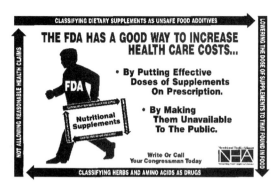

FIGURE 23. Industry groups distributed this poster to health food stores during the 1993 campaign to overturn the FDA's restrictions on health claims for dietary supplements. Posters like this encourged people to lobby Congress to protect their "constitutional rights" to take supplements.

$250,000 for a supplement trade group, and to have said that "Utah companies are dominant players in the supplement industry and . . . there's no senator alive who wouldn't want to do what he could for that industry."[29]

Other supplement industry groups also warned their members that the FDA wanted to limit access to the products. An industry group called the Health Freedom Task Force produced a television commercial featuring a well-known actor displayed as arrested and handcuffed, presumably by FDA enforcers, for possessing a bottle of vitamin C.[32] Although the FDA termed those images "absolutely false," its ongoing activities were not reassuring. The FDA had just conducted a survey of claims made for supplements sold in health food stores in which investigators asked leading (and perhaps entrapping) questions like these of store personnel: "I am feeling kind of weak, do you have anything to help fight infection or help my immune system?" "Do you have anything that works on cancer?" Of 129 such requests, 120 had elicited recommendations for specific products. The report of this investigation also listed many agency enforcement actions against supplements for which people had reported adverse reactions.[33] From 1989 to 1992, the FDA had taken 290 actions against supplement makers, most of them just warning letters. Among the actions, 250 were for making unsubstantiated "drug" claims and the others for reasons of safety or improper labeling, leading the FDA Commissioner to conclude that "the marketplace is awash with unsubstantiated claims. . . .

[W]e are literally back at the turn of the century when snake-oil salesmen made claims for their products that could not be substantiated."[34]

THE INDUSTRY'S "INCREDIBLE WAR" OVER FIRST AMENDMENT FREEDOMS

With the FDA position apparently locked in place, the supplement industry intensified its lobbying efforts. In October 1993, the FDA offered one compromise; it proposed to authorize a health claim that supplements of folic acid could reduce the risk of neural tube defects.[35] The agency seemed unlikely to be setting a precedent favorable to the supplement industry, however, because its stringent substantiation requirements for claims were about to become law. The Dietary Supplement Act of 1992 had granted supplements a one-year exemption from labeling rules applied to foods, but this extension was due to expire on December 15, 1993. When Congress did not pass any of the introduced dietary supplement bills by the end of 1993, the rules for labeling of conventional foods automatically applied to supplements, and the industry would have to follow those rules starting in June 1994. This meant that health claims for supplements—other than the two approved for calcium and folic acid—would have to be authorized in advance by the FDA and shown to meet each term of the substantiation criteria that applied to conventional foods.

In December board members of the Council for Responsible Nutrition met with FDA officials to "underscore the need for a one-year extension of the effective date on . . . labeling regulations and the necessity to revise the agency's proposed rules." The council's president said its members believed that "FDA sees the need to be responsive to our concerns . . . and we will continue to work to get our member company's [sic] views accepted." The council informed its membership that it would continue to work with members of Congress to obtain legislation that "fully addresses the concerns of the dietary supplement industry."[36]

Senator Hatch also continued to take the lead in developing legislation to block the FDA's restrictions on supplement health claims which, in his view, had caused this

> incredible war over our First Amendment freedoms. . . . [A]t issue is the right of millions of Americans to products that have been used safely for millennia. On one side is a tenacious bureaucracy, the Food and Drug Administration (FDA), which by most accounts has shown a 30+ year animosity to dietary

supplements. . . . [O]n the other side are 65 United States senators, 240 representatives, and a legion of citizen activists who are united behind the Dietary Supplement Health and Education Act . . . which will protect their right to unrestricted access to dietary supplements and information about their positive health benefits.[37]

The senator viewed as "frightening" FDA's 1993 supplement-labeling proposals; he said they meant that "purchase of high potency vitamins and minerals should be limited, access to herbal products should be restricted, and amino acids should be available only by prescription." The senator surely knew better—the proposals suggested doing so only when the products were labeled with unauthorized health claims—but he said, "If we let the FDA get away with this, next time it will be even easier for the agency to overregulate another industry. . . . You have to wonder what interests the FDA is protecting when it holds up the regulatory shield to block the public from receiving potentially life-saving information in the name of good science."[37]

Consumer groups, on the other hand, viewed the proposed supplement bills as placing "an intolerable burden on the general public to ferret out reliable scientific information from unreliable marketing hype and worse." Interestingly, the food industry also opposed the early versions of the legislation on the grounds that supplements and foods should be permitted to "compete on a level playing field" without a "double standard based on whether a nutrient is added to a processed food or sold as a dietary supplement."[38]

SUPPLEMENT INDUSTRY WINS DSHEA; FDA COMPROMISES

These arguments continued into the next year, until Congress passed DSHEA and the President signed it into law on October 25, 1994. Industry officials hailed the bill as a "move forward for the 100 million consumers who rely on dietary supplements . . . and the millions more who could benefit from these products. . . . [We were] happy we were able to get the bill through Congress this year. . . . We achieved most of our legislative goals."[39] DSHEA passed when the FDA agreed to a compromise; the agency would now permit structure/function statements for supplements just like the ones the industry had proposed a decade earlier. Unauthorized claims that a product could prevent or treat a disease, however, would still cause products to be regulated as drugs. The *New York Times* called DSHEA a "retreat for the FDA" and noted how few issues during that congressional session "generated as much grass-roots emotion, largely because the supplement industry waged a well-financed scare campaign that had many health-minded Americans convinced, wrongly, that the Food and Drug Administration was about to ban these popular products. . . . [T]he compromise measure . . . is probably the best that could be hoped for given widespread congressional support for weaker, industry-backed legislation."[40]

During the following year, industry groups pressed for removal of the remaining restrictions on health claims as "burdensome" and a "disincentive." They asked Congress to enact further legislation to compel the FDA to use the truthful-and-not-misleading substantiation approach of the Federal Trade Commission (FTC). They also continued to find grounds for challenging the FDA in the courts.

Such demands were supported by the report of a "dialog" among about 40 industry and government leaders and a sprinkling of academics and consumer advocates who met from 1993 to 1995 to reach consensus on the best ways to use health claims to promote sales of foods that "advance health." From the outset, this group assumed that health claims were beneficial. With this assumption, and with at least half of the participants having overt ties to the food industry, the group's consensus predictably favored a more "responsive" interpretation of scientific standards by the FDA, greater opportunities for food companies to make health claims, and public–private partnerships to "assist and encourage the food industry in the creative use of dietary guidance tools . . . in labeling and advertising."[41] Such recommendations supported the supplement industry's agenda.

The Commission on Dietary Supplement Labels also supported a more flexible standard for scientific substantiation of health claims. The commission, which had been established under a specific provision of DSHEA, met from 1995 to 1997 to recommend ways to implement the bill's provisions. According to its report, the existing FDA standard "serves the public interest . . . [but] should not be so strictly interpreted as to require unanimous or near-unanimous support. FDA should ensure that broad input is obtained to ascertain the degree of scientific agreement that exists for a particular health claim. The use of appropriate panels of qualified scientists from outside of the agency is encouraged, and the views of other government agencies should be given considerable weight in determining whether significant scientific agreement exists."[42]

CONGRESS ALLOWS HEALTH CLAIMS
FOR FOODS: FDAMA, 1997

Three years after approving DSHEA, Congress passed another law that indirectly affected health claims for dietary supplements, the FDA Modernization Act of 1997 (FDAMA). The main purpose of this legislation was to speed up FDA's approval processes for drugs and devices, but one provision addressed health claims for foods. It required the FDA to authorize nutrient-content and health claims for conventional foods whenever such claims were substantiated by (1) an authoritative statement (2) currently in effect (3) published (4) by a U.S. government scientific body or the National Academy of Sciences.[43] Under FDAMA, the FDA had to deal with petitions for health claims within 120 days; if it missed the deadline, the claim would automatically be authorized. Thus a July 1999 advertisement by General Mills that "The FDA agrees that eating whole grain foods like Cheerios, Wheaties and Total . . . may reduce your risk of heart disease and some cancers" is not precisely correct. All that is certain is that FDA chose not to deal with the claim within the allowed time period.[44] Table 31 summarizes this and other claims subsequently authorized, some of which apply to supplements.

Given congressional intent, the FDA had little choice but to apply the provisions of FDAMA to supplements as well as to foods. Thus supplement makers requesting authorization of a health claim also would need to notify the FDA 120 days in advance and include documents demonstrating that the claim met the substantiation criteria. They would then be free to use the claim, *unless* the FDA—within the 120-day period—issued an "interim final regulation" prohibiting its use or filed a lawsuit.[45] The FDA interpreted congressional intent to mean that it should continue to apply science-based standards to the definition of "authoritative statements" and should require manufacturers to document that claims reflected (1) consensus, (2) deliberative review of the scientific evidence, and (3) significant scientific agreement.

Holding supplements to even these standards soon embroiled the agency in new disputes. In 1998 the FDA explained how it intended to apply the standards to dietary supplements when it proposed rules to help manufacturers distinguish permissible structure/function claims from prohibited disease claims. The FDA proposed to deny claims implying that a supplement could have a beneficial effect on a disease, condition, symptom, or response to a stage of life (such as menopause)—a stricter definition than that allowed by DSHEA. Industry officials found such distinctions illogical: "FDA's attempt to separate the symptoms of a disease from the disease itself falls short, raising more questions than it answers."[46] Other groups were even less restrained; an industry-supported "Save DSHEA" campaign hoped to generate 100,000 letters criticizing the latest proposals.

Just 2 months later, within the prescribed 120-day waiting period, the FDA denied a petition from Weider Nutrition International to authorize nine health claims that the company wanted to use to market its omega-3 fatty acid, garlic, and nutritional products. According to the FDA, the proposed claims did not meet one or another element of FDAMA or of the agency's substantiation criteria. For example, the FDA rejected the claim that "antioxidants are thought to help prevent heart attack, stroke and cancer" because the statement came from a USDA research announcement, not from a *deliberative* USDA review. It rejected another claim, that "calcium consumption by adolescents and adults increases bone density and may decrease the risk of fractures," because calcium increases bone density only in adolescents (in adults it reduces bone loss) and because "risk of fractures" is not equivalent to osteoporosis or to fractures related to osteoporosis.[47]

Such a precise interpretation of the criteria was certain to be perceived by the industry as nit-picking and to reinforce its suspicions that the FDA would continue to hold health claims to the letter of the law regardless of congressional demands for greater flexibility. In particular, critics now accused the FDA of undermining the intent of DSHEA as well as of FDAMA. Early in 1999, the House Committee on Government Reform held hearings on precisely this point: "DSHEA: Is the FDA trying to change the intent of Congress?" In his opening statement, the committee chairman, Dan Burton (Rep-IN), explained that Congress clearly intended DSHEA to give Americans more open access to supplements: "The American people demanded to be heard on this issue and Congress listened to them. More letters and faxes were received on this topic than any other single piece of legislation in history."[48] These hearings also were notable for the appearance of the actress Raquel Welch, who testified on behalf of the National Nutritional Foods Association against the proposed rules.

THE COURTS INTERVENE: *PEARSON V. SHALALA*

As indicated in the previous chapter, the next step in the recurring cycles of supplement regulation is to take the FDA to court. The industry's most impressive court victory was a challenge to the FDA's "significant scientific agreement" standard in the landmark case *Pearson* v. *Shalala*. In the words of the 1999 appeals court,

> dietary supplement marketers Durk Pearson and Sandy Shaw, presumably hoping to bolster sales by increasing the allure of their supplement's labels, asked the FDA to authorize four separate health claims . . . (1) consumption of antioxidant vitamins may reduce the risk of certain kinds of cancers, (2) consumption of fiber may reduce the risk of colorectal cancer, (3) consumption of omega-3 fatty acids may reduce the risk of coronary heart disease, (4) .8 mg of folic acid in a dietary supplement is more effective in reducing the risk of neural tube defects than a lower amount in foods of common form.[49]

Pearson and Shaw were supported by an organization of health professionals who use supplements in their practice and by Citizens for Health, a group of proponents of supplements. Citizens for Health was represented in the case by the chairman of its board, Jim Turner, a lawyer with a decades-long career opposing FDA policies on supplement regulation; he was the author in 1970 of *The Chemical Feast* (Penguin edition, 1976), a report by Ralph Nader's group that was highly critical of those policies.

On appeal, the court ruled that lack of support for "significant scientific agreement" was no reason to deny a health claim. Such a denial would be unconstitutional on First Amendment (freedom-of-speech) grounds: The phrase lacked "definitional content." The court called the FDA's requirements for scientific substantiation "almost frivolous" and ruled that "it simply will not do for a government agency to declare—without explanation—that a proposed course of private action is not approved." Furthermore, the court chided the FDA for its unsound and "simplistic view of human nature or market behavior" in arguing that health claims might mislead consumers. Such concerns, it ruled, could easily be handled through use of a disclaimer on the package label. This decision cleared the way for less restrictive rules on health claims for supplements and encouraged makers of conventional foods to insist that *Pearson* v. *Shalala* meant that they were entitled to precisely the same First Amendment rights.

Also in 1999 a Utah court interpreted DSHEA to mean *unambiguously* that dietary supplements are to be regulated as foods, not drugs, and that they can be sold even when they contain active ingredients identical to those in prescription drugs. In *Pharmanex* v. *Shalala*, the court ruled that the FDA had no right to restrict sales of Cholestin, a "milled red yeast rice" supplement, even though it contained a chemical indistinguishable from lovastatin, the active ingredient in cholesterol-lowering prescription drugs.[50] Although such cases and others in progress were sure to be interminably litigated, they suggested that the supplement industry had achieved an environment in which *all* policies for health claims—whether for conventional foods or dietary supplements, for labels or advertising—would be forced by Congress or the courts to converge toward the less scientifically demanding approach of the FTC.

THE "TENACIOUS BUREAUCRACY" CONCEDES

By this time, the FDA had little choice but to compromise its science-based approach. In January 1999, the agency announced program priorities for the coming year, with supplement claims high on the agenda. The FDA held meetings to solicit public input on how supplement labels could make claims that were truthful and not misleading, and it produced a guide for the food and supplement industries to explain just what was meant by the term *significant scientific agreement*. This guide, based on a report to the FDA from its Food Advisory Committee, is remarkable for its length (18 pages of single-spaced text), complexity, and impenetrability. In addressing inherent problems of nutrition research—that studies vary in methods and reliability, are confounded by behavioral and environmental factors (such as cigarette smoking, level of education, and poverty), require judgment in interpretation, and hardly ever yield unambiguous results—the FDA then defined *significant scientific agreement* as an apparent tautology:

> Significant scientific agreement refers to the extent of agreement among qualified experts in the field. In the process of scientific discovery, significant scientific agreement occurs well *after* the stage of emerging science, where data and information permit an inference, but before the point of unanimous agreement within the relevant scientific community that the inference is valid. The . . . standard is met when the validity of the relationship is not likely to be reversed by new and evolving science, although the exact nature of the relationship may need to be refined over time.[51]

The FDA seemed to be saying that it would consider the evidence for each product on a case-by-case basis and would give greatest weight to claims supported by federal advisory committees such as that appointed to review the *Dietary Guidelines*. If so, the FDA would have difficulty dealing with health claims that were not covered by the *Dietary Guidelines*, such as those that had been litigated in *Pearson* v. *Shalala*.

In September 1999, the FDA announced that it would begin complying with the decision in *Pearson* and was seeking information about scientific studies to substantiate claims such as those linking supplements of antioxidant nutrients to reduced risk of cancer, or omega-3 fatty acids and reduced risk of coronary heart disease. In November the agency denied health claims that had been filed by plaintiffs in *Pearson v. Shalala* and another linking saw palmetto (an herbal supplement) to reduced risk for benign prostate disease. It also denied a claim linking supplements of vitamins B_6 and B_{12} to reduced risk of vascular disease. These denials caught the attention of Representative Peter DeFazio (Dem-OR), who complained that the FDA "may not with impunity deny or delay fulfillment of the First Amendment obligations defined in *Pearson*."[52] A group of scientists who conduct research on heart disease weighed in to support a claim for omega-3 fatty acids, as did an association of makers of fish meal and oils, arguing that "if the FDA wants to show that they respect the scientific community more than the political community," the agency should authorize this claim, which, they said, was supported by rigorous clinical trials.[53] Greater pressures on the FDA to authorize a wider range of health claims could only be expected.

The FDA launched the new millennium in January 2000 by outlining a 10-year plan for implementing the provisions of DSHEA and the requirements of *Pearson v. Shalala,* a plan "built on the 'twin pillars' of law and science." The plan stated that by 2010, the FDA would have in place a science-based regulatory system that would provide the public "with a high level of confidence in the safety, composition, and labeling of dietary supplement products." In response to this plan, Representative David McIntosh (Rep-IN) asked the FDA to "please explain why it will take 16 years [from the 1994 DSHEA to 2010] to implement *Pearson*, when the court held that FDA's health claims policy suppresses free speech protected by the First Amendment."[54]

Also in January 2000, the FDA issued final rules for structure/function claims for dietary supplements. Writing this notice must have been a thoroughly miserable experience. The FDA had received more than 235,000 comments on the proposed rules, many of them as form letters, but at least 22,000 from individuals. Nearly all of the industry comments said that the FDA was unnecessarily restricting health claims, whereas the comments from health groups argued that the rules were not nearly restrictive enough. The FDA's compromise was to permit structure/function claims—provided that they did not imply that the product could diagnose, mitigate, treat, cure, or prevent a disease, terms taken to mean "damage to an organ, part, structure, or system of the body such that it does not function properly" Thus the FDA was backing off from the more encompassing definition it had proposed earlier. In a clear concession to the industry, the agency said that it would not object to structure/

function claims for "common conditions associated with natural states or processes that do not cause significant or permanent harm." This meant that supplement makers could now legally claim their products were beneficial for a whole host of mild conditions: hot flashes, menstrual symptoms, the mild losses of memory, hair, and sexual function associated with aging, and—most controversially—the morning sickness that can accompany pregnancy.[55]

Some advocacy groups were outraged that the FDA would allow such claims and considered the action a "snake-oil exemption . . . a complete cave-in to industry."[56] In response to strenuous objections from leading experts in birth defects that structure/function claims might encourage pregnant women to take potentially dangerous supplements, the FDA quickly issued a statement advising supplement makers "not to make any claims related to pregnancy on their products," announced public meetings to discuss safety concerns, and urged "all pregnant women to consult their health care provider before taking any dietary supplements or medication."[57] As for industry, its representatives either applauded the FDA's ruling on structure/function statements or complained that the agency had not conceded nearly enough: "Through bureaucratic encroachment, they're going to rob the structure/function claim of its validity. . . . [I]t's just an outrageous power grab really . . . the First Amendment is supreme law, not the agency's regulations."[58]

The FDA's ongoing struggles to maintain scientific integrity in the face of pressures from the industry, Congress, the courts and, presumably, the public are best illustrated by its dealings with requests for supplement health claims. In October 2000, the agency issued a "letter" announcing a new dimension in health claims—a "qualified" claim in which supplement producers could link omega-3 fatty acids (the "good" fats from fish oils and some plants) to reduced risk of coronary heart disease. In a 36-page review of research on omega-3 fats and health, the FDA concluded that use of such supplements was safe and lawful, but that the weight of the evidence required the label to include this qualification: "The scientific evidence about whether omega-3 fatty acids may reduce the risk of coronary heart disease (CHD) is suggestive, but not conclusive. Studies in the general population have looked at diets containing fish and it is not known whether diets or omega-3 fatty acids in fish may have a possible effect on a reduced risk of CHD. It is not known what effect omega-3 fatty acids may or may not have on risk of CHD in the general population."[59]

From a scientific standpoint, this statement is a balanced summary of the current state of knowledge. From a marketing standpoint, however, it is hard to imagine how it might fit on a supplement label, let alone whether anyone might read or understand it. Perhaps for this reason, toward the end of 2000 the FDA gave a million dollars to the Institute of Medicine to develop a scientific framework to help the agency evaluate the role of dietary supplements in health.

Although the FDA's plan for 2001 also kept health claims for dietary supplements on its "A list" for action, it seemed doubtful that the "incredible war" would soon end, not least because the courts were so sympathetic to suits related to *Pearson v. Shalala*. The *Pearson* legal team sought and won separate court actions forcing the FDA to permit claims that supplements of folic acid, vitamin B_6, and vitamin B_{12} could reduce the risk of vascular disease, and that "0.8 milligrams of folic acid in a dietary supplement is more effective in reducing the risk of neural tube defects than a lower amount in common form." In this last case, "*Pearson II*," the judge announced that "the philosophy underlying *Pearson I* is perfectly clear: that the First Amendment analysis . . . applies in this case, and that if a health claim is not inherently misleading, the balance tilts in favor of disclaimers rather than suppression. . . . [T]he FDA has again refused to accept the reality and finality of that conclusion."[60] With such enthusiastic encouragement, the *Pearson* plaintiffs could be expected to litigate any claim denied by the FDA, one after another.

IN THE WAKE OF DSHEA: THE CYCLES CONTINUE

While the supplement industry continued to press the FDA for more lenient regulations, mainstream publications began looking more seriously at the consequences of DSHEA. Late in 1998, for example, the *New England Journal of Medicine* published several accounts of people who had become ill as a result of taking herbal supplements, along with an editorial scathing in its criticism of such unscientific practices:

> We see a reversion to irrational approaches to medical practice, even while scientific medicine is making some of its most dramatic advances. . . . Since [DSHEA] these products have flooded the market, subject only to the scruples of their manufacturers. They may contain the substances listed on the label in the amounts claimed, but they need not . . . labeling has risen to an art form of double-speak. . . . It is time for the scientific community to stop giving alternative medicine a free ride. There cannot be two kinds of medicine—conventional and alternative. There is only medicine that has been adequately tested and medicine that has not, medicine that works and medicine that may or may not work.[61]

The *New York Times* agreed and called on Congress to "revisit its ill-advised decision in 1994 to insulate pills and powders sold as 'dietary supplements' from Federal regulation." Noting that "an industry-financed scare campaign convinced health-minded Americans that the Food and Drug Administration was about to ban conventional vitamins and other popular products from supermarket shelves," the *Times* continued, "Many in Congress may be unwilling to challenge the political power of the supplement industry. . . . But surely Congress can find a way to let . . . vitamins remain on the market while reinstating the F.D.A.'s power to require systematic testing of more exotic or risky products."[62]

In response, an industry group called the Corporate Alliance for Integrative Medicine announced itself "alarmed and concerned" about the newspaper's "disservice to its subscribers and the public."[63] It joined other industry groups in a $5 million public relations campaign to create the Dietary Supplement Education Alliance to "put a positive face on the industry." "Without this public relations offensive," explained the Alliance's chairman, "product sales will further erode to dangerous levels due to an onslaught of mainstream news media stories that say the industry is unregulated and question the efficacy and safety of many of its products." As another industry spokesman put the matter, "You can never let your guard down. . . . It's never over. Even if you win, it's still not over."[64]

The director of the supplement industry's Council for Responsible Nutrition also recognized the high-profile commentaries as a new challenge: "Given the ever louder anti-DSHEA drumbeats, we must recognize that the law may not last forever." To meet the challenge, he said, the industry would need to be vigilant in policing itself: "We no longer can remain silent when maverick companies market untested new ingredients, make unproven or overstated claims, and use inadequate quality controls. We must ensure that any ingredient we market is safe. . . . We must adequately substantiate all claims we make. And we must be sure that what's on the label is what's in the bottle."[65]

For the moment, the supplement industry had won just about all of the concessions it had so long been seeking. It had succeeded in removing the government from any meaningful control over its products. Now it would have to police irresponsible companies or risk repeal of DSHEA. Thus the long-sought deregulation of dietary supplements had consequences—some expected, others less so. The next chapter examines some of these consequences and their risks and benefits to the public.

CHAPTER 12

DEREGULATION AND
ITS CONSEQUENCES

FOLLOWING ENACTMENT OF THE DIETARY SUPPLEMENT
Health and Education Act of 1994 (DSHEA), the results of its lowest-common-denominator regulatory approach were apparent almost immediately. Most evident was the remarkable growth of the supplement industry; this, of course, had been the point of the industry's efforts in pushing for the legislation. As this chapter relates, however, DSHEA led to additional consequences, some intentional and some unintentional. Food companies seeking similar increases in growth began to produce supplement-enhanced foods that could be marketed using health, nutrient-content, and structure/function claims. Pharmaceutical companies began adding herbal and vitamin supplements to over-the-counter drugs. Furthermore, companies attempted to position both foods and drugs as *supplements*, expressly to take advantage of the more relaxed regulatory requirements for health claims on those products. The ability of the Food and Drug Administration (FDA) to respond to this situation was severely compromised as it was flooded by requests for review or authorization of claims, was overwhelmed by legal requirements to respond quickly, and was heavily challenged by the lawsuits that inevitably resulted when it denied a petition. As health claims proliferated, public concerns about the composition, safety, and efficacy of supplements increased, as did public confusion about diet and health. Finally, DSHEA further polarized the gulf between people who viewed supplements as useful even without proof of efficacy and those who wanted supplements held to science-based standards.

STIMULATING AN EXPLOSION IN SALES

There seems little question that DSHEA achieved industry objectives; it helped stimulate investment in dietary supplements. In the first 5 years after its enactment, supplement sales in the United States grew from $4 billion to nearly $15 billion, with herbals alone earning $4 billion. Sales of dietary supplements, as pills and as added to foods, were expected to exceed $30 billion by the year 2005 and to reach $49 billion by 2010. Worldwide, the market for supplements was nearly $40 billion in 1997, with herbals accounting for nearly $17 billion of that amount. Herbal supplements were a particularly good investment; their sales increased by 18–20% annually during the late 1990s according to one source, and by 269% from 1996 to 1999 according to another. Such growth rates greatly exceed the 10–12% annual increase for nutritional supplements—and both exceed the 1% growth rate typical of conventional foods.[1] Figure 24 shows some examples of supplements readily available at any local drugstore early in 2001.

Prior to DSHEA, investment in herbal and botanical supplements had been largely restricted to small, local health food stores. With such encouraging increases in sales, mainstream pharmaceutical companies—American Home Products, Bayer, and Warner-Lambert, for example—began investing in these products and selling them through mass-market channels. Pharmaceutical companies tended to pick supplements that were backed by at least some scientific evidence of safety and efficacy and to use drug-level quality-control methods to ensure more consistent composition, thereby adding a bit of respectability to an otherwise marginalized market. The relaxed rules for health claims allowed supplement marketers to target messages to the specific concerns of the 80 million "baby boomers" who, as they reached middle age, became even more interested in self-care, more distrustful of conventional medicine, and more resentful of the increasingly impersonal nature of the managed care health system.

MARKETING FOODS AND DRUGS AS SUPPLEMENTS

In addition to providing a bonanza for supplement makers, DSHEA also led to a blurring of the distinctions among foods, supplements, and drugs. As we shall see in Part V, major food companies began to invest heavily in research and development of products designed just so that they could be marketed using health claims. Food companies viewed the entire category of nutritionally enhanced foods (inconsistently termed

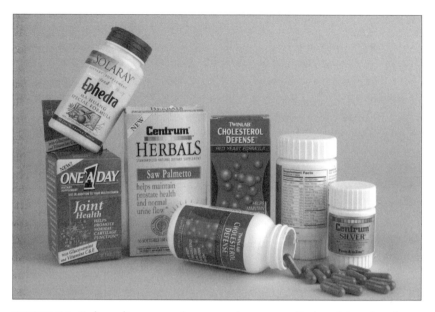

FIGURE 24. By law, dietary supplement packages may display claims that the products support body structure or function. These supplements are labeled with claims for promotion of normal cartilage function, prostate health, and healthy cholesterol levels. The "Silver" product implies special benefits for older adults. The Ephedra package gives no information about its purpose; presumably, its buyers know what it is supposed to do for them. (Photo by Enrique Caballo, 2001)

designer foods, functional foods, nutraceuticals, or—as I like to call them—techno-foods) as an unparalleled opportunity to achieve growth rates for food products as impressive as those for supplements. The new food products included not only the familiar vitamin-enriched breakfast cereals but also such innovations as tortilla chips supplemented with St. John's Wort and calcium-supplemented chocolates. The only conceivable explanation for development of such products was to present them as dietary supplements so that they could be marketed using health claims. By the time DSHEA was enacted, health claims were well understood as an effective stimulant to sales.[2]

Food companies understood the decision in *Pearson* v. *Shalala* (discussed in the previous chapter) to mean that the same permissive rules about health claims that applied to supplements also should be applied to foods as well. If so, food companies could market a product as a dietary supplement and avoid difficult approval processes for new ingredients. They could use structure/function claims, and they could list herbal and other non-nutrient constituents on product labels even if the amounts of these ingredients were too small to have any noticeable health benefit. The labeling rules for supplements require the "Supplement Facts" label to list nutrients the same way they might appear on food labels. Other individual dietary ingredients (such as herbs or phytochemicals) must be listed by weight, but mixtures of herbal substances may be listed by the weight of the total blend, not by the amounts of their separate ingredients. Even more, the label does not have to compare the amounts of herbs that are present to doses known to be effective, a regulatory omission that is a great advantage when the quantities of "active" ingredients are infinitesimal. With such advantages, it is understandable why the Grocery Manufacturers of America threatened its own lawsuit to force the FDA to grant food companies the right to use health claims that had been won for dietary supplements in *Pearson* court decisions.[3]

Drug companies also were eager to enter the food-as-supplement market because they could sell foods with "therapeutic" benefits without having to go through lengthy and expensive drug-approval processes. As I explain in the next chapter, a division of Johnson & Johnson developed a cholesterol-lowering margarine, Benecol, and planned to market it as a dietary supplement. When the FDA balked at this strategy, the company successfully petitioned to have Benecol approved as a food considered GRAS—generally recognized as safe. When drug companies began taking advantage of this new marketing niche by adding vitamins to aspirin and other over-the-counter drugs, the FDA had to warn them not to do so until the agency had reviewed the regulatory status of such products.[4]

Other products also crossed the line between supplements and drugs. A product called Cholestin, for example, contains an extract of milled rice fermented with red yeast; this food has been used in East Asia for more than 2,000 years as a colorant, flavor enhancer, and herbal remedy. In the United States, however, Cholestin is sold as a capsule. In a study funded in part by its manufacturer, investigators found the product's active ingredients to include at least nine compounds that inhibit cholesterol biosynthesis in the body, thereby lowering the level of cholesterol in blood.[5] Because one of these compounds is virtually identical to lovastatin, a prescription drug approved for cholesterol lowering since 1987, the FDA understandably viewed Cholestin as a drug and moved to prevent further importation of red yeast rice. As noted in the previous chapter, the courts overruled this action in *Pharmanex* v. *Shalala* and allowed

Cholestin to be sold as a dietary supplement (although a federal court later overturned this decision).

Researchers have confirmed that Cholestin reduces blood cholesterol levels by about 10%, but they note that it is formulated to contain higher levels of active ingredients than traditional red yeast rice. As a prescription drug, lovastatin has been studied extensively, but hardly any research has been done on the eight other cholesterol-lowering ingredients in Cholestin. Marketed as a dietary supplement, Cholestin may contain ingredients present in prescription drugs, and its manufacturer does not have to adhere to the quality, safety, or testing standards for such drugs. Consequently, it can be priced well below its prescription counterpart. Early in 2001, I bought 50 capsules of the "cholesterol defense" red yeast formula shown in Figure 24 for $10.69. At the recommended dose of 4 capsules per day, a month's supply would cost about $27, a considerable savings over the $120–$350 that taking prescription lovastatin would cost.[6] Whether Cholestin offers any other advantages is uncertain, because makers of supplements are not required to reveal doses or side effects. Given this situation, it is understandable that drug companies might want to compete with such "supplements" by advertising their own products directly to the public and claiming benefits that federal agencies might otherwise consider false or misleading. In short, as a result of DSHEA, both food and drug manufacturers now demand the same regulatory advantages as those granted to producers of supplements.

DISCOURAGING ENFORCEMENT

Supplement deregulation thoroughly preoccupies FDA staff, who must write proposed, interim, and final rules; respond to thousands—and sometimes hundreds of thousands—of public comments; deal with requests for new health claims; monitor announcements of structure/ function claims; and address legal challenges. As just one example, the FDA filed 23 *Federal Register* notices related exclusively to supplement regulation, many of them quite detailed, just from April 1995 to September 1997.[7] Structure/function notifications alone create much work. From late 1994 to late 1998, supplement companies filed information on more than a thousand claims for products designed to improve mental health or relaxation, to increase energy, to improve cholesterol levels and cardiovascular function, to improve digestion, to boost the immune system, or to prevent colds, allergies, and infections. The FDA wrote "courtesy" letters objecting to about one-fourth of these claims. In a few cases, it issued warnings against products that seemed demonstrably dangerous, and occasionally it asked companies to issue a recall.[8]

Since DSHEA, however, the FDA has not banned a single supplement—not even the few products it believes harmful. The legislation traps the agency in an impossible situation. On the one hand, the FDA is strongly criticized for failing to respond promptly to adverse effects associated with supplements. On the other hand, Congress, annoyed with the FDA's strict regulatory approach to drugs and tobacco as well as to supplements, has reduced the agency's autonomy and funding levels to the point where its resources are demonstrably inadequate for the work it is expected to perform. Although the FDA's budget was about a billion dollars in 2001, Congress had earmarked most of that amount for specific programs, and its entire allocation for dietary supplement regulation included just $6 million and fewer than five full-time employees. Employees, exhausted by relentless pressures from members of Congress or their staff, leave the agency in droves, further depleting its resources. Even if it were accorded adequate funding, the FDA would have difficulty performing the kinds of analytical research needed for determining supplement safety, because the methods that are useful for testing and evaluating nutrient supplements do not apply to most herbals and botanicals, and methods specific to those products are still being developed.[9]

Perhaps because it bears considerable responsibility for so severely undermining the FDA's regulatory authority, the supplement industry is beginning to recognize that overburdening the agency may be counterproductive to industry interests. Dr. Annette Dickinson, the vice president for scientific and regulatory affairs at the supplement trade association, the Council for Responsible Nutrition (CRN), testified to this effect before a congressional committee in March 1999: "DSHEA is working. It could work even better if FDA has sufficient resources to complete some of its remaining obligations under DSHEA. . . . FDA does not have adequate staff or other resources to properly evaluate the adverse event reports. . . . This puts every company at risk of being held 'guilty until proven innocent' without investigation."[10]

The situation is not much better at the Federal Trade Commission (FTC). Although the FTC's stated policy is to defer to FDA's standards for scientific substantiation of claims, and although it has filed hundreds of actions against dietary supplements over the years, it took action against just eight supplement makers in 1998. Apparently, a product must be as egregiously fraudulent as "Vitamin O," a supplement of bottled seawater marketed as a disease treatment, before the FTC will issue one of its rare injunctions. The FTC does send electronic-mail warnings to firms that make "incredible" claims; by early 1999 it had sent 1,200 such messages. The agency also conducts "health claims surf days" during which it reviews Internet advertisements. So many Web sites promote unproven remedies, however, that the agency does not have the resources necessary to investigate more than a tiny fraction of them. This explains the rare cooperation between the FTC and the FDA on "Operation Cure All," a joint campaign that began in 2001 to enforce rules against fraudulent claims made for supplements and other products marketed on the Internet. Two of the earliest actions were against companies promoting St. John's Wort as a treatment for tuberculosis, influenza, and other infectious diseases that were unlikely to be cured by this herb.[11]

ELICITING CONCERNS OVER SAFETY AND EFFICACY

In the absence of firm regulation, the proliferation of supplements and of the claims for them has heightened concerns about safety and efficacy and has subjected the products to increasing scrutiny. Most concerns focus on supplements other than vitamins and minerals, but even these common nutritional products have been subject to questions about whether they are needed or cause harm in excessive amounts.

Vitamin and Mineral Supplements

Supplement trade associations go to great lengths to defend the safety of vitamins and minerals over a wide range of doses, arguing that nutrients rarely produce adverse effects except when consumed at exceedingly high levels.[12] Taking single nutrients in moderately high doses may not be a good idea, however. Because many different nutrients are involved in every aspect of human physiology, high doses of just one nutrient can create imbalances that adversely affect the absorption or metabolism of other nutrients. The potential for high doses of vitamins A and D to induce toxic symptoms, for example, has been a source of concern for decades and was a principal reason for the FDA's historical interest in controlling the doses of supplements.

More recently, clinical trials of cancer prevention using supplements of beta-carotene (a precursor of vitamin A found in many brightly colored fruits and vegetables) further illustrate the hazards of taking high doses of single nutrients. Because previous clinical trials revealed that cigarette smokers who ate diets rich in fruits and vegetables had lower rates of lung cancer, researchers thought that beta-carotene might be responsible for cancer protection. They compared the effects of a high-dose beta-carotene supplement against those of a placebo in men who smoked cigarettes. To their dismay, the men who took the supplements had *more* lung cancers than those who took placebos.[13] Although the supplement industry argued that the results applied only to people who smoked cigarettes, most observers interpreted the trial results as confirming the potential hazards of consuming single nutrients in high doses. The results also were interpreted as demonstrating the health advantages of consuming foods—not supplements.

In 1997 the *New York Times* columnist Jane Brody summarized these and other potential hazards of the excessive intake of vitamin and mineral supplements. Apparently, the idea that nutritional supplements might produce adverse effects was *news*. In a *Time* magazine interview, Ms. Brody said, "My major hope was to awaken the public to the fact that vitamins and other supplements are not always innocent. . . . [T]oo many people are taking huge doses without much evidence that they will do any good and without considering the harm they might cause."[14]

And just how much good do supplements do? Trade associations argue that the benefits are substantial. The Council for Responsible Nutrition (CRN), for example, insists that research studies support the benefits of taking nutritional supplements in amounts over and above those needed to prevent deficiencies or those that can be obtained from food: "A large and rapidly expanding body of research suggests that increasing intakes of specific nutrients may be helpful in protecting against . . . debilitating and deadly diseases and conditions. . . . The available evidence overwhelmingly favors the conclusion that a generous, balanced intake of essential nutrients is essential for optimal health and that supplements are safe and beneficial in helping to achieve such intakes."[15] On this basis, the CRN raises a dietary supplement flag over the USDA's *Food Guide Pyramid* and promotes a dietary supplement pyramid of its own, as shown in Figure 25.

Makers of nutritional supplements also maintain that if more people took their products, hospital costs would be reduced by 40–60% and medical expenses by $20 billion or so annually.[16] It is difficult to know whether such assertions are correct. As discussed in the Appendix, taking supplements is a health behavior that "tracks" with other characteristics that predict good health. People who take supplements are less likely to smoke cigarettes or abuse alcohol and are more likely to follow dietary recommendations and to exercise; they also are more likely to be educated,

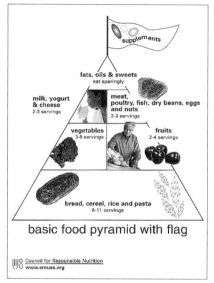 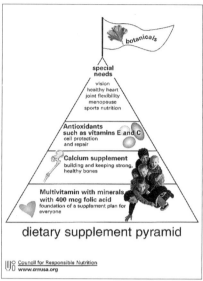

FIGURE 25. Supplement trade associations promote their members' interests by suggesting that diets would promote better health if they topped off the USDA's *Food Guide Pyramid* with nutritional supplements, and nutritional supplements with botanicals. (Courtesy Council for Responsible Nutrition, Washington, DC)

financially well off, and—no surprise—healthier. Only recently have the results of well-designed studies convinced mainstream scientists that the supplement industry may be right about the benefits of higher-than-recommended levels of nutrients—but only for a few nutrients, and only within limited ranges of intake.[12] Many scientists and clinicians, aware of the precept "first do no harm," remain uncomfortable about the idea of taking large amounts of one or another single nutrient or of using any nutritional supplement without clear evidence of need.

Considering issues of need, safety, and efficacy, most nutritionists continue to prefer foods to supplements for the reasons given in Table 29. The government's *Dietary Guidelines* issued in 2000 say, "Don't depend on supplements to meet your usual dietary needs," but they do suggest that certain groups of people—pregnant and other young women, older adults, and people on restricted diets—may need specific supplements for special purposes.[17] When government and professional groups do advise that the general public use supplements, they tend to recommend a daily multivitamin/multimineral product that provides nutrients in amounts close to recommended intakes. For example, with the caveat that more is not better and that "supplements are not magic bullets and won't fix lousy diets," the Center for Science in the Public Interest (CSPI) recommends an ordinary daily vitamin and mineral supplement that contains the protective nutrients most likely to be deficient in average diets.[18] This advice seems quite reasonable, especially given that extra vitamins and minerals are so readily available from nutrient-enriched and fortified foods, as we shall see in the next chapter.

Herbal Supplements

But what about the value and safety of the 1,500 to 1,800 non-nutritional herbal, botanical, and other classes of supplements now available? Little is known of the chemical composition, active ingredients, or mechanism of action of most of these products, and only a very few have been subjected to controlled clinical testing.[19] As interest in this field has grown, studies have begun to demonstrate—albeit modest—benefits for some traditional herbal remedies. Small improvements, for example, have been observed in studies of saw palmetto for prostate problems and taking feverfew for migraine headaches.[20] In some cases, as might be expected, studies funded by companies that make the products tend to show benefits for the supplement, whereas independent studies find no such benefits; studies of ginkgo biloba for memory loss in the elderly are a prime example of such research inconsistencies.[21]

Although most scientists consider studies that suggest benefits of herbal supplements as preliminary and inconclusive, the products may well help people with conditions that cannot be treated successfully with conventional medicines even if they do so simply through placebo (or other self-healing) effects. As discussed in the Appendix, such effects can be very powerful and are often neglected in conventional medical practice.

Nearly all published studies on the health effects of herbal supplements recommend further research, but makers of herbal products have little incentive to test their products. Research is expensive, time-consuming, and not always conclusive; unless the product can be patented, which traditional herbs cannot, the companies are likely to have difficulty recovering the costs of clinical trials. In the absence of a solid body of research, however, it is not possible to apply the usual scientific criteria to decide whether a supplement really does improve health.

As for the safety of herbal supplements, the industry maintains that problems are rare. *Rare*, however, is a comparative term. From 1993 to 1998, the FDA received 2,621 reports of serious problems related to taking supplements, including 101 deaths—numbers that can be viewed as reassuring or alarming, depending on one's point of view.[8] One difficulty with interpreting safety data is that people assume that dietary supplements are benign and may not associate health problems with taking the products. On the other hand, medical journals and newspapers tend to give disproportionately dramatic coverage to isolated reports of harm caused by taking supplements.

Furthermore, safety is especially difficult to assess in products of inconsistent composition. An evaluation by *Consumer Reports* of echinacea and ginkgo supplements, for example, identified considerable variation in the contents of different brands, as well as among different samples of the same brands. One testing laboratory reported that half of the glucosamine/chondroitin (antiarthritis) products it sampled did not contain as much chondroitin as was listed on the label, perhaps because this substance costs four times as much as glucosamine. Although the combination of the two substances is advertised widely as beneficial, the "joint health" product shown in Figure 24 only contains glucosamine. The testing laboratory also found supplements of saw palmetto, ginkgo biloba, and echinacea to contain less of those substances than listed on the product labels.[22] So little is known about the interactions among herbal supplements and conventional drugs that anesthesiologists warn patients to stop taking supplements before undergoing surgery. Pharmacists at major drug chains also have begun asking customers about supplement practices and advising them about possible interactions that might be harmful. The uncertainties reinforce the opinion of some scientists that taking supplements is like playing a lottery and provide grounds for more extreme critics to argue that the supplement industry is surely "the most dangerous and the least regulated . . . in America today."[23]

Example: Ephedra

The industry argues that deregulated or not, safety concerns about supplements are overstated. But are they? Less than reassuring is the regulatory history of ephedra (ma huang), an herbal supplement that is said to stimulate the central nervous system, elevate mood, and relieve coughs but is used most frequently for weight loss. The active ingredients in ephedra supplements are ephedrines—amphetamine-like alkaloids related to "uppers" as well as to components of over-the-counter cough and cold medications. As prescribed by doctors, doses of 100 milligrams of ephedrine per day do indeed induce weight losses of 1 to 2 pounds per week. Ephedra supplements, however, vary widely in the amounts of the alkaloids they contain. Of particular concern is that the products may contain too much ephedrine, because overdoses cause a wide range of unpleasant and sometimes dangerous side effects: headaches, nausea, irregular heartbeats, sleeplessness, dependency, and—in extreme instances—death. Despite the potential hazards, ephedra products are promoted as "herbal phen-fen" in tribute to the combination of phentermine and fenfluramine drugs that used to be prescribed for obesity until they were banned for their potentially dangerous side effects.[24] As an example of the size of the market for such products, the industry estimates that two *billion* doses are consumed annually and that one of the more popular ephedra-based supplements generated sales of $900 million in 1999.[25]

From 1993 to 1997, the FDA received more than 800 reports of adverse effects and 20 to 30 documented reports of deaths associated with the use of more than 100 different kinds of ephedrine-containing supplements, and it received at least 400 more reports of adverse effects during the next two years. Many of the problems occurred soon after the first use among young adults who would not otherwise be expected to be at such high risk.[26] On this basis, the FDA proposed to regulate ephedra supplements as drugs if a single "serving" contained more than 8 milligrams of ephedrine alkaloids and the daily dose contained more than 24 milligrams (an amount much lower than the prescribed dose) and to require labels to state, "Do not use this product for more than 7 days . . . taking more than the recommended serving may result in heart attack, stroke, seizure, or death."[27]

In response, dietary supplement companies argued that the FDA's approach to the regulation of ephedra was flawed and would have a devastating effect on small businesses. They induced the House Science Committee to investigate the method used by the FDA to demonstrate the supplement's harmful effects. This method relied on people's unverifiable self-reports.[28] To the industry, regulations based on self-reported problems "appeared to be breaking new ground" because they were not based on controlled clinical studies. Encouraged by supplement manufacturers, the House ordered a General Accounting Office (GAO) investigation of the scientific validity of the adverse event report system. After a nine-month investigation, the GAO said that the FDA's use of this system was incomplete and inconsistent and that the agency's cost/benefit justification for using it "was not fully transparent" (translation: the basis of the FDA's decisions was unclear). An even tougher assessment from the Health and Human Services Inspector General scolded the FDA for failing to identify the ingredients of 32% of the products mentioned in reports or to obtain 58% of the medical confirmations it had requested.[29] How the FDA was expected to produce such information from a voluntary system based on self-reports remained unclear.

Futhermore, the FDA had stopped collecting reports of adverse reactions to supplements more than a year earlier as a result of "budget constraints."[30] Nevertheless, in April 2000, the FDA responded by withdrawing the parts of the proposed rule that were related to the dose of ephedra, asking for public comment, and making the adverse event reports available for public inspection.[31] The supplement industry and its supporters took the GAO report as a license to attack the adverse report system. The Council for Responsible Nutrition contracted with "independent" toxicologists to evaluate the risk of ephedra, did its own review of the FDA's adverse event reports, and announced that the supplement is safe when used correctly. Its president told the New York City Council that "ephedra dietary supplements are appropriately marketed to consumers, in a manner consistent with federal, state, and local laws."[32]

The industry also induced members of Congress to demand extensions to the comment period on the ephedra proposals. As an example of the tone of these actions, the plaintiffs in *Pearson* v. *Shalala*, building on their success in that case, also entered into this new debate. They filed "their characteristically lengthy comment," one that pulled no punches: "The era of FDA regulation of truthful speech is coming rapidly to an end . . . [making] the FDA appear to be arrogant fools pretending that somehow only the FDA can access and interpret scientific information for consumers."[33]

While the FDA held its ephedra docket open for further reports and comments, independent investigators reviewed 140 of the adverse event reports and concluded that 31% of them were "definitely or probably related" to use of ephedra supplements and that another 31% were "possibly related." Nearly half of the events involved cardiovascular symptoms, and nearly one-fifth involved the central nervous system. Of these events, 13 had resulted in permanent disability and 10 had caused death.[34]

Despite such evidence, ephedra products continue to be available anywhere supplements are sold. A clerk at my local health food store sold me the product shown in Figure 24, although he warned me to be cautious about taking it. Its label states that the daily dose should not exceed 100 mg of ephedra alkaloids and that the pills should not be taken for more than 12 weeks—a dose 4 times higher and that a course of application 12 times longer than the standards proposed by FDA. The label warns, "This product should NOT be used by individuals with heart disease, high blood pressure, thyroid disease, diabetes, or those who have difficulty urinating. It should NOT be taken concurrently with antihypertensive drugs or antidepressants containing MAO inhibitors. . . . [I]mproper use of this product may cause nervousness, rapid heart beat, or may otherwise be hazardous."

In the political climate of the late 1990s, Congress was willing to tolerate the relatively small number of serious side effects and the even fewer fatalities caused by supplements as a small price to pay for giving the public the "freedom to choose." Congressman Burton was quite explicit about this relative-danger concept during his 1999 hearings on DSHEA: "106,000 people die a year from prescription drugs, 42,000 a year from automobile accidents. It is more likely that you will be struck by lightning and die in this country than it is that you will die from using a dietary supplement with just 16 deaths reported last year."[35]

Even if this low figure is correct, it is unlikely to comfort the families of the deceased or to reassure customers who assume that any supplement they buy is natural, safer than any drug they might take, and government-approved. With Congress unwilling to regulate these products and the FDA unable to take action, issues related to the potential harm of dietary supplements will be left increasingly to the courts to resolve. In 1999 the family of a woman with hypertension who died of a stroke after taking ephedra supplements sued a health club that had recommended the product. Other such cases are sure to follow. Thus another evident but presumably unintended consequence of supplement deregulation has been the transfer of regulatory authority from the FDA, an agency established for that purpose, to the courts.

CONFUSING THE PUBLIC

As I explained in the Introduction, the cacophony of nutrition news and advertising has caused even further public confusion about diet and health—to the great advantage of food producers. To many people, messages about single nutrients seem so contradictory as to thoroughly obscure the basic principles of healthful food choices. Presumably, health claims are supposed to help resolve confusion by "educating" the consumer about the benefits of certain food products and, as a consequence, stimulating purchases of those products. People opposed to health claims suspect that commercial reasons predominate and that the messages not only lack significant educational value but also mislead the public into thinking that the products convey special health benefits when, in fact, they do not.

Health Claims for Foods

The 1984 Kellogg's campaign to promote eating cereals high in fiber as a way to reduce cancer risk (Chapter 10) demonstrated beyond question that health claims increase the market share of specific products, at least in the short term, and subsequent studies have confirmed this observation. Whether health claims improve public knowledge of diet and disease prevention is a more difficult question to answer, because so many factors other than supplements also influence health. As noted earlier, people who take supplements typically eat better diets, and they also share other health-promoting characteristics and attitudes that affect responses to health messages. All of these factors must be considered and distinguished from any effects of the messages themselves. In addition, health claims occur in an environment of newspaper and magazine advertising and of peer and medical discussions of nutrition issues—these too affect opinions about health matters. Finally, as health and nutrition educators are only too well aware, improved knowledge does not necessarily lead to improved attitudes toward healthful eating or to behavioral changes to improve dietary intake.

Researchers, therefore, have attempted to isolate the effects of health claims—as distinct from all other factors—on the nutrition knowledge, attitudes, and behavior of consumers. Early studies examined the responses to nutrient-content claims that began appearing in product advertisements in women's magazines in the mid-1970s. These studies indicated that women who read the claims developed favorable impressions of the advertised products whether or not they actually understood the information.[36] The reason? They believed that if the nutrition information appeared in print, it had to be correct.[37] Studies like this one convey the impression that nutrient-content claims increase awareness of the nutritional benefits of products but do not yield much in the way of improved knowledge or better food choices.

Federal Trade Commission (FTC) economists and FDA social scientists independently analyzed the effects on consumer behavior of the

1984 Kellogg's fiber-and-cancer campaign. Their quite different interpretations of the results make an interesting case study, for their conclusions reflect the distinct policy approaches of the two agencies. Researchers from both agencies agreed that before the start of the campaign, high-fiber cereals were more likely to be eaten by people who were white, more highly educated, nonsmokers, and users of vitamin supplements. They also agreed that sales of Kellogg cereals and other high-fiber products increased in the months following the campaign. Differing, however, were their interpretations of *why* the sales increased. Soon after the campaign, the FDA analysts cautiously observed that the sales increase was

> consistent with the successful educational impact of the Kellogg diet and health campaign: consumers seemed to be making an apparently thoughtful discrimination between high and low fiber cereals. The clearest evidence of a successful consumer education campaign would be increased sales for high fiber products that were not promoted. However, in the competitive marketplace, successful product promotions are quickly emulated, and consumer education effects are difficult to identify confidently.[38]

Later FDA reports viewed the effects of health claims on consumers as "complex and not easily summarized," mainly because survey responses seemed to be specific to the product as well as to the claim. FDA researchers concluded that even prominent claims on labels conveyed only limited information and were ignored by the vast majority of consumers. Health claims, they concluded, "led consumers to believe that the product was likely to have positive health effects that it did not have. The effect . . . was to reduce the likelihood consumers would read the nutrition information on the back of the package." Such findings, they said, made it "hard to conclude that the impact of health claims is to produce more accurate perceptions of products' health benefits."[39]

Further FDA studies reinforced doubts about the educational value of health claims compared to other sources of nutrition information. Researchers collected data on the proportion of people who were aware of the links between fiber and cancer before, during, and after the Kellogg campaign and compared this information to the number of newspaper and magazine articles that were appearing on the subject. The reactions to the claims seemed to depend most on what people *already* understood about diet and health. Any increase in overall awareness of the connection between dietary fiber and cancer risk occurred during periods when the news media most frequently discussed such issues; awareness fell in parallel with a decline in news accounts. The FDA researchers interpreted these results as consistent with consumer confusion and with the "relatively low level of credence" given to health information provided by food companies.[40] From the FDA interpretation, it appeared that the public was suspicious of the credibility of health claims on food package labels.

In contrast to the FDA's skeptical view, FTC researchers were (and remain) enthusiastic about the educational benefits of health claims. Their post-Kellogg 1989 studies identified significant increases in the use of high-fiber cereals among women who were least educated, smoked cigarettes, and were nonwhite—precisely the groups that might benefit most from dietary improvements and that were least likely to be reached by government advice. These impressive results led the FTC researchers to conclude that the FDA's restrictions on health claims were counterproductive.

> Legal restrictions on manufacturers' ability to communicate the health effects of fiber cereals appear to have limited the public's knowledge of the fiber/cancer issue and restricted the information's spread to certain groups within the population. Our evidence suggests that had producer advertising never occurred, fewer individuals would be eating cereal, and those eating cereal would be eating lower fiber cereals. This effect would be most pronounced for nonwhites, smokers and women who lived in female-headed households.[41]

Furthermore, in response to the FDA's focus on news media as the source of consumer information, the FTC researchers countered that data from several sources appeared to support the value of the Kellogg campaign: "Of course, it is difficult to assess the precise effect that health claims have contributed to improvements in diet . . . [but] all the evidence presented here suggests that augmenting these sources of information with truthful producer health claims is likely to benefit consumers."[42]

These somewhat different interpretations, each reflecting the stance of the particular agency, are most likely to be resolved—if resolution is possible—by independent investigators. That both views have some merit is indicated by one third-party survey of the results of the Kellogg campaign. In that study, researchers assessed awareness and understanding of the health claims on cereal boxes among middle-to-upper-income, college-educated, female homemakers in Utah. The results: Women who knew the most about fiber most liked and understood the health claims. As a group, however, these women exhibited little understanding of how much fiber was recommended, of what foods contain it, or of the meaning of the claims. The study also showed that the results of surveys about health claims also depend on who is asked; in this one, the participants thought that the government—not Kellogg—was responsible for the health messages and, therefore, found them more credible. The investigators concluded that many consumers misunderstood health claims and thus might buy products for the wrong reasons. They interpreted their findings as a clear signal that policymakers should "exercise caution to ensure that health messages on food labels are responsible and accurate."[43]

Health Claims for Supplements

The consumer surveys just reviewed were conducted prior to DSHEA, and none dealt directly with health claims for supplements. In 1996, however, the FTC conducted a test of consumer understanding of the nutrition information conveyed by health claims in food and supplement advertising. The agency was especially interested in finding out whether people understood *qualified* claims—those that attempted to account for undesirable as well as desirable characteristics of the products. The design of this study was exceptionally complex (respondents were shown multiple versions of similar claims) and the written report is densely written and not easy to interpret. FTC investigators, for example, evaluated the reactions of consumers to several types of advertising statements for a fictitious cheese that was high in calcium but also high in saturated fat. From some—but not all—statements, some people understood that the cheese was high in both desirable and undesirable nutrients, but many people did not. In general, the qualified health claims led respondents to "seriously underestimate" the level of undesirable ingredients in products. People also tended to interpret advertisements stating that a product was "lower" in an undesirable nutrient as meaning that it was "low" in that nutrient (which was not necessarily the case).

In a part of the study that posed by far the most difficult analytical challenges and required "compromises in the precision of the tested hypotheses and the analytical rigor with which they were developed," FTC researchers also evaluated reactions to an unauthorized disease claim for a fictitious supplement that they called "ACE Vitamins." The test claim read as follows: "What we know about antioxidants and cancer: scientists have known for some time about the special health benefits of fruits and vegetables that are rich in antioxidants like vitamins A, C, and E. Eating plenty of these foods can reduce the risk of certain kinds of cancer." The FTC researchers also measured the way people responded to a control message: "Now you can get the antioxidant vitamins you want everyday in just one tablet!"

They compared reactions to these messages to reactions in response to four additional test messages that offered differing assessments of the strength of the scientific evidence linking antioxidant supplements to prevention of cancer: (1) "Scientists have now proven . . . ," (2) "Some medical studies are now finding . . . ," (3) "It looks promising, but . . . ," and (4) "Some medical studies are now suggesting, but it's too early to tell for sure." As if these messages were not confusing enough, still another test message explained the harm caused by oxygen-induced damage to the body: (5) "It's hard to believe, but the same thing that rusts the paint off your car may also wear down your body."

The perhaps unsurprising result: The various messages showed little difference in conveying the extent of scientific uncertainty. Uncertainties were best communicated by a second exposure to the most highly qualified statement (statement 5), perhaps because it was most dramatic. But no matter how strong the qualifier, respondents still wanted to take the supplement and believed the advertisements. They uniformly interpreted the messages to mean that scientists were at least somewhat confident about the claim that antioxidant vitamins might reduce cancer risk. The FTC investigators concluded that unless warning statements are utterly explicit, most people will miss the point and will think that supplements produce greater health benefits than can be demonstrated by existing scientific studies.[44]

In their own exploration of this point, researchers at the FDA asked groups of consumers to discuss their reactions to claims for several dietary supplements. The results of these focus-group studies were especially revealing from the "two-culture" standpoint. Participants liked to see information about health benefits on labels, but, as might be expected from perusal of Table 28, they saw no meaningful distinction between structure/function claims and FDA-authorized health claims. Furthermore,

> Most participants were cavalier about the idea of scientific certainty. They expressed less concern about the truth value of the health claim than about the likely efficacy of the product for them. They did not equate the two ideas. The claim might be scientifically valid, but the product might not work for them, or the truth value of the claim might fail to meet some scientific standard, but the product might still work for them. . . . Most participants thought it was self-evident that a supplement product would not work the same for everybody. . . . The practical implication . . . was that you needed to try the product for yourself to see if it would work for you.[45]

This "try it" attitude derived from the implicit assumption of most of the survey participants that supplements are inherently safe.

Taken together, such studies confirm that health claims sell products, make products appear healthful whether or not they are, and are understood by some people (those who are better educated, etc.) but may confuse others. Since the advent of DSHEA, surveys have demonstrated increasing public confusion about diet and health.[46] Whether health claims for dietary supplements have added to the confusion remains to be determined, but it is difficult to imagine that they contribute in any meaningful way to public understanding of nutrition issues.

POLARIZING TWO CULTURES

In the entire history of the influence of private enterprise on federal nutrition policy, the actions of the dietary supplement industry must surely rank among the most effective. Over the years, industry groups relentlessly and successfully opposed any attempt by federal agencies to restrict the contents, dosages, or claims of benefit that could be made for dietary supplements. Whenever the FDA attempted to impose regulations, it faced massive opposition. Invariably, the net result was a loss of the agency's credibility and erosion of its ability to regulate foods and drugs, let alone supplements. As summarized by one commentator, "Time and again the FDA has proposed comprehensive regulations to monitor dietary supplements, and at each juncture the agency has been met by lobbying and grass roots efforts, led by supplement manufacturers, health food stores, and food faddists, all of whom have convinced Congress to block the FDA's efforts. Even the comparatively minor regulations the FDA has issued face waves of hostility in the courts."[23]

Supplement marketers succeeded in opposing the FDA because they were able to take advantage of popular beliefs in the value of natural remedies and widespread distrust of modern science and medicine. They also successfully exploited the division of regulatory responsibility between the FDA and the FTC, agencies with quite different missions and philosophies. Finally, because most supplements are "safe," they were able to convince Congress and the courts that little regulation is required. I put "safe" in quotation marks because 12% of all consumers who report using herbal supplements—nearly 12 million people—have reported experiencing adverse reactions.[1] Many herbal remedies are known to produce allergic reactions, toxic reactions, mutagenic effects, and drug interactions, and because most such problems are unsuspected and underreported, our recognition of the harm that such supplements may cause surely reflects just the "tip of the iceberg."[47]

The supplement industry's effectiveness can be explained in part by a political environment that has increasingly favored a government that is smaller, less intrusive, and less responsible for the welfare of individuals. Supplement deregulation may appear as just one more conflict between business interests and consumer protection, but it is notable in the industry's use of the "freedom of choice" approach to oppose science-based standards. This approach, of course, also figures prominently in discussions pertaining to the use of more demonstrably hazardous products, such as cigarettes and firearms.

Dietary supplements are a good example of C. P. Snow's two-culture analysis of perceptions of science. How the general public decides whether or not to take supplements is quite different from the way a science-based regulatory agency makes decisions about a product's safety or effectiveness. People choose to take supplements for conscious or unconscious reasons that do not necessarily depend on science. This explains why, during hearings on barriers to implementation of DSHEA, Congressman Burton implied that the FDA insufficiently recognizes the "importance of spirituality in healing and the important role of botanical products and nutrition in healing."[35] Reasons based on personal beliefs—spirituality among them—have convinced about half the adult population of the United States to use dietary supplements, if for no other reason than as a form of nutritional insurance. The supplement industry deliberately appeals to such beliefs when it argues for the right of people to choose to consume more or less safe products without government interference—whether or not these products have been proved effective through clinical trials.

Science-based belief systems, on the other hand, explain why federal and private health agencies rarely recommend nutritional supplements as a replacement for foods. The 1995 *Dietary Guidelines* advised consumers that "daily vitamin and mineral supplements . . . are considered safe, but are usually not needed by people who eat the variety of foods depicted in the *Food Guide Pyramid*." In recognition of the widespread use of supplements and the studies that show benefits for some of them, the 2000 *Dietary Guidelines* allowed that "some people need a vitamin–mineral supplement to meet specific nutrient needs."[17] Science-based arguments, however, have convinced many professionals of the need for skepticism, if not outrage, about the lack of evidence for the safety and efficacy of herbal and botanical supplements, as well as about their deregulated status. As explained by a science-minded lawyer concerned that FDA policies had become too *lenient* about health statements, "The FDA proposal recognizes as an appropriate 'structure and function' statement for a dietary supplement a claim that the product 'improves absentmindedness.' . . . *There are no foods that affect absentmindedness"* [emphasis added].[48]

The depth and passion of the opposing views cannot be overstated. For example, the *Journal of the American Medical Association's* publication of studies indicating possible benefits from certain dietary supplements appears to have contributed to the abrupt dismissal of its distinguished editor; factions of the American Medical Association opposed to alternative medicine were said to have worked to undermine his position.[49] People may feel better when they take supplements, but should health officials use feelings as a basis for regulatory decisions? Or should the FDA instead "take the lead in reenergizing a crucial phase of its basic mission, to promote honest, rational, scientific medicine by vigorously combating its opposite?"[50] The issues of safety and efficacy raised by this deregulated marketplace should force us to consider carefully whether we should permit so great a reduction in the enforcement ability of the one government entity devoted to a science-based regulatory approach, unpopular though it may be. Yes, the FDA's current stance may appear too economically threatening to the supplement industry and too intrusive to some segments of the public. And yes, relatively few of these products do overt harm. Our society tolerates far more damage from handguns and automobiles than supplements are ever likely to cause, and we handle the demonstrably greater hazards of cigarettes and alcohol with warning labels.

What really is at stake here is whether irreparable damage has been done to the ability of our federal regulatory system to ensure the safety of foods and supplements and to balance public health interests against the economic interests of corporations. Is it not in the public interest to demand that there be some federal system to guarantee that all those products on the shelves are safe and effective? Shouldn't there be some regulatory framework to control patently absurd or misleading claims? The resolution of differences of opinion about the value of dietary supplements is not well served by destroying the ability of a science-based agency to remove harmful products from the marketplace. A return to the pre-1906 days of rampant quackery hardly seems in the best interests of the country.

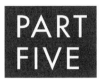

PART FIVE

INVENTING TECHNO-FOODS

AS WE SAW IN THE LAST CHAPTER, THE NUTRITIONAL attributes of foods are a natural selling point, and the advertising of health benefits increases sales. Food companies are vitally interested in the ways that they might take advantage of three approaches used by government and health officials to promote better diets: education, supplements, and fortification or alteration of foods to make them "healthier." Part I of this book explained how the food industry protects its interests by influencing federal dietary advice to the public. Part IV discussed how makers and sellers of dietary supplements worked the system to obtain a free hand in marketing their products. Part V focuses on the third approach: strategies for improving the marketability of foods as "healthy" by adding nutrients or other supplements or by subtracting undesirable components. These days, food products constructed for this purpose are classified in their own special category and are variously called "functional foods," "designer foods," or, sometimes, "nutraceuticals." I much prefer the designation "techno-foods" which, as my colleague Greg Drescher once explained, works well "for want of a better pejorative term."[1] Collectively, these designations refer to foods and beverages that have been constructed to confer health benefits *beyond* the nutritive value of the foods themselves. In developing techno-foods, manufacturers deliberately take advantage of the increasingly liberal regulatory environment for health claims to appeal to the public's desire for uncomplicated ways to follow dietary advice and achieve optimal health.

By the definition used here, techno-foods encompass an enormous range of products: foods enriched or fortified with vitamins, minerals, protein, fiber, amino acids, or fatty acids, as well as herbs, plant phytochemicals, and even wood pulp derivatives. They also include "lesser-evil" foods that have been formulated to be low in calories, fat, sugar, salt, caffeine, or allergens or to contain artificial substitutes for unwanted ingredients such as sugar or fat. As explained in Chapter 13, fortification clearly yields some health advantages although most of the benefits claimed for this approach are uncertain. In part as a result of fortification strategies—the addition of vitamins and minerals to basic foods such as milk and flour—nutrient deficiencies now rarely occur among Americans, hardly ever cause noticeable symptoms, and are observed mainly among people who consume patently inadequate diets or are ill. The increasingly common addition of vitamins and minerals to products as diverse as breakfast cereals, candy, and water, however, is unlikely to provide additional increments in health and raises concerns about the possible hazards of too much of a good thing.

Chapter 14 addresses issues related to the addition of herbal and other non-nutritional dietary supplements to conventional foods. It also covers the lesser-evil foods reduced in unwanted fat, sugar, or other factors. Such products, many of which would otherwise be relegated to the top of the *Food Guide Pyramid*, were developed expressly to take advantage of the nutrient-content, health, and structure/function claims permitted by various acts of Congress. Because manufacturers developed these products precisely so that people would eat more of them, it is not surprising that the burgeoning availability of apparently "healthy" foods has had little effect on overall consumption of fat, sugar, or calories. As we have seen, recommended dietary *patterns*—not single nutrients or foods—are associated with good health. Unless we change our overall diets and eat less, techno-foods will not help us lose weight or reduce risk factors. As a final ironic twist, as explained in Chapter 15, "healthy" techno-foods such as those made with the no-calorie fat substitute olestra appeal most to people who are *already* following dietary and other recommended health practices.

It should be evident that the philosophical rationale for techno-foods is flatly reductionist; the value of a food is reduced to its single functional ingredient. Underlying this philosophy is the conviction that if diets rich in fruits and vegetables protect against cancer and heart disease, then some component of those foods must be responsible. If a single component is responsible for the benefit, the argument continues, then that component will be even more beneficial if isolated, purified, and used in larger amounts. This logic is flawed in that it fails to consider the complexity of food composition and the interactions among food components. Throughout evolution, food plants developed hundreds of chemicals to ward off unwanted insects and predators, and a great many of these have been shown to stimulate detoxifying enzymes in people who eat them. Thus almost any food plant—and oats, flaxseed, soybeans, tomatoes, carrots, garlic, onions, broccoli, cabbage, sprouts, citrus fruits, cranberries, grapes, and tea are only the best-studied examples—seems to protect against disease in clinical studies. The nutrients and other plant chemicals that occur in greatest amounts in these foods become candidates for use as "magic bullets," but numerous other possibilities have barely been explored. Potentially protective components also have been isolated from fish, fermented dairy foods, and even beef. The complexity of food composition means that no single nutrient is likely to work nearly so well as a diet rich in the fruits and vegetables from which that nutrient was isolated.

We shall see in these chapters that because techno-foods offer manufacturers a genuine opportunity to promote sales, food and beverage companies go to extraordinary lengths to protect the marketing environment for such products. Thus the development of these foods has produced at least three undesirable results: a further blurring of the distinctions among foods, supplements, and drugs; a further erosion of the ability of federal regulators to protect the public from harmful substances in foods; and, most important, a further increase in public confusion about how best to achieve recommended diets.

CHAPTER 13

GO FORTH AND FORTIFY

IN DEVELOPING TECHNO-FOODS FORTIFIED WITH ESSENTIAL nutrients and designed to be "healthier," food companies were responding not only to the marketing advantage of such products, but also to the demands of federal health officials, in what appeared to be a win–win situation. By the late 1980s, consensus about the health benefits of recommended diets—those that followed the *Dietary Guidelines*—seemed almost universal. Because Americans were spending an ever-increasing proportion of their food dollars on products and meals prepared outside the home, nutritionists and health officials believed that the industries responsible for pre-prepared foods should join homemakers as primary targets of policy recommendations. Many of us believed that if we could influence the food industry to improve the nutritional quality of its products by creating foods reduced in fat, saturated fat, cholesterol, sugar, and salt, but higher in fiber, then people would buy them enthusiastically, and everyone—industry and the public alike—would benefit.[1] We could not imagine that the food industry indeed would respond to this idea, but with a vengeance. In their quest to promote "eat more," food·and beverage companies rushed to create products that could be marketed as more healthful, whether or not they really would improve patterns of dietary intake. This chapter reviews the ways in which food companies added vitamins and minerals to foods at all levels of the USDA's *Food Guide Pyramid*, top as well as bottom. We shall see, however, that fortification does not automatically make diets better and that it raises questions about potentially harmful effects.

THE IMPETUS FOR "HEALTHIER" FOODS

The first formal demands for creation of "healthier" food products appeared as early as 1980 when, as part of its first ten-year plan for improving the nation's health, the U.S. Public Health Service called for a 20% reduction in sodium levels in processed foods to be achieved by 1990. Those who devised this plan anticipated that to promote overall improvements in nutritional status, "major food processors and distributors will incorporate nutrition principles and concepts into their food and marketing strategies and messages," presumably to the extent then possible under Food and Drug Administration (FDA) and Federal Trade Commission (FTC) regulations.[2]

A stronger impetus to develop "healthy" food products came in the form of policy recommendations in the 1988 *Surgeon General's Report on Nutrition and Health*. The report's principal conclusion was that "overconsumption of certain dietary components is now a major concern for Americans. While many food factors are involved, chief among them is the disproportionate consumption of foods high in fats, often at the expense of foods high in complex carbohydrates and fiber that may be more conducive to health."[3] Because the main contributors of fat to American diets are meat, poultry, dairy products, and fried and processed foods, the report issued a challenge to the food industry: "Food manufacturers can contribute to improving the quality of the American diet by increasing the availability of palatable, easily prepared food products that will help people to follow the dietary principles outlined here. Because the public is becoming increasingly conscious of the role of nutrition in health, development of such products should also benefit the food industry."[3]

In 1990 the Public Health Service's second ten-year plan made even more explicit requests. It called on food companies to offer for sale by the year 2000 at least 5,000 processed food products lower in fat and saturated fat. In 1986 about 2,500 such products were on the market, and this goal was designed to double their number.[4]

In recognition of the potential for increased sales that might be generated by responding to this mandate, food companies quickly accelerated development of fat substitutes, and produced items such as reduced-calorie cheesecake mixes and McDonald's McLean hamburgers, which replaced some of the beef fat with agar derivatives, vegetable proteins, and water. By 1991 the industry already had exceeded the goal for the year 2000 and was marketing 5,600 reduced-fat products.

From 1992 on, about 2,000 new reduced-fat products were introduced annually, along with hundreds of other products that were lower in calories, salt, cholesterol, or sugar or contained added fiber or calcium. By 1996, 38% of new food products were designed for some nutritional purpose, and 40% of these nutritionally modified products were lower in fat.[5]

To the food industry and some federal officials, such products offered a pragmatic solution to a fundamental dilemma: Most people interested in following dietary advice will not do so unless they like what they are eating, and the food industry has no interest in creating products it cannot sell. One way to address the dilemma is to concede that people are going to eat "junk" foods anyway and encourage the food industry to create "healthier" versions. This idea seemed especially attractive because food companies consider new products the key to expanding sales. Nutritional enhancements might give new products a favorable edge in the fiercely competitive marketplace for processed foods, even though labeling a food as "healthy" was no sure guarantee of success; the McLean burgers, for example, failed miserably and were soon taken off the market. Nevertheless, food marketers recognized that the success rate was higher for innovative products, and the success of even a few nutritionally enhanced foods would provide a strong incentive to produce others. From 1989 to 1993, nutritionally enhanced foods and beverages in 37 categories rose from 26% to 30% of all sales, an increase much better than that for regular versions of the products.[6]

There was every reason to think that such products would do even better if health claims could be made for them. Indeed, the changes in federal laws that permitted statements about health benefits on package labels stimulated further interest in creating food products for specific nutritional purposes. A final impetus derived from the way such products could be marketed. Nutritionally enhanced foods could be advertised in positive terms—for their beneficial attributes rather than for the absence of undesirable factors: "Industry is betting that consumers, after years of being bombarded with negative health messages to cut back on fat, cholesterol, and sodium, are ready to warm up to foods that emphasize the positive benefits of newly added ingredients, even if the scientific community has not yet concluded that they are truly beneficial."[7] These kinds of societal pressures gave food manufacturers just the rationale they needed to create even more nutritionally enhanced techno-foods, beginning with the addition of vitamins and minerals.

"NUTRIFICATION": FORTIFYING AND ENRICHING FOODS

Like much else in nutrition, fortification has an eventful history. The very first techno-foods were fortified or enriched. To explain the difference: vitamins and minerals are added to white flour to compensate for the loss of nutrients that occurs when whole grains are milled. For example, unfortified white flour contains 25% or less of vitamin B$_6$, magnesium, and zinc and less than 10% of the vitamin E found in the whole grain. The white flour sold in stores is considered fortified because vitamins (thiamin, niacin, riboflavin, and, more recently, folic acid) and one mineral (iron) are added at *higher levels* than those found in the original grain. In contrast, enrichment is the restoration of nutrients to their *original level* in the unprocessed food. Despite these technical distinctions, the term *fortification* usually refers to any addition of vitamins or minerals to food.

As a public health approach, fortification was designed to overcome widespread deficiencies of certain key nutrients in the diets of the general population. The practice dates to the early 1830s, when a French chemist advocated the addition of iodine to table salt to prevent goiter (enlarged thyroid glands). Europeans began adding iodine to salt in the early 1900s, but large-scale additions of other nutrients did not become possible until later in the century when scientists identified vitamins and learned how to purify and synthesize them in large quantities. In the United States, a 1918 survey found one-third of the population of Michigan (where soils are particularly deficient in iodine) to have enlarged thyroid glands; in some areas, the prevalence exceeded 60%. Within just ten years from the time iodized salt was introduced in 1924, officials were iodizing more than 90% of the salt sold in Michigan. The happy result was that goiter had all but disappeared, in Detroit, for example, the prevalence of goiter fell from 47% to 2% among school children and to about 1% among adults.[8] This remarkable achievement encouraged the use of iodized salt throughout the country and virtually eliminated iodine deficiency as a public health problem.

Vitamin D was first added to milk in 1931, but fortification truly took off just prior to World War II when the FDA established a *standard of identity* for enriched flour that went into effect in 1942. A standard of identity is a recipe for the nutrient composition of a specific food such as enriched bread; the food must contain each of the elements of that recipe in order to be marketed under that designation. The FDA soon established standards of identity for other foods: cornmeal and grits in 1943, pasta in 1946, enriched bread in 1952, and rice in 1958.[9]

In the 1950s, manufacturers began to fortify cereals with additional vitamins, minerals, and protein at levels higher than in the original foods. The initial purpose of fortifying cereals and grains was to raise the intake of the four nutrients then considered most deficient in the diets of the population: thiamin, niacin, riboflavin, and iron. To ensure adequate intake, the standard specified higher amounts than in the original grain. Even though losses of all of the other vitamins and minerals in whole grains were just as substantial, nutritionists considered those nutrients less critical to public health. As a public health strategy, fortification and enrichment ("nutrification") seemed to make good sense because they were "the most rapidly applied, the most flexible, and the most socially acceptable intervention method of changing the intake of nutrients without a vast educational effort and without changing the current food patterns of a given population. The principle of nutrification challenges a long-standing belief that the consumer must consciously desire and be involved in nutritional change."[10]

Fortification strategies especially appeared to make sense because nutrient deficiencies occurred most commonly among low-income populations without enough money to buy a variety of foods or enough education to make the most nutritious choices. Because nutrient deficiencies were still observed in areas with much poverty, the 1969 White House Conference on Food, Nutrition, and Health strongly recommended the accelerated use of fortification, particularly of breakfast cereals and other foods likely to be basic sources of calories for ethnic, cultural, socioeconomic, and regional groups at especially high risk of inadequate nutrient intake.[11] In response, the FDA raised the levels of thiamin, niacin, and riboflavin in the standard of identity for grain foods and more than doubled the iron standard. The amounts of these nutrients in the food supply immediately increased. Indeed, the availability of iron rose so quickly that health officials began to be concerned that the food supply contained too much of it; the FDA reduced the standard, but then increased it again some years later. During the 1970s, various groups used data indicating that a significant proportion of the population was deficient in one or more nutrients as a basis for proposals to expand enrichment formulas to include up to ten vitamins and minerals, but the FDA rejected these out of fear that they might lead to excessive, unbalanced, and potentially harmful intake of essential nutrients.[12]

Folic Acid Fortification: Panacea or Techno-Fix?

The interweaving of the scientific and commercial issues that arise in any discussion of fortification is best exemplified by the addition of folic acid to grain products. In 1996 the FDA announced that it would require food companies to add this vitamin, which is also known as folate, to enriched grain products by January 1998.[13] The objective was to reduce the number of infants born with seriously debilitating brain and spinal cord defects (such as spina bifida) that result from incomplete closure of the neural tube during the first month of fetal development. Studies had revealed that mothers who consumed adequate amounts of folic acid and other vitamins during early pregnancy reduced the odds that they might bear a child with a neural tube defect by 50% or more. Although the doses used in the studies varied by more than ten-fold, and few studies distinguished the benefits of folic acid from those of other supplementary vitamins, most (but not all) experts viewed this research as definitive evidence of the need for women of childbearing age to consume more of this vitamin. Because risk factors for neural tube defects are poorly understood, and because the fetal neural tube closes before a woman might have any idea that she was pregnant, the FDA chose fortification—rather than advice to eat better diets or take supplements—as the method most likely to raise folic acid intake among women "at risk" of pregnancy.

Unlike the other nutrients used in fortification, which were added to the food supply to prevent deficiencies in large segments of the population, folic acid was expected to prevent about half of the 4,000 cases of neural tube defects that occurred each year, a very small proportion of the 3 million or so babies born in the United States annually. To prevent these few—albeit devastating—cases, fortification would be likely to raise the folic acid intake of 260 million Americans, among them many who were already obtaining adequate amounts of the vitamin from foods. Indeed, raising folic acid intakes would produce one additional benefit: it would reduce blood levels of homocysteine, a by-product of protein metabolism associated with higher rates of coronary heart disease and stroke. The potential benefits, however, would need to be balanced against a possible hazard. Excessive amounts of folate interfere with the ability to diagnose deficiencies of vitamin B_{12}, a problem noted with increasing frequency among the elderly. Overall, the benefits of fortification were expected to outweigh the risks, but many questions remained unanswered.[14]

At the time the FDA called for folic acid fortification, the incidence of neural tube defects had been declining at a steady rate for many years and was already quite low. If the incidence declined further, it would not be obvious whether it did so as a continuation of ongoing trends or as a result of an increase in intake of the vitamin. Thus, in this one respect, folic acid fortification could be considered a techno-fix likely to promote the proliferation and consumption of more expensive processed foods, and not necessarily by the people who needed them most. As a member of the FDA Food Advisory Committee at the time, I saw this particular situation as a missed opportunity for developing a nationwide education campaign to encourage everyone to eat more fruits and vegetables—the primary dietary sources of folate as well as of so many other health-promoting nutrients and components. Federal officials considered this idea unrealistic, however, not least because of the substantial cost of such a campaign. I also was concerned that the masking of vitamin B_{12} deficiency might lead to yet another techno-fix: the addition of vitamin B_{12} to the standard of identity for enriched grains. To skeptics, myself among them, folic acid fortification was almost certain to lead to calls for the addition of larger numbers of essential nutrients—whether needed or not—to the general food supply.[15] As explained later in this chapter, subsequent evidence supports some benefits of folic acid fortification but leaves questions about other possible benefits unanswered.

Beyond Standards of Identity: Voluntary Fortification

By the late 1970s, Hoffman-La Roche, a leading producer of bulk vitamins, had demonstrated the technical feasibility of adding nutrients to cereals and other foods. The company took pains to justify the need for doing so. It argued that even well-off Americans consume inadequate diets, that processing and cooking deplete foods of vitamins, and that the health benefits of vitamin sufficiency were well established—arguments identical to those used by supplement manufacturers (see Table 29). On this basis, the company urged food manufacturers to fortify their products voluntarily, an action that would seem to benefit the public and to be good for business.

> Roche believes that nutrition is good business . . . food fortification, technologically feasible at low costs, opens up new marketing possibilities for food manufacturers and enables them to provide adequate nutrition levels through the food products that consumers most often choose . . . food manufacturers

can not only serve the public need by improving nutrition among American consumers, but they can also succeed in selling their products to a broader section of the buying public.[16]

The company's 1978 position paper emphasized the low cost and high profitability of fortification. For example, Roche said that adding 12 vitamins at 100% of the RDAs (Recommended Dietary Allowances, defined as standards for levels of intake that meet the nutritional needs of practically everyone in the population) would cost just over half a cent per ounce, or just 7 cents for a 12-ounce box of cereal. As it happens, I still have two General Mills cereal box tops that I bought in 1979 to illustrate the economic benefits of fortification. One is from a box of Wheaties, a cereal then made from grain enriched to its standard of identity, but nothing else; it is stamped with a retail price of $0.93. The other is from its multiply-fortified counterpart, Total, which cost $1.29 in those halcyon days. Thus the addition of 7 cents worth of nutrients permitted the retailer to charge 36 cents more per box for an otherwise identical cereal. Clearly, fortification presented an attractive marketing opportunity. As we shall soon see, it still does.

With a national policy mandate to "go fortify," the technical ability to do so, and a substantial price incentive, manufacturers began to expand voluntary fortification of food products. Some nutritionists feared that as people became more aware of nutrition and recognized the value of nutritionally enhanced products, food manufacturers would engage in a vitamin and mineral "horse race" and fortify every product on the shelf. Indeed, they did, at least with respect to breakfast cereals. In 1969 manufacturers voluntarily fortified about 11% of all ready-to-eat cereals, but the proportion leaped to 92% by 1984. This rapid change led Gilbert Leveille, then president of the Institute of Food Technologists and a science director at General Foods, to urge his colleagues to develop an overall nutrition policy rather than using fortification indiscriminately: "The addition of nutrients to a product just so they may be listed on the label is not a sound nutritional philosophy."[9] Few, however, paid attention to this sensible advice.

When chronic diseases began to replace nutrient deficiencies as the leading diet-related health problems, they were seen as yet another incentive to develop fortified foods that would improve public health and enhance the quality of life. Citing the growing body of research on the protective effects of antioxidant nutrients, food technologists increasingly promoted fortification with vitamins A, C, and E as a means to prevent or delay certain cancers, heart disease, cataracts, arthritis, diabetes, and even Alzheimer's disease. Fortification, in the view of food manufacturers, could be used to support a range of preventive strategies for children as well as adults, particularly if the government could be induced to relax restrictions on health claims.

> Governments are investigating how to get children and young adults to consume more calcium . . . a logical option is to enhance products containing sugar with calcium; products like candy, soft drinks and other sweet products that appeal to this younger audience. . . . It is now expected that legislation affecting these types of products will become more lenient, allowing for specific claims on product labels in the future. This is a quickly evolving market and exciting new possibilities lay ahead for manufacturers.[17]

This single-nutrient approach to dietary "improvement" increased pressures to fortify foods, as did federal legislation in 1990. As discussed in previous chapters, the Nutrition Labeling and Education Act of 1990 made it possible for manufacturers to make a few claims for the nutrient content and health benefits of their products on package labels, and the Dietary Supplement Health and Education Act of 1994 allowed structure/function claims for nutritional supplements and, by inference, foods. The ability to make nutrient-content claims—to promote the fact that foods are high, rich, or good sources of one or another vitamin or mineral—encouraged manufacturers to add these nutrients to their products.

Yet another impetus to fortify was the replacement of the former standards of dietary adequacy, the RDAs, with Dietary Reference Intakes (DRIs). An RDA for any particular nutrient was a level of intake "adequate to meet the known nutrient needs of practically all healthy persons."[18] This population-based definition meant that the RDA is higher—sometimes significantly higher—than the amount needed by 97% of individuals. In the late 1990s, the Food and Nutrition Board of the National Academies' Institute of Medicine replaced the RDAs with new DRI standards that, confusingly, maintained RDAs as one component. The DRIs were designed to promote "biologic–physical well-being" and prevention of diet-related chronic diseases, as well as prevention of the traditional nutritional deficiencies addressed by the former standards. For some nutrients, the Food and Nutrition Board established new standards at such high levels that people could not possibly meet them just by eating conventional foods.[19] For example, the RDA for calcium had been 800 mg/day for middle-aged adults, but the DRIs increased the standard for "adequate intake" (for adults aged 31–50 years) to 1,000 mg/day.

Food manufacturers interpreted this increase as a strong incentive to add calcium to their products.[20] Similarly, "to provide antioxidant protection," the board raised the RDA for vitamin C by about 50% and by even more for cigarette smokers. This increase also provided a rationale for increasing the number of products fortified with antioxidant nutrients, as well as the levels of fortification.[21]

As if RDAs and DRIs are not complicated enough to understand and distinguish, the FDA uses yet a third standard—the Daily Value—for evaluation of nutritional content on food labels. The FDA's derivation of Daily Values is especially obscure, but the values for most vitamins and minerals are based on RDAs issued in 1968, although a few are based on standards established in 1980 or 1989. In general, the Daily Values are an average of the RDAs for adult men and women combined.[22] Food manufacturers routinely add nutrients to breakfast cereals at levels that provide 25% or more of the Daily Values for a dozen vitamins and minerals in a 1-ounce serving. Cereals such as General Mills' Total contain 100% or more of the Daily Value for 12 nutrients per serving and amounts ranging from 4% to 25% for 5 others. Manufacturers produce not-from-concentrate orange juice fortified with vitamins A, C, and E, or with added calcium—additions applauded in the business pages of daily newspapers: "Tropicana is getting back to its roots, and segmenting the juice business along health lines instead of flavor lines. . . . They're going after the most profitable part of the orange juice market."[23]

Although most fortification is used in breakfast cereals and juice drinks, manufacturers also have produced items of less evident desirability, such as vitamin-supplemented Gummi bears, sweetened juice "drinks," and doughnuts, and, in what has been termed "the first fast-food nutraceutical," a vegetarian burrito fortified with 100% of the Daily Value for 23 vitamins and minerals.[24] Between January and August 1998 alone, manufacturers introduced 31 new calcium-fortified products, many of them of candy, snacks, or sweetened drinks of otherwise questionable nutritional value.[25] Figure 26 shows some examples of nutrient-fortified but otherwise largely top-of-the-*Pyramid* foods. Food technologists—people who develop such products for food companies—consider such products to make eminent good sense. Americans eat about 27 pounds of candy a year per capita, for example, and annual sales amount to $22 billion. From the manufacturers' point of view, consumers want convenience, good taste, and good nutrition, and "candy laced with functional ingredients can offer the whole package."[26]

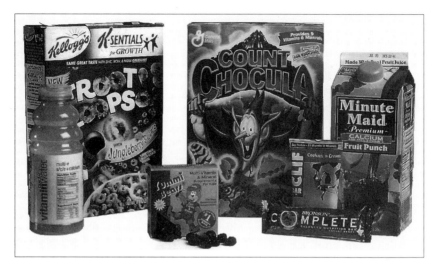

FIGURE 26. The nutrient-fortified products illustrated here are marketed as nutritious, even though they are high enough in sugars and sweeteners to be classified as top-of-the-*Pyramid*. The nutrient-fortified water replaces a one-a-day capsule with a more expensive alternative. (Photo by Shimon and Tammar Rothstein, 2000)

Breakfast Cereals: Sugar and a Vitamin Pill

Fortification permits manufacturers to market foods of dubious nutritional quality as health foods—even to health professionals. Here, for example, is an excerpt from an advertisement that appeared in the *American Journal of Public Health* in July 1999:

> When parents ask you for nutrition advice, can you look them straight in the eyes and say "Froot Loops cereal"? . . . presweetened cereals are a major source of nutrients for kids in the U.S. . . . What if, we reasoned, the cereals kids love were fortified with the things that dietitians, pediatricians, and nurses love? Introducing K-SENTIALS from Kellogg's. Put simply, they're kids' cereals with a very special prize inside: Like the added calcium in our Froot Loops, Cocoa Krispies and Apple Jacks. And the B vitamins in Kellogg's Frosted Flakes and Corn Pops. So do K-SENTIALS mean that kids will no longer have to eat their brussels sprouts or peas? (Sorry kids, not by a long shot.)

Not by a long shot, indeed. The advertisement fails to mention that Froot Loops cereal ("Marshmallow-Blasted") contains no fruit and no fiber and provides 53% of the calories from added sugar. The New Froot

Loops ("same great taste with zinc, iron, & now calcium"), reduces the sugar to 50% of calories and offers all of 1 gram of fiber per serving. Nevertheless, the company advertises Froot Loops as a health food. A comic strip on the back of the package explains: "Kellogg's Froot Loops is what you need for the good stuff that helps you grow." "Wow! calcium helps grow strong bones." "Zinc and iron help me study better." The comic character on the box of Frosted Flakes, a cereal that supplies a mere 47% of its calories from sugar, says, "With B-vitamins to help release energy from the carbohydrates in foods you eat . . . Kellogg's Frosted Flakes is great fuel for your body."

Kellogg's $20 million campaign to convince health professionals that its sugar-laden cereals are essential to children's health followed an earlier $20 million campaign directed at the general public ("With Kellogg's, a healthier life is within your reach"). The campaign featured full-page, bright red advertisements in major newspapers headlined with such questions as "Did you give them vitamins they need this morning?" "Did you help them grow to their potential this morning?" "Right now, are you giving your unborn child the folic acid she needs?" The answer? "Eating these Kellogg's cereals."[27] Kellogg also advertises its cereals to dietitians who work in food service: "When it comes to great taste and nutrition, your sales are in the balance. Your customers want balance. Balance between what's good for them and what tastes good to them. Any products you offer that are both will naturally be consistent sellers. . . . Help your customers get the balanced nutrition and great taste they're looking for. With Kellogg's, a healthier life—and healthier profits—are within your reach!"[28]

Such campaigns can best be explained as a valiant attempt by cereal companies to deal with declining market shares, price wars, and marketing costs as high as 35–40% of sales. Kellogg, for example, was attempting to reverse the 10% decline in market share it had endured since the late 1980s. Business analysts viewed Kellogg cereals as in trouble, because they had been "upstaged" by bagels, breakfast bars, muffins, and generic products. The company seemed far too dependent on cereals. Its only hope was to "try to tune in to today's tastes by . . . pitching its cereal as a nutritional part of a healthy diet."[29]

For the public, however, fortified cereals are an expensive way to obtain supplemental nutrients; they cost more—sometimes much more—than unfortified versions. In the summer of 1999, for example, General Mills' Total cost up to 40% more than its merely enriched counterpart, Wheaties. By winter 2001, however, General Mills was adding 15 nutrients to Wheaties at half the RDA levels, and the price differential had dropped below 20%. From the standpoint of the consumer, any one-a-day supplement would provide a more extensive complement of nutrients at much less expense. Such price issues are considered one of the key factors responsible for Kellogg's chronically declining market share, disappointing financial results, management instability, plant closures, and worker dismissals—even in its hometown of Battle Creek, Michigan.[30]

Kellogg abandoned the K-Sentials advertising late in 1999, when the campaign proved "too complicated" for the public and failed to improve sales.[31] Instead, the company tried another tack and began selling Special K and other cereals with a structure/function claim on the label: "Adequate intakes of folic acid, vitamins B_6 and B_{12} may promote a healthy cardiovascular system." As I explained in Chapter 5, the company placed an advertisement in the *Journal of the American Dietetic Association* asking, "Have you heard the good news? Now many of your patients' favorite Kellogg's cereals are fortified with 100% of the daily value of folic acid B_6 and B_{12}." The journal displayed this advertisement on the page opposite a Kellogg-sponsored fact sheet on the role of these vitamins in pregnancy and heart disease, thereby implying an endorsement by the American Dietetic Association of a health claim that had not yet been authorized by the FDA. With this kind of support, companies continued to press for increased fortification and invoked health claims as useful strategies for boosting sales.

DOES FORTIFICATION WORK?

An important question is whether fortification really does improve health. For some nutrients, the answer is an unequivocal yes, but for others it is less certain. Today, the laws of about half the communities in the United States require water to be fluoridated to help prevent tooth decay. FDA standards of identity require salt to be iodized, milk to contain vitamin D, margarine to be fortified with vitamin A, and grain products to contain added thiamin, niacin, riboflavin, iron, and, more recently, folic acid. Fortification demonstrably raises the quantity of nutrients available in the food supply; amounts of iron, thiamin, niacin, and riboflavin are about 50% higher than they were prior to fortification and 20%–30% higher than they were in 1970.[32] As a result of increasing fortification, grain products contributed 37% of the iron in the U.S. food supply in 1970 but 51% in 1994, and they also contributed major proportions of the other fortifying nutrients.[33] These increases surely help prevent deficiencies of the particular nutrients used in fortification.

The actual proportion of vitamin or mineral deficiencies eliminated as a result of fortification, however, is not easy to determine. On the one hand, the almost complete elimination of rickets, goiter, and pellagra, invariably attributed to fortification of foods with vitamin D, iodine, and niacin, respectively, is considered one of the great public health achievements of the twentieth century, as is the 40%–60% reduction in tooth decay that followed the introduction of fluoridated water.[34] In some cases, however, factors other than fortification may have been equally or more important in eliminating nutrient deficiencies. The relationship of niacin fortification to pellagra best illustrates this point. Death rates from pellagra were declining well before the initiation of mandatory niacin fortification, and the rates consistently fell by half every four years from 1938 (when there were 3,200 deaths) to 1954 (when there were fewer than 200). Congress mandated niacin fortification in 1943 but repealed it in 1946, and only 22 states required it by 1948. Under these circumstances, the proportion of pellagra deaths prevented by niacin fortification is difficult to disentangle from the changes in food prices, income, food availability, food habits, and economic growth that also were taking place at that time. People were eating better and more varied diets that could prevent pellagra as well as deficiencies of all other essential nutrients—those that are used in fortification and those that are not.[35]

This point brings us to the question of the role of single nutrients in overall diets. In that context, the effect of folic acid fortification is of great current interest. In deciding to what level grain products should be fortified with folic acid, the FDA estimated that everyone who ate fortified foods would increase intake of the vitamin, particularly those who ate the largest amounts of fortified grain products.[36] Indeed, once folic acid was added to grains, increases in average levels of folate in blood across the population became evident almost immediately. By mid-1999, it was apparent that blood levels of folate had doubled among adults who ate fortified grain products and that low levels had been almost completely eliminated. As an added benefit, blood levels of homocysteine, a risk factor for cardiovascular disease, also had decreased. Fortification of folic acid appears to increase its availability in the food supply, its dietary intake, and its level in the blood of people who eat foods fortified with folic acid—all in proportion to the amount of grain products consumed. Whether it also leads to fewer babies born with neural tube defects (the purpose of its addition to grains) remains questionable.[37] Nevertheless, food companies are increasingly adding folic acid to their products and using that fact in marketing. A 1999 box of General Mills' Total cereal, for example, proclaimed, "100% folic acid," and its rear panel contained this message: "Saving babies together: a message from the March of Dimes . . . [H]elp spread the word about folic acid and help save a baby."

Whether higher levels of folic acid fortification improve the health of babies or adults is difficult to determine, in part because people who already eat the best diets—those who are wealthier, better educated, and more concerned about their health—are the most likely to increase their nutrient intake by eating fortified foods. They also are the most likely to be consuming additional nutrients from dietary supplements. Whether fortification confers additional health benefits on such people is difficult to say with certainty and requires more sophisticated kinds of research studies than are currently available.

Furthermore, fortification raises some concerns about the safety of voluntary fortification. When the FDA establishes standards of identity for fortified products, it does so on the assumption that consuming nutrients in multiples of RDAs, whether or not beneficial, would at least be harmless. No such determinations apply to voluntary fortification, however. That it is overly optimistic to assume the inherent safety of nutrients added to the food supply is best illustrated by the case of iron fortification.

Iron deficiency and its most severe consequence, anemia, have long been the most prevalent conditions of undernutrition among Americans, but current rates are quite low except among low-income and minority toddlers, adolescent girls, and women of childbearing age.[38] Too much iron, however, is toxic. Most people are protected from taking in too much iron because this mineral is poorly absorbed. Indeed, absorption usually acts as a firm control over the amount of iron in the body; more iron is absorbed when body iron stores are low, less when stores are adequate. Because humans do not have any way to excrete much iron (other than through menstrual and other blood losses), poor absorption protects most of us against accumulating toxic levels of iron in the body. Perhaps as many as a million Americans, however, have a genetic condition, known as hemochromatosis, that causes them to absorb slightly more iron than they need. Over time, iron stores build up to toxic levels, and unless treated (by bleeding), iron overload can lead to liver and heart problems and, in severe cases, can cause death. For people with this condition (usually male adults and postmenopausal women), excess iron in the food supply represents an ongoing hazard.[39]

As a result of food fortification, the amount of iron in the food supply increased by about one-third from 1970 to 1994 and is now more than double the amount necessary to maintain adequate iron status in the population. This increase has helped reduce rates of iron-deficiency anemia to their present low levels. Listings of hemochromatosis on death certificates, however, increased by 60% from 1979 to 1992. This percentage seems high to some investigators, but others believe that it underestimates the actual number of deaths because the condition is routinely "underdiagnosed, often misdiagnosed, and probably underreported."[40] The trade-off between the competing risks of iron-deficiency anemia and iron overload has led some health officials to recognize that it is quite possible to have too much of a good thing, and several have called for a reevaluation of current fortification policies. Industry-initiated additions of iron to the food supply may well be contributing to a condition harmful to at least a million adult Americans—far more than the 2,000 or so infants conceived with neural tube defects. The discrepancy in these rates raises questions about the scientific basis of fortification policies.[32] The exceedingly high intake of calcium and other nutrients now obtained from fortified foods and supplements also raise the possibility of undesirable health consequences unknown at this time.

Given the complexities of this situation, do the potential benefits of fortification outweigh the potential risks? For product manufacturers, the answer is an unequivocal yes. They need only look at the greatly increased sales to women concerned about osteoporosis of calcium-fortified juices and fruit drinks made by Tropicana, Minute Maid, and Campbell.[41] Whether widespread fortification produces real health benefits, however, is less evident. It might seem intuitively obvious that a food supply that contains more vitamins and minerals is better for health than one that contains fewer of them (and food marketers take full advantage of this idea), but this relationship is not easy to demonstrate in economies where food intake is sufficient or in excess. Once a food supply contains enough nutrients, more will improve health only among people whose intake is less than optimal. Because fortified foods cost more, they may be beyond the reach of people who run the greatest risk of deficiencies; instead, they tend to benefit most the people who need them least. Furthermore, fortification has long been suspected of undermining efforts to educate the public about the need to follow recommended dietary patterns rather than increasing the intake of single nutrients or foods:

> Can we really accept that super-fortification will eliminate our need to select widely from conventional foods to balance nutrient intake? Americans are intrigued with the notion that a pill or a potion can settle all nutritional needs. Thus, we regard fortified cupcakes and synthesized orange juice as necessary steps in achieving that goal. . . . Dumping nutrients into such foods will not neutralize their detrimental effects or make them more healthful. Furthermore, fortification schemes serve primarily to add to the public's confusion about nutrition. By their nature, fortification practices discourage the most desirable modifications in food selection behavior.[42]

This point is important because the nutrients used in fortification make up only a small fraction of the total number of nutrients known to be essential in human diets. Those nutrients, and other key components—the numerous types of fiber and phytochemicals, for example—can be obtained only from foods. People who eat fruits and vegetables obtain vitamins, minerals, fiber, and other food components that are not covered by the rules governing standards of identity. These missing ingredients make fortification a techno-fix with inherently limited impact, because this method fails to address fundamental causes of inadequate dietary intake, such as poverty or insufficient education.

In the most successful examples of the use of fortification—the elimination of goiter by adding iodine to salt and the reduction in tooth decay by adding fluoride to drinking water—the added nutrients replace minerals that are missing or insufficient in local soils and water supplies. In these cases, fortification benefits everyone who lives in geochemically deprived areas. In these few instances, fortification is by far the best approach to improving overall public health. With regard to other nutrients, however, the issues are more complicated. The fortification of cereals, milk, and margarine, for example, addresses vitamin and mineral deficiencies that are caused largely by poverty or other socioeconomic conditions that affect a relatively small proportion of the American population. In an ideal world, nutritional deficiencies among such groups would be corrected through education, jobs, or some form of income support—all better overall strategies than fortification. In the real world, however, it is easier to fortify foods than to eliminate underlying economic disparities, which explains why fortification so often appears to be the most sensible option for dealing with dietary deficiencies.[43] Such broader issues also apply to the marketing of the new functional techno-foods, as described in the next chapters.

CHAPTER 14

BEYOND FORTIFICATION

MAKING FOODS FUNCTIONAL

BECAUSE ALL FOODS AND DRINKS INCLUDE INGREDIENTS (calories, nutrients, or water) that are essential for life, any one of them has the potential to be marketed for its health benefits. Many vitamins and minerals participate in energy-yielding biochemical reactions, and the phrase "contains vitamins essential for energy" would accurately describe just about any food except pure sugar, starch, or alcohol (which have calories, but no nutrients). Accordingly, when Congress in 1990 instructed the Food and Drug Administration (FDA) to consider authorizing certain claims for the health benefits of conventional foods and then in 1994 demanded that it permit less restrictive claims for dietary supplements, companies immediately began to market foods for their favorable nutritional properties. Indeed, the Grocery Manufacturers of America insisted to the FDA that the decision in *Pearson* v. *Shalala* (Chapter 11) meant that the same standards that governed health-related claims for supplements also applied to foods.[1]

Table 32 gives some examples of the ways in which conventional foods are marketed on this basis. Tropicana, for example, promotes regular orange juice—unfortified—for its content of potassium ("as much as a banana") and vitamin C ("a full day's supply") and for its natural lack of saturated fat or cholesterol (which are found mainly or only in foods of animal origin). Under the rules for authorized health claims, the manufacturers of soy- and oat-based cereals proclaim these products' ability to reduce risks for heart disease or cancer. Table 32 also gives examples of the ways in which manufacturers use health, nutrient-content, and structure/function claims to market their products.

TABLE 32. Examples of conventional foods and of fortified, supplemented, and other techno-foods that claimed special health-promoting benefits on package labels in the late 1990s

---

Conventional foods (no added nutrients)

Orange juice (Tropicana): *As much potassium as a banana, a full day's supply of vitamin C, naturally fat free, cholesterol free, & sodium free. A good source of folate.*[a,b]

Oats (Quaker): *Three grams of soluble fiber from oatmeal daily, in a diet low in saturated fat and cholesterol, may reduce the risk of heart disease. This cereal has 2 grams per cup.*[b,c]

Breakfast cereal (Kellogg): *Nutri-Grain cereals are made with whole grains and are a good source of fiber . . . a low fat diet rich in foods with fiber may reduce the risk of some forms of cancer.*[b,c]

Nutrient-fortified

Total breakfast cereal (General Mills): *100% Daily Value of 10 vitamins and minerals. 100% folic acid.*[d] *Healthful diets with adequate folic acid may reduce a woman's risk of having a child with a brain or spinal cord defect.*[c]

Calcium-enriched orange juice (Tropicana): *With as much calcium as milk . . . builds stronger bones in children and adolescents. Helps maintain bone mass in adult women.*[b,c]

Chromium High Beverage (Saratoga Fruit for Thought): *Apple, guava, and banana mixed with chromium picolinate, a naturally occurring element believed to have metabolizing and energizing qualities.*[d]

Chocolate Almond Fudge Bar (Clif): *Formulated supplementary sports food. Source of antioxidants. The natural energy bar.*[d]

Herbal-supplemented

Ginkgo Biloba Rings (Robert's American Gourmet): *Herbal snack. Yes, a memory snack . . . Gingko biloba has been shown to increase blood flow to the brain which can increase MEMORY AND ALERTNESS.*[d]

Ginseng Crunch Cereal (New Morning): *Low fat. A cholesterol free food. Low sodium.*[a] *An herbal dietary supplement. Ginseng for energy & antioxidant.*[d]

Kitchen Prescription Chicken Broth and Noodles with Echinacea (Hain Pure Foods): *Herbal supplement. We've . . . blended our soup with natural Echinacea, creating a delicious and satisfying herbal supplement . . . Support your immune system* * *with a cup of Kitchen Prescription today!*[d,e]

Cranberry Echinacea (Rocket Juice): *traditional herbal defense with vitamin C.*[d]

In addition to using health claims to sell conventional foods, food manufacturers also are developing "functional" foods—products created just so that they can be marketed using health claims. Food technologists develop these products by *adding* desirable components, such as vitamins, minerals, herbals, fiber, or other ingredients that might reduce disease risk factors, or by *reducing* undesirable components, such as fat, saturated fat, *trans*-saturated fatty acids, sugar, or salt. This chapter

TABLE 32. *(continued)*

Fiber-supplemented
Ensemble cheddar baked potato crisps (Kellogg): *made with a natural soluble fiber that actively works to promote heart health (as part of a diet low in saturated fat and cholesterol).[f]*

Cholesterol-blocking
Benecol spread (McNeil Consumer Healthcare): *Benefits cholesterol. Just three servings a day . . . together with a low fat, low cholesterol diet and exercise will benefit your cholesterol level.[f] The unique dietary ingredient in Benecol products, plant stanol ester, is derived from plants.*
Take Control spread (Lipton): *Helps promote healthy cholesterol levels (as part of a diet low in saturated fat and cholesterol).[f]*

Techno "lesser-evils"
Trans Fat Free! Super Light Margarine (Heart Beat Foods): *Great taste! Lactose Free. The small amount of partially hydrogenated soy oil has a dietically* [sic] *insignificant level of trans fatty acids which we round to zero.*
WOW potato chips (Frito-Lay): *All the taste. Fat free. Half the calories.*

---

[a]FDA-authorized nutrient-content claim.

[b]Also labeled with a check mark from the American Heart Association and the statement *Meets American Heart Association food criteria for saturated fat and cholesterol for healthy people over age 2. While many factors affect heart disease, a diet that is low in total fat, saturated fat and cholesterol combined with a healthy lifestyle may reduce the risk of heart disease.*

[c]FDA-authorized health claim.

[d]Structure/function claim permitted under provisions of the Dietary Supplement Health and Education Act (DSHEA) of 1994.

[e]The asterisk refers to the DSHEA disclaimer: "*This statement has not been evaluated by the Food and Drug Administration. This product is not intended to diagnose, treat, cure or prevent any disease.*"

[f]Structure/function claim used because the product is too high in fat to meet requirements for an FDA-authorized health claim.

explains how the food industry came to consider functional foods as an avenue to new sales opportunities, one made possible by the increasingly liberal regulatory environment for health claims.

THE REGULATORY QUAGMIRE

Soon after the Nutrition Labeling and Education Act (NLEA) of 1990 forced the FDA to consider authorizing certain health claims that companies could put on food labels for marketing purposes, the National Cancer Institute (NCI) initiated a new $20 million research program to develop "designer foods" enriched in cancer-fighting phytochemicals—substances such as lycopenes, indoles, flavonoids, and sterols—that are typically found in food plants, but in minute amounts. As Jane Brody explained in the *New York Times*, the idea of adding beneficial plant chemicals to existing foods was intended to speed up the annoyingly long and expensive process required to obtain the FDA's approval for new food additives or supplements.[2] Because phytochemicals occur naturally in fruits and vegetables, the FDA could consider foods supplemented with these substances as generally recognized as safe (GRAS) for human consumption and would not require them to undergo premarket testing or authorization. Because functional foods include those to which desirable components are added, as well as those from which undesirable components are removed, they do not fit neatly into the traditional regulatory categories established by the FDA. From 1990 to 1994, manufacturers had three choices for marketing functional foods. If the products were *GRAS*, they could be marketed immediately. If they were considered *food additives*, manufacturers would have to demonstrate that the ingredients were safe. But if they wanted to claim that their products affected a *disease*, manufacturers would need to demonstrate that the product qualified for an authorized health claim or would have to meet the requirements of drug regulations and prove safety and efficacy.[3] Obviously, manufacturers preferred the GRAS alternative. They also hoped that the remaining restrictions on health claims for conventional foods would soon disappear or be applied more leniently.[4]

FUNCTIONAL FOODS AS DIETARY MEDICINES

Food manufacturers had every reason to be optimistic. The Dietary Supplement Health and Education Act (DSHEA) of 1994 permitted supplement companies to market their products with statements of structure/function that could hardly be distinguished from FDA-authorized health claims (Table 28, page 229). DSHEA also provided a new regulatory opportunity for functional foods: they could now be marketed as *dietary supplements* using such claims. The benefits of this alternative were self-evident. For example, in response to the announcement of its designer foods project, the NCI received "an eight-inch stack of telephone messages, mostly from industry officials."[2] The potential market for foods with drug-like effects could easily encompass the entire adult population, because conditions such as obesity, diabetes, heart disease, arthritis, and cancer might be expected to affect almost everyone who lives long enough.

The pressure to develop therapeutic foods derived directly from food company imperatives to overcome the infamously slow growth (a mere 1% to 2% annually) of the food industry as a whole. The companies could see that low-fat products and dietary supplements were doing much better than the industry average. Thus functional foods presented a most welcome opportunity. Using the broadest definition—one that includes supplements, organics, health foods, and "lesser evils"—functional foods were estimated to have earned $86 billion in sales in 1996, with a growth rate of nearly 8% more than in the previous year, and to have risen to $91.7 billion just one year later. Together with supplements, "functional" conventional foods were said to be worth $14.7 billion in 1998 and were projected to be worth $49 billion by 2010.[5]

The size of this potential market encouraged virtually every large food or drug company—Johnson & Johnson, Cargill, DuPont, Unilever, and Monsanto, for example—to establish functional-foods divisions. Marketing opportunities also have spawned a thriving consulting industry that offers frequent seminars and conferences on growth opportunities in this area and ways to build value and profits. Best of all, the new foods could be marketed with "eat more" messages. Although food companies had long been producing fat substitutes and sweeteners, foods made from them, and lesser-evil foods lower in fat, cholesterol, sugar, and salt, they could now take a less puritanical approach. Manufacturers could shift the emphasis from "removing the bad" to "enhancing the good," thereby opening up "a vast array of commercial possibilities."[6] The sections that follow illustrate some of these possibilities.

Herbal-Supplemented Everything

The search for a "magic bullet" is behind most of the new functional-food products marketed to date. Surely, the prize for the greatest "triumph of marketing ingenuity" goes to the vast array of herbal-supplemented cereals, snack foods, and drinks sold in the guise of dietary supplements just so that they can be labeled with structure/function claims. Figure 27 shows some examples of such products. The variety of herbs used in these products is extensive and is becoming more so, whether or not there is any evidence that they are safe or that they do any good when added to foods. Although the products must comply with the rules for labeling supplements, these rules do not require disclosure of ingredients present in minute amounts or of the amounts of ingredients in mixtures.[7] The New Morning company's breakfast cereals, Ginseng Crunch ("for extra energy") and GinkgOs ("Improves blood flow to the brain . . . to sustain memory"), each of which is labeled explicitly as "an herbal dietary supplement," say that they contain 60 mg of the active

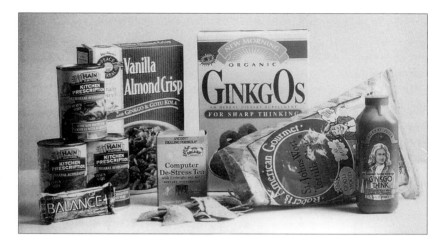

FIGURE 27. Herbal-supplemented foods such as those illustrated here could be found in regular supermarkets as well as health food stores in 1999 and 2000. To take advantage of the relatively relaxed rules that apply to health claims for supplements, they were marketed more as supplements than as foods. (Photo by Shimon and Tammar Rothstein, 2000)

ingredient per serving but give no indication of the significance of such a dose. Similarly, a Rocket Juice Cranberry Echinacea drink, a "traditional herbal defense with vitamin C," is simply said to contain 100 mg of the herb; no further explanation follows. Because a 16-ounce serving of this beverage contains 2 ounces of sugar (from juice extracts) as the principal source of its 230 calories, it is difficult to view this product as anything more than yet another heavily sweetened soft drink.

The overburdened FDA has taken a dim view of such products and deals with them as best it can. In early 2000, the agency issued a warning to Robert's American Gourmet about label violations for its Spirulina Spirals (because they did not contain enough vitamin B_{12} to claim that they are a "good source"), for its Echinacea Shells (because saying that this food can be an effective antibiotic constitutes a drug claim), and for other products considered misbranded because of misleading or illegal label statements. Reportedly, the FDA warning letter stated, "We note that ingredients such as echinacea, *Ginkgo biloba*, St. John's wort, cat's claw, kava kava, and spirulina are listed on the labels of several of your products. FDA has not issued a food additive regulation authorizing the use of these ingredients in food. Additionally, we are not aware of a basis for concluding that these ingredients are GRAS for use in conventional food."[8] The FDA also had issued similar warnings to Hain's about its Kitchen Prescription soup line (shown in Figure 27).

As if not enough products were already supplemented, producers of hard liquor were reported to be exploring the marketing potential of alcoholic beverages supplemented with ginkgo, ginseng, and other herbs. Such innovations, designed particularly to appeal to people aged 25 to 35, were certain to attract the attention of the relevant regulatory agency, in this case the Bureau of Alcohol, Tobacco and Firearms (BATF).[9] In February 2001, overwhelmed with the number of herbal-supplemented foods and beverages that were appearing on the market, the FDA issued a blanket warning letter to the food industry that botanicals could not be assumed to be approved food additives or GRAS, that health claims for foods containing such supplements were governed by legal requirements, and that companies would be well advised to "contact the agency regarding the regulatory status of ingredients and claims they intend to use for foods." When the FDA began sending letters warning individual companies that marketing supplement-containing products as conventional foods defied federal law, the industry reacted with outraged surprise. A representative of the National Nutritional Foods Association said that such letters were "part of an FDA effort to stop an inevitable flow of products that have already bypassed an antiquated regulatory scheme. Dietary supplements are foods for every purpose but one, which is structure/function claims. . . . And that distinction has worn away. So there really is no viable distinction."[10] When companies as large as Procter & Gamble and Coca-Cola began collaborating to produce a functional drink containing glucosamine, (a supplement said to help relieve symptoms of arthritis) and Pepsi "playfully" began advertising a new drink as "liquid liposuction," it was even more apparent that the FDA would have no end of difficulty regulating this market.[11]

Fiber- and Soy-Supplemented Foods

In response to petitions from Quaker Oats, Kellogg, and Protein Technologies International, respectively, the FDA authorized health claims for soluble fiber from oats in 1997, for psyllium husk in 1998, and for soy protein in 1999 (see Table 31 in Chapter 11). As we shall see, the purpose of these requests was to increase market share. In substantiating the claims, the companies drew on studies of single foods or food components in isolation from their dietary context. Despite the ambiguity of the results of such studies, the FDA authorized each claim. It had to: under the various laws and court decisions governing the FDA's actions in this area, the agency must approve claims backed up by well-conducted studies, no matter how out of context they may be or how quickly contradicted by further research. The health claims for oat bran, psyllium fiber, and soy proteins illustrate these problems.

Oat Bran   In January 1996, when the FDA first proposed to approve the Quaker Oats request for a claim for oat fiber, the company placed a full-page newspaper announcement in the *New York Times*: "Why is this man smiling? FDA proposes first food-specific health claim: diets high in oatmeal and low in saturated fat and cholesterol may reduce the risk of heart disease." When the FDA issued its final rule in January 1997, the company again announced the news in full-page advertisements: "Now he has another reason to smile . . . Quaker oatmeal. Oh what those Oats can do." General Mills also bought full-page advertisements: "FDA announces heart healthy news. So go ahead. Eat to your heart's content . . . the one and only Cheerios." An additional reason for smiling was the "pretty good 'pop' in sales" now expected and the immediate jump in the prices of shares of stock in Quaker, General Mills, and Kellogg, all of which would be using the claim to promote their products.[12]

In authorizing the oat fiber claim, the FDA required the qualifying phrase *as part of a diet low in saturated fat and cholesterol* so as not to mislead people into thinking that eating oatmeal was sufficient to reduce the risk of heart disease. Although cereal makers include that phrase on boxes, they do so grudgingly. For example, the Cheerios box says, "*as part of a heart-healthy diet, the soluble fiber in Cheerios May Help Reduce Cholesterol.*" The Quaker Oat Bran label splits the message into three distinct parts: soluble fiber from oat bran (large type) *as part of a low saturated fat, low cholesterol diet* (small type) may reduce the risk of heart disease (enclosed in a red heart).

Quaker Oats advertisements promote the research basis of the cholesterol-lowering effects of oat cereals. A full-page color advertisement in the *New York Times Magazine* of September 27, 1998, pictured 100 smiling people in Lafayette, Colorado, holding boxes of Quaker Oats because, according to the copy, after 30 days of eating the product, 98 of them lowered their cholesterol—the ad doesn't say by how much— thereby "redefining oatmeal as a soul food."[13] Indeed, research studies suggesting that oat fiber reduces blood cholesterol levels by 5–10% have appeared since the early 1960s, and Quaker submitted 37 such studies, conducted between 1978 and 1994, in support of its health-claim petition.

A Quaker Oats advertisement in the March 1999 *Journal of the American Dietetic Association* asserted that such studies "documented the cholesterol-lowering effect of soluble fiber (beta-glucan) from oats. . . . Some studies have attributed a 4–8% decrease in total cholesterol to the addition of oatmeal to a healthy diet. Other studies included oatmeal in a specific low-fat diet which resulted in a 10–12% decrease in total cholesterol."

The FDA said, however, that just 20 studies produced statistically significant reductions of blood cholesterol levels. Of the remaining 17, it disqualified one for poor methods and found the rest to have yielded equivocal effects at best. Despite these discrepancies, the FDA agreed that the preponderance of evidence supported a cholesterol-lowering effect—although a small one—from eating oat fiber as part of an otherwise low-fat diet.

These actions took place a decade after the oat bran craze of the late 1980s and were expected to restore some of the losses in sales that had occurred when the oat bran bubble burst. The craze began as a result of 11 studies that by 1988 had demonstrated reductions in blood cholesterol ranging from 3% to 26% as a result of eating from 1 to 5 ounces of oatmeal or oat bran daily. This widely publicized "single-food" research generated immediate commercial attention in the form of "eye-popping" sales that quickly drained national oat supplies and depleted retailers' shelves of oat cereals. At the time, manufacturers added oat bran to *everything*, even beer. The label of Robert's American Gourmet potato chips read, "Now with oat bran! The potato chip that's good . . . and good for you! You can enjoy these treats to your heart's delight!" Because the peak of interest in oat bran occurred in 1989 during the hiatus when the FDA was not regulating health claims, the companies were particularly eager to take advantage of this situation; they would not have to prove that their products actually lowered cholesterol or, for that matter, have to put much oat bran into them. According to one review of the studies, up to 35 servings of some products would be needed to achieve a 3% drop in blood cholesterol levels.[14]

The craze ended a year later, however, when Harvard researchers reported that oat bran appeared to be no better than any other high-fiber cereal in lowering levels of cholesterol in blood.[15] Quaker Oats officials immediately objected that the study was too small, uncontrolled, and atypical to be considered significant—a view that also received support from other, presumably less partisan sources. The question of partisanship in interpretation of the science is particularly relevant to this case, because Quaker Oats had paid for the studies reporting the most impressive

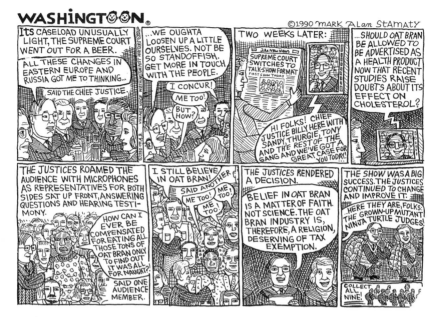

FIGURE 28. The political cartoonist Mark Alan Stamaty used conflicting research on the health benefits of oat bran to point out how the public ignores science in deciding whether foods are "healthy" and how the U.S. Supreme Court permits popular opinion to influence its decisions. The drawing was published in the *Washington Post* and the *Village Voice* in 1990. (Courtesy ©Mark Alan Stamaty)

benefits of oat fiber, as well as for an influential analysis of the combined results of 20 clinical trials.[16] The less favorable 1990 study was one of the few conducted by independent investigators. Figure 28 illustrates one political commentator's understanding of the religious, commercial, and legal issues raised by the conflicting scientific studies of the health benefits of oat bran.

Does oat fiber lower blood cholesterol levels? Of course it does—conditionally. Like any other whole grain cereal, oats are high in fiber and contribute to the cholesterol-lowering effects of diets low in fat, saturated fat, and cholesterol. Whether oats are sufficiently different from other fiber sources to merit their own special health claim is far less evident. The potential marketing benefits—not the science—explain companies' persistent attempts to obtain FDA authorization for health claims.

Psyllium Husk   Similar issues of science as opposed to commercial pressures apply to functional foods supplemented with psyllium husk, the dried seed coat of the stemless annual herb *Plantago ovata*. Psyllium is grown in India, where it is commonly used as a household remedy for constipation, and it is the active ingredient in over-the-counter laxatives such as Metamucil. Its bulking action in part explains its ability to cause cholesterol to be excreted rather than absorbed from the intestine.

When Kellogg succeeded in convincing the FDA to approve a health claim for psyllium fiber, it created a $65 million functional-foods division to introduce an entire line of food products called *Ensemble* ("Great food that does great things") designed to provide an easy way for the huge number of American adults with elevated cholesterol levels to lower them.[17] Because it takes three daily servings of psyllium-based products to lower blood cholesterol levels, and people were unlikely to eat that much cereal, Kellogg's designed the line to include 22 different food items in several categories: breads, cereals, potato chips, mini-cakes, and pastas. The company wanted to appeal to what might seem like a relatively narrow target audience: people who look for health foods in regular supermarkets. To reach this audience, the company gave the packages a "European-style" design; the name was spelled out as en-sem-ble on a box with understated graphics, plenty of white space, and green borders (see Figure 29). Ensemble products came with "a fee-for-service cholesterol management solution": private nutrition counseling services that would be conducted in six coaching sessions (over the telephone) for $150. The products were expected to sell for premium prices.

Ensemble packages displayed two types of claims. Labels for products that qualified for FDA-authorized health claims, such as fettuccine primavera and blueberry mini-loaves, said, "Made with a natural soluble fiber that actively works to lower cholesterol" followed, in small print, by "Soluble fiber from psyllium husk, as part of a diet low in saturated fat and cholesterol, may reduce the risk of heart disease." Products too high in fat or too low in nutrients to qualify for that claim instead displayed a structure/function claim. The packages of oatmeal cookies, fettuccine Alfredo, and carrot cake mini-loaves, for example, said, "Made with a natural soluble fiber that actively works to promote heart health" followed, in very small print, by "as part of a diet low in saturated fat and cholesterol." The fine distinction between "may reduce the risk of heart disease" and "actively works to promote heart health" would surely be lost on anyone other than a federal regulator or food company attorney.

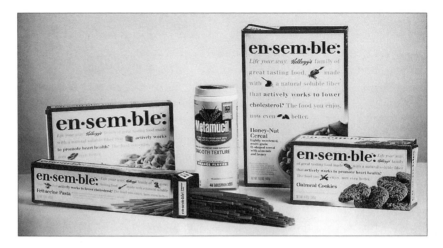

FIGURE 29. Kellogg's line of foods supplemented with psyllium fiber and Procter & Gamble's psyllium-containing Metamucil made identical claims on their labels for promotion of heart health. Kellogg withdrew the Ensemble product line in 1999 when it failed test-marketing. (Photo by Shimon and Tammar Rothstein, 2000)

As it happens, the Ensemble line was a *second* attempt by Kellogg's to introduce psyllium fiber into its cereals. In 1989 the company had introduced Heartwise, "the natural, multi-grain psyllium cereal: According to medical research, a diet low in fat and high in soluble fiber can help lower cholesterol. At the Kellogg company, we believe that Heartwise can be part of that diet." This statement, of course, addressed a medical condition and therefore constituted a drug claim, but the product appeared during the period when FDA was not taking action against unauthorized health claims. Instead, six states filed lawsuits against Kellogg to prevent the claim's use. In 1990 Texas banned sales of Heartwise because its package label did not alert buyers that psyllium husk caused laxative and allergic effects in some people. The allergic reactions were particularly alarming. Reportedly, a nurse who had given psyllium-containing laxatives to several of her patients developed life-threatening symptoms the first time she ate Heartwise cereal; other such cases also had been reported.[18]

When Kellogg finally added a warning statement, a Texas legal official called it "backhanded . . . in 'mice' type" and said that "Kellogg constantly lies about its products. . . . Companies under investigation by states these days feel they have First Amendment rights to lie to their customers."[19] These statements elicited outraged denials by company officials and a further exchange of lawsuits. Texas sued Kellogg over health claims, and Kellogg sued the Texas official for slander: "It has taken 85 years to build one of the best corporations in the world and we will not allow an arrogant, irresponsible public official to attack our reputation."[20]

Objections to the cereal were likely to come from another source as well. Prior to the introduction of Heartwise, the Procter & Gamble (P&G) company had objected to similar disease claims made for Benefit, a cereal made by General Mills and advertised in the *New York Times* on September 12, 1989, as containing "a natural blend of oat bran, rice and psyllium grain. What makes Benefit so remarkable is the psyllium grain. Ounce for ounce, this natural grain contains 8 times more soluble fiber than oat bran. . . . Reduce cholesterol, Get the Benefit."

P&G is the maker of the psyllium-containing laxative Metamucil. In the late 1980s, the company had asked the FDA to authorize a cholesterol-lowering claim for its product because it was inconsistent to allow the "new cereals to make cholesterol-reduction claims while Metamucil cannot."[21] The FDA rejected this request on the grounds of insufficient data and instead asked Kellogg and General Mills to submit scientific data demonstrating that their products were safe. It seemed likely that P&G's objections also would apply to Heartwise, but the issue became moot when both cereals failed to sell. General Mills withdrew Benefit soon after the test-marketing, and Heartwise disappeared a year or so later.

For the Ensemble line, Kellogg maintained that it had corrected the problems that plagued Heartwise. Whereas the psyllium used in Heartwise was crude and likely to have been contaminated with allergenic proteins from the whole seed, the Ensemble line was supplemented with preparations of 95% pure psyllium husk. Just to be on the safe side, the Ensemble products all displayed a warning notice (in very small type): "For individuals with food allergies: This product contains psyllium, wheat, almond and soybean ingredients." Finally, P&G's concern about unfair competition also was resolved; boxes of Metamucil now display a heart health claim: "Diets low in saturated fat and cholesterol that include 7 grams of soluble fiber per day from psyllium husk, as in Metamucil, may reduce the risk of heart disease by lowering cholesterol." Thus authorization of the health claim for psyllium husk led to a thorough blurring of the distinctions among claims for the health benefits of foods, supplements, and over-the-counter drugs.

Perhaps for this reason, and because they were aware of the fate of Heartwise, some early commentators were less than optimistic about the Ensemble line's chances of success. Advertising industry observers thought that the $2 million that Kellogg spent for promotion in the first half of 1999 was not nearly enough. I also was dubious that these products could succeed: I had encountered them that spring at a Kellogg-sponsored breakfast for heads of nutrition departments, and I thought they tasted chalky. As it turned out, Ensemble products never reached supermarkets. During 1999 Kellogg withdrew the line from all but one test market, accepted the resignation of the executive in charge of the project, and abandoned the Ensemble line.[22] In this instance, the small reduction in blood cholesterol promised by these products was insufficient to overcome consumer concerns about cost, taste, and (perhaps) an association with an over-the-counter laxative product.

Soy Protein   In May 1998, Protein Technologies International, a division of DuPont that manufactures isolated soy proteins for commercial use, petitioned the FDA to permit claims that soy protein could help reduce the risk of coronary heart disease. By August, the FDA had completed its initial review, and it published the proposed rule in November.[23] This rapid response reflected pressure from Congress and industry to authorize health claims quickly, and it also reflected the FDA's acceptance of the validity of studies suggesting that about an ounce of soy protein per day can reduce blood cholesterol by about 10% in people with high cholesterol levels.

The soy story requires a brief digression into soy science. To begin with, soybeans and their derivatives—miso, soy sauce, soy milk, tofu, and tempeh—are traditional foods in Asian diets. Asians who consume soy foods display lower rates of coronary heart disease, breast cancer, and other conditions than North Americans. On this basis, researchers have examined the effects of isolated soybean components (proteins, isoflavones, and fiber) on such conditions. Isoflavones are phytochemicals, in this case estrogen-like compounds that accompany the proteins after they are extracted. Investigators wondered, for example, whether isoflavones separately or with proteins might be responsible for the low rates of menopausal symptoms and breast cancer among Asian women. They also suggested that American women should eat more soy foods in order to gain such benefits.[24]

As early as 1981, researchers reported that soy proteins reduced blood cholesterol levels, and soon proposed soy proteins as a means of treating high blood cholesterol.[25] When a review paper concluded that soy protein—with isoflavones—lowered blood cholesterol levels, the *New York Times* warned readers to "prepare for the onslaught: soy cookies, soy bread, soy muffins, soy milkshakes, soy pretzels, soy soups and a new, surely improved version of that old unfavorite, the soy burger."[26] In September 1998, the Center for Science in the Public Interest welcomed its Nutrition Action Healthletter subscribers to "the overblown—and under-substantiated—world of soy claims," warning that most of the claims came from the companies' marketing departments.[27] This skepticism was soon justified by independent studies suggesting that substituting soy for other proteins in the diet might have little effect on the coronary risk of North Americans. Studies also suggested that soy might have some disadvantages, such as increasing the risk of coronary heart disease or of breast cancer.[28] Despite such concerns, the FDA "tentatively" concluded that soy protein—independent of its isoflavone content—reduced coronary risk and merited a health claim: "25 grams of soy protein, combined with a diet low in saturated fat and cholesterol, may reduce the risk of coronary heart disease." To qualify for this claim, a product would need to contain about a teaspoonful (6.25 grams) of soy protein per serving. To reap the benefit, people would need to eat four servings per day.

Many products on the market were expected to meet the 6.25 gram requirement. Soy proteins—in the form of isolated proteins, concentrates, or flour—already were common ingredients in food products, where they served as extenders and stabilizers. A 1995 estimate suggested that 12,000 products containing soy proteins were on the market, and more were soon to follow.[26] New functional soy foods were rapidly joining this market: breads, cereals, power bars, drinks, and even potato chips. As soon as the FDA authorized the claim, soy food companies announced the decision in the usual full-page *New York Times* advertisements. One published on October 24, 1999, from a soy "veggie" burger company (owned by Kraft Foods/Philip Morris) said, "It's official—soy is heart healthy!" The new health claim was expected to stimulate creation of even more new products, especially because other giant food companies such as Kellogg, ConAgra, General Mills, and Campbell Soup all were pursuing ways to take advantage of the claim. Archer Daniels Midland, the world's dominant processor of soybeans, also was planning to cash in on this marketing opportunity by entering into partnerships with pasta and cereal makers.[29]

Would such products succeed? They might, if people could be induced to view soy as mainstream rather than as a health food. Even if the scientific justification for the soy claim raised questions, marketers were optimistic about its economic justification, and with good reason. Sales of soy beverages, for example, grew more than 82% in 1999, leading Bestfoods to back its NutraBlend product with a $20 million advertising budget: "As consumers become more open to the message of soy health benefits . . . they're looking for these products; and now is the time to advertise."[30]

Cholesterol-Blocking: Margarines

Driving the creation of psyllium-supplemented and other classes of functional foods is the idea that food products with therapeutic benefits can be sold without having to be subjected to lengthy and expensive drug-approval processes. In May 1999, the FDA permitted two companies, Unilever and Johnson & Johnson, to market margarines containing different types of ingredients, both of which could reduce blood cholesterol levels by about 10%. For both companies, the margarines represented first entries into the functional-foods marketplace. From a nutritionist's standpoint, making a high-fat, high-calorie table spread appear to be a health food seems a pessimistic approach to dietary change; it assumes that consumers will ignore advice to cut down on high-calorie table fats, so these might as well be made "healthier."

For Johnson & Johnson, the economic issues must have been compelling. Its interest in the product began in 1997 when one of its subsidiaries, McNeil Consumer Healthcare, bought the marketing rights to a Finnish margarine. Business analysts viewed the company's purchase as "breaking a nutraceutical barrier with its much-anticipated U.S. introduction of what could become a blockbuster new product, cholesterol-reducer Benecol."[31] The enthusiasm derived from the outstanding success of Benecol margarine in Finland, a country where coronary heart disease is rampant. Since Benecol's 1995 introduction, an estimated 165 million servings had been sold in that country, even though the margarine was priced six times higher than regular brands.[32] The potential for a similar reception in the United States, home to a much larger number of people with high cholesterol levels, seemed even more favorable. Immediate sales were predicted to be in the hundreds of millions of dollars, and annual revenues were expected to reach $2.5 billion within just a few years.[31]

The active ingredient in Benecol is sitostanol ester (plant stanol ester), a cholesterol-like substance obtained from pine tree pulp or canola oil. Sitostanol is not itself absorbed by the body, but it blocks the absorption or reabsorption of about half the cholesterol present in the intestine. Industry-supported clinical trials in Finland and Canada demonstrated that people who ate low-fat diets *and* substituted Benecol for other spreads lowered their blood cholesterol readings by about 10%. Later studies showed Benecol to reduce cholesterol further in people who already were taking cholesterol-lowering drugs.[33]

Initially, the McNeil company insisted that sitostanol met the congressional definition of a dietary supplement and wanted to market Benecol as a "supplement in a spread."[34] In addition to desiring the greater flexibility in health claims granted to dietary supplements, the company assumed that this strategy would enable Benecol to be marketed ahead of a competing product, Take Control, produced by Lipton (a division of Unilever). This strategy failed, however, when the FDA interpreted Benecol as a food with a new ingredient, which meant that the company would have to file a food additive petition to prove that sitostanol was safe at its expected level of use—a process guaranteed to be long and costly.

Lipton's Take Control also contains cholesterol-like substances, in this case sterols derived from soybeans. Unlike the sitostanol ester in Benecol, bean sterols are partially absorbed by the body, but they block cholesterol absorption and reabsorption and reduce blood cholesterol levels by about the same amount under similar conditions.[35] Lipton requested FDA approval of Take Control as a soybean-derived food considered GRAS; the FDA agreed and approved it before approving Benecol, an action considered "a blow for Johnson & Johnson." According to FDA officials, the agency wanted to maintain a level playing field between the two firms: "The key here is that this company chose to market this product appropriately under the food provisions of the law, and they've met those provisions."[36] McNeil therefore switched strategies and asked the FDA to consider Benecol a food with a GRAS ingredient. The FDA did so, just two weeks after approving sale of Take Control. A three-quarter-page advertisement in the *New York Times* on May 27, 1999, announced Benecol's arrival in stores: "Introducing a revolution in managing cholesterol (you'll find it right between the butter and eggs)."

For these margarines to be effective in lowering cholesterol, people need to eat two servings a day of Take Control or three of Benecol, and this makes price an issue. As expressed by a skeptical European, "eating four daily teaspoons of Finnish wood pulp disguised as a margarine may lower cholesterol, but it will cost as much as the rest of your breakfast."[37] In American markets, the initial cost of these products induced sticker shock. Early in July 1999, my local market was selling an 8-ounce tub or 16 individually packaged servings of Take Control for $4.69, or $9.38 per pound. The Benecol spreads (regular and light) were even more expensive: $5.69 for 21 individual servings weighing 5.9 ounces. These prices made Benecol eight times more expensive than the least expensive stick margarine, and made Take Control five times more expensive. Neither would be likely to be purchased by low-income individuals with high cholesterol who might benefit from its use.

The price differential—and the innovative concept—presented marketing challenges. Because the margarines are high in fat, they do not qualify for health or nutrient-content claims under the "jelly bean rule" discussed in Chapter 11. They can, however, be marketed with structure/function statements. The Take Control product uses "helps promote healthy cholesterol levels," followed by the required disclaimer in fine print, "as part of a diet low in saturated fat and cholesterol." The Benecol products just say, "benefits cholesterol."

Benecol, however, would get plenty of promotion. Its advertising budget was expected to be $35 million for the initial launch alone, much of it for television commercials.[31] As might be expected, promotional efforts also focused on health professionals. A two-page advertisement that appeared several times in the American Dietetic Association's journal during 1999, for example, displayed color photographs of toasted English muffins with and without Benecol margarine, with the headline, "Guess which one helps promote healthy cholesterol levels?" The second page provided a coupon for ordering copies of relevant scientific studies and information about how the product worked: "By substituting Benecol 3 times a day for butter, margarine, or spreads, your patients will quickly discover that diet can make a meaningful change in their cholesterol levels." It also explained the difference between Benecol and its competitor: "Plant *stanol* esters are different from plant *sterols* in an important way. The *stanol* component of Benecol is virtually unabsorbed, whereas *sterols* are absorbed to a greater degree." The advertisement did not mention whether this distinction makes any difference in lowering cholesterol levels or in any other aspect of health.

Advertising methods included the usual coupons, Web sites, telephone "coaching" of consumers, and doctor's-office tie-ins. They also included one program-length television "infomercial" that raised questions of journalistic ethics because it was narrated by a reporter for the station.

Observers who were distressed by that ethical breach said the program was "not real news, but it looks and tastes just like real news" (the reporter was fired).[38] The principal marketing method, however, was—and continues to be—through physicians. The approach to doctors was based on Johnson & Johnson's existing network of drug detail people who could suggest that physicians recommend Benecol to their patients if for no other reason than the margarine is much less expensive than cholesterol-lowering drugs. The company was reported to have unleashed "its more than 300 salespeople to storm doctors' offices touting the cholesterol-lowering effects of consuming stanols."[39]

In the year ending in August 2000, Benecol and Take Control sales were about $27 million each, numbers considered disappointing in comparison to expectation. Although Benecol held more than 12% of the market share of margarine in Finland, it and Take Control each reached just 2.2% of the U.S. market.[40] Some analysts attributed consumer resistance to the high cost of the products, but taste may also have been a contributing factor. A taste panel judged Benecol to have a waxy, Crisco-like texture and found Take Control to turn toast damp and soggy. By the end of 1999, McNeil had withdrawn its projected $100 million television campaign for Benecol but was continuing to market the products to physicians who would recommend them to their patients. In July 2001, I had a hard time finding Benecol products in local supermarkets, although Take Control was usually available. Even so, *Advertising Age* had been calling them "dysfunctional foods" for some time.[41]

"Lesser Evils": Lighter Fats, Fat Substitutes

Much current research on functional foods focuses on fats and oils either reduced in unwanted saturated or *trans*-saturated fatty acids, or enriched in desirable monounsaturated or omega-3 fatty acids or vitamins (see the Appendix). By the late 1990s, omega-3–enriched infant formulas, noodles, margarines, beverages, and eggs were widely available in Japan and Europe; American companies still were trying to solve technical problems and had not released products to U.S. markets.[42] I first saw "omega-3 eggs" in American markets late in 2000. According to package inserts, the "cage free" hens laying these eggs had been fed organically grown flaxseed or an unspecified "all natural, vegetarian feed." The labels also state that the eggs are certified organic and contain no growth hormones, medications, antibiotics, or pesticides. The package insert for one brand claims that egg omega-3, like that in fish oil, helps maintain normal blood pressure, supports brain and eye function, and provides important nutrients for pregnant women and nursing infants. Like other eggs, these contain about 70 calories each, along with 1.5 grams of saturated fat and more than two-thirds the Daily Value of cholesterol, 215 milligrams. In early 2001, a half-dozen such eggs cost more than two dollars in my local Manhattan market.

Also at this time, the "spread" sections of supermarkets were filled with lighter margarines and those reduced in *trans*-saturated fatty acids. Light margarines are stabilized mixtures (emulsions) of oil and varying amounts of water. "*Trans* fat–free" margarines are made from vegetable oils that have not been hydrogenated. The mixtures are not particularly stable, and these products cannot be used in standard recipes for cooking or baking. The most important development in this field, however, was the late 1990s introduction by Procter & Gamble of its new fat substitute, olestra, to which the next chapter is devoted.

FOOD AS A TECHNO-FIX: HEINZ KETCHUP

As discussed in the introduction to Part V, techno-foods offer a reductionist approach to choosing healthful diets. That such approaches can lead to even more absurd consequences than those already mentioned is illustrated by the attempted transformation of Heinz ketchup into a functional food. Early in 1999, Heinz placed the advertisement shown as Figure 30 in the *New York Times Magazine*. It shows a bottle of Heinz ketchup with the headline "Lycopene may help reduce the risk of prostate and cervical cancer.*" The asterisk refers readers to a review article on the health benefits of lycopene.[43] At the time, I was surprised to see an advertisement with so blatant a claim for disease protection, because the FDA had not authorized a lycopene-and-cancer claim for package labels, and the Federal Trade Commission usually defers to guidelines of the FDA in such matters. Furthermore, ketchup contains processed tomatoes, sugar, and salt (in that order) and could hardly be considered a health food, not least because it typically is used as a garnish for hamburgers and fried potatoes. The advertisement singled out one component of ketchup, lycopene (a plant pigment naturally present in tomatoes and other fruits and vegetables), and it clearly associated ketchup with cancer prevention by including a prominent endorsement from the Cancer Research Foundation of America.

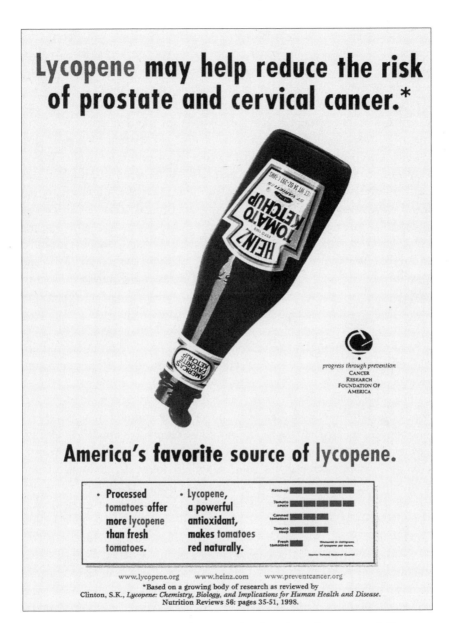

FIGURE 30. This advertisement for Heinz ketchup from the *New York Times Magazine* (January 10, 1999) made an unauthorized health claim for lycopene and cancer risk. Heinz withdrew the advertisement under challenge by the Federal Trade Commission.

Eating tomatoes is demonstrably good for health, as all fruits and vegetables contain a variety of components protective against disease. Ketchup, however, seems a bit of a stretch. Under the FDA's rules, support in a single scientific publication fails to meet the criteria for scientific substantiation of health claims because it does not reflect significant scientific agreement as a result of a deliberate review by a government or private health agency. Before DSHEA, so blatant a disease claim would have promptly attracted the attention of both FDA and FTC. In response to my queries, however, an FDA official reminded me that this was an advertisement, not a label, and hence was not a concern of his agency; he referred me to the FTC. An FTC official said the matter was not public information and could not be discussed. Nevertheless, the FTC was reported to be investigating the claim and to be especially interested in what was being said on a Heinz-sponsored Web site (**www.lycopene.org**); it dropped the investigation when Heinz discontinued the claims. Heinz, in the meantime, reported a 4% increase in market share as a result of media accounts of the virtues of lycopene, especially when this phytochemical is present in cooked tomatoes.[44] This sales advantage was enough of an incentive to marketers to continue using single scientific articles as a basis for health claims in advertisements, and more such attempts were sure to follow.

From this selection of examples, it should be evident that functional foods are more about marketing than health. By adding functional ingredients to foods, marketers are attempting to transform "junk" foods into health foods or to give foods already classified at the base of the *Pyramid* a bit more of an edge. Despite weak or ambiguous evidence for significant health benefits from functional ingredients, the public will buy foods perceived as healthier—provided that they taste good and are reasonably priced. Overall, the evidence for an economic benefit of health claims is convincing, except when cost and taste considerations interfere.

With so many companies now claiming health benefits, the industry is beginning to be concerned that the market will become oversaturated with such claims. If people become accustomed to viewing foods as medicines, the functional-foods approach could backfire. People might stop eating such foods if they do *not* feel better when they eat them (because the products do not work) or if they *do* feel better (because the products are no longer needed). As already noted, taste and cost are also important considerations; restaurant critics tend to give "thumbs down" reviews to techno-foods, and cost is always an issue in food choice, especially when people are expected to pay premium prices for uncertain health benefits. Overall, functional foods reinforce the misleading idea that health benefits depend on single ingredients, and they divert attention from the need to promote healthful dietary patterns. As we will see in the next chapter, reductionist approaches, issues of taste and cost, and the extraordinary efforts taken by companies to obtain approval for techno-foods are illustrated by Procter & Gamble's decades-long persistence in seeking FDA approval to market its fat substitute, olestra, for use in snack and other foods.

CHAPTER 15

SELLING THE ULTIMATE TECHNO-FOOD

OLESTRA

I WAS NO LONGER A MEMBER OF THE FDA'S FOOD ADVISORY Committee during the years when it was considering approval of Procter & Gamble's (P&G) fat substitute, olestra, but I followed its deliberations closely. On June 17, 1998, the committee confirmed a judgment that it had made more than two years earlier. Once again, it agreed that olestra was reasonably certain to cause no harm as a food additive. The members did, however, advise the FDA that foods containing this substance should carry a warning statement: "This product contains olestra. Olestra may cause abdominal cramping and loose stools. Olestra inhibits the absorption of some vitamins and other nutrients. Vitamins A, D, E, and K have been added."[1]

This peculiar decision—judging olestra "safe" while alerting consumers to its potential hazards—was the culmination of P&G's 30-year struggle to convince the FDA to approve olestra for marketing. The company's persistence in that effort is easily understood. Olestra is P&G's name for the ultimate in "lesser-evil" fat substitutes, sucrose polyester. Sucrose polyester is a sugar-based compound that retains the sensory and physical properties of natural food fats but is neither digested nor absorbed by the human body and therefore yields no calories. In theory, substitution of olestra for natural fats could help people reduce their intake of calories, fat, saturated fat, and cholesterol and thus reduce risks for obesity and diseases related to it: coronary heart disease, certain cancers, and diabetes.[2] The potential uses of olestra in food preparation—and the potential economic returns to P&G investors—could be very large indeed.

The reasons why the FDA took so long to approve olestra also are readily understood. The use of olestra raises health issues that are not easy to resolve. Olestra is an oil-like compound that is not digested. As such, it might be expected to behave in the body like mineral oil, which has laxative effects and interferes with the absorption of nutrients (vitamins A, D, E, and K), phytochemicals, and drugs that are soluble in fat. A second concern is quantity. As a substitute cooking fat, olestra might be eaten in very large amounts. Although P&G had conducted many studies of olestra, these lasted only a few weeks or months, not nearly long enough to reveal any long-term effects on digestive function or on depletion of essential vitamins. Furthermore, P&G itself, rather than independent investigators, had conducted nearly all of the studies on olestra. The company was responsible for the studies because food additive laws require *petitioners* to demonstrate that substances are safe before the FDA approves them. Congress does not grant the FDA a mandate or funds to conduct independent evaluations of additives under review.

An additional problem is that food additive regulations require only that companies demonstrate safety and technical effects. The companies do not have to prove that their products improve health. Thus the FDA could not require P&G to demonstrate that olestra really does help people reduce caloric intake, chronic disease risk, or obesity, and the company made no attempt to do so during the approval process. If olestra indeed produced long-term benefits, there was no way to know about them.

With questions about long-term safety and benefits impossible to resolve with the information available, the FDA approved olestra but required a warning notice. Unlike drugs, which also are approved on the basis of limited testing by manufacturers and must carry warnings of any side effects, olestra does not require a doctor's prescription. Unlike other food additives that carry warning notices, such as sulfites, artificial sweeteners, or even psyllium husk, olestra was the first additive likely to be consumed in large quantities; a 1-ounce serving of potato chips contains up to 2 teaspoons (10 grams). In contrast, diet soft drinks contain only milligram amounts of artificial sweeteners, and Kellogg's Ensemble cereals were designed to contain 2.4 grams of psyllium husk per serving. On quantitative grounds alone, olestra raised unprecedented public health and regulatory issues.

It should be evident from even this brief introduction that the case of olestra is well worth attention. Olestra is the most ironic of techno-foods; it is designed to encourage people to eat more top-of-the-*Pyramid* snack foods. Made with olestra, such foods may be fat-free, but they are not calorie-free. And health-conscious consumers, the group most likely to be enthusiastic about olestra products, might be paying a price for their concern about fat reduction in the form of a loss of protective vitamins and phytochemicals, just because these are soluble in fat.

A 30-YEAR REGULATORY SAGA

P&G researchers discovered sucrose polyester accidentally during an unsuccessful 1968 search for fats that could more easily be digested by premature infants. Conventional fats are composed of a "backbone" of a small sugar (glycerol) to which three fatty acids are attached, one to each of *three* linkage sites on the sugar. P&G scientists replaced the glycerol with sucrose (common table sugar) to which up to *eight* fatty acids could be attached. The resulting olestra molecule is so much larger than natural fats that it cannot be broken down either by normal digestive processes in the small intestine or by bacterial digestion in the large intestine. The molecule is too big to be absorbed across the intestinal wall to any appreciable extent; it cannot be metabolized and therefore produces no calories. In addition, P&G scientists were able to manipulate the fatty acid composition of olestra to give it the thickness, cooking properties, and taste of natural fats and oils. Hence it could substitute for any conventional oil to prepare fast foods, restaurant meals, or, for that matter, foods cooked at home. Table 33 lists the impressive array of potential commercial and home uses of olestra.

"Learning Together" with FDA

The possibility that olestra might be eaten in amounts far greater than any other food additive explains the FDA's regulatory predicament. Food additives usually are consumed in tiny amounts but tested in animals at hundred-fold higher levels. This method could not be used to find out whether olestra induced diarrhea or depleted fat-soluble vitamins, because animals could not be forced to eat enough of it. P&G needed to develop different types of methods for evaluating safety, and the FDA needed to establish new regulatory standards for a product that could not be tested in routine ways. Over the years, P&G and FDA "learned together" how to approach these tasks.[3]

The 30-year saga of bringing olestra to market begins with P&G's first discussions with the FDA in 1971. Table 34 summarizes the key events in

TABLE 33. Examples of potential uses of olestra

Snack Foods	Restaurant Foods	Home Use	Table Spreads
Potato chips[a]	French fries	Fried chicken	Margarines[b]
Corn chips[a]	Fried chicken	Grilled meats and vegetables	Cheeses[b]
Cheese puffs[a]	Fried fish	Sautéed meats and vegetables	
Crackers[a]	Onion rings	Baked desserts and snacks	
Doughnuts			
Pastries and pies			
Cakes and cookies			
Ice cream[b]			

[a]Use of olestra in savory (salty and spicy) snacks was approved by the FDA on January 24, 1996.
[b]Table spreads and ice cream were not included in P&G's 1987 petition to the FDA.

this history. Just before publishing the earliest scientific studies on olestra, P&G obtained its first patent and met with the FDA to discuss what the company would need to do to obtain approval. P&G's initial idea was to propose olestra as a new food additive, which meant that the company would have to prove that the substance was safe under conditions of expected use. Company scientists then went to work. In the course of their studies, they found that substituting olestra for natural dietary fats appeared to cause a decline in blood cholesterol levels. This felicitous finding raised the possibility that the company could market olestra as able to lower blood cholesterol levels—a disease claim. If so, the FDA would consider olestra a drug and would require the company to demonstrate the product's safety and efficacy. P&G filed a drug-approval petition with the FDA in 1975. Under FDA drug rules for efficacy, P&G would have to demonstrate at least a 15% reduction in blood cholesterol levels. When its studies did not confirm a reduction this large, P&G abandoned the drug-approval strategy and returned to its initial plan to obtain approval of olestra as a food additive.

The food additive approach seemed especially attractive when, in 1984, the FDA tacitly permitted Kellogg to claim that its high-fiber cereals helped reduce the risk of cancer, an event discussed in Chapter 10. The Kellogg claim led P&G to hope that the FDA would also allow health claims for olestra, tacitly or otherwise. After three years of further studies, the company filed its food additive petition. It requested approval of olestra as a substitute for up to 35% of the natural fats used in home cooking and up to 75% of the fats used for commercial purposes.

TABLE 34. Key events in the history of the approval and marketing of olestra, 1968–2000

1968	Procter & Gamble (P&G) researchers develop sucrose polyester (olestra); conduct animal studies.
1971	P&G discusses approval criteria with FDA; obtains first patent.
1973	P&G initiates human feeding studies; conducts further animal studies.
1975	Olestra found to reduce blood cholesterol levels. P&G petitions FDA for drug approval.
1977	U.S. Senate committee recommends lower fat intake to reduce risk of chronic disease.
1984	Kellogg advertises high-fiber cereals for cancer prevention. FDA relaxes some restrictions on health claims.
1987	Olestra fails to reduce cholesterol levels by 15%. P&G changes strategy and petitions FDA for food additive approval. Center for Science in the Public Interest (CSPI) raises safety objections.
1988	Initial patent expires; three others are due to expire in 1994. *Surgeon General's Report on Nutrition and Health* identifies fat reduction as a major priority for public health.
1989	FDA requires additional safety tests for olestra.
1990	P&G limits food additive petition to savory snacks. Nutrition Labeling and Education Act requires FDA to consider health claims on food labels.
1991	Congress considers bills to revive the expired olestra patent and to extend three others for 10 years after FDA approval; holds hearings; asks the General Accounting Office (GAO) to report on reasons for delay in FDA approval.
1992	GAO attributes delay to P&G's indecisiveness and to FDA's unprecedented regulatory requirements. Congress holds patent hearings; adjourns without taking action.
1993	Olestra patent bills reintroduced. Congress enacts generic law that extends one olestra patent until January 25, 1996, with two more years possible if FDA approves marketing by that date.
1994	Dietary Supplement Health and Education Act permits claims for dietary supplements and health-related conditions.
1995	CSPI issues White Paper opposing FDA approval of olestra. FDA Food Advisory Committee recommends approval. Frito-Lay obtains exclusive supply agreement for a limited term after start of national marketing.
1996	FDA approves olestra for use in savory snacks on January 24. P&G begins test-marketing; brands olestra "Olean;" petitions FDA for less explicit warning notice. CSPI petitions FDA for more prominent warning notice; petitions Federal Trade Commission to halt deceptive olestra advertising.
1997	P&G, Frito-Lay, and Nabisco conduct further market tests.
1998	P&G and Frito-Lay announce nationwide release of Olean products. FDA Food Advisory Committee reaffirms olestra approval with warning notice.
1999	Frito-Lay sales disappointing; Company petitions FDA to eliminate label warning notice.
2000	P&G petitions FDA to eliminate warning notice; test-markets crackers made with olestra. CSPI petitions FDA to revise, not eliminate, the warning.

Because the petition did not ask the FDA to approve use of olestra for table spreads and ice cream, P&G considered the request "a conservative first step."[4] The FDA, however, viewed the vast scope of potential uses outlined in Table 33 as raising safety issues that required further testing. Therefore, to expedite approval, P&G again changed strategies. This time, it asked only for authorization to use olestra in savory (salted and spiced) snacks.

In support of this petition, P&G submitted 150 animal and human studies and 150,000 pages of data related to the effects of olestra on absorption and excretion of drugs, vitamins, carotenoids (plant precursors of vitamin A that have antioxidant properties), and minerals, as well as on hormone levels, intestinal function, and certain gastrointestinal diseases.[5] Late in 1995 the FDA provided a summary of this information to a subcommittee of its Food Advisory Committee and to the parent committee itself. The FDA also gave these committees a detailed critical analysis of P&G's research, prepared by the Center for Science in the Public Interest (CSPI).

CSPI had been organizing opposition to olestra since 1987 when it first challenged the safety of the product in response to P&G's food additive petition. Its 1995 analysis dealt with several potential effects of olestra on health and intestinal function. These are listed in Table 35 along with additional concerns about the quality of the scientific studies examining such effects. CSPI's interpretation was that olestra depleted carotenoids and fat-soluble vitamins and caused noticeable gastrointestinal disturbances. On that basis, and because olestra appeared to be associated with precancerous liver lesions in animals, CSPI maintained that the FDA should deny approval.[6]

Studies conducted or supported by P&G, however, invariably found olestra to pose no health risks.[7] The company has a vested interest in such results, of course, and critical scientists were troubled by the fact that the FDA was unable to require confirmation of company-sponsored results by disinterested investigators, especially because P&G's study methods appeared to be "years behind" research designs used by others.[8] They argued that the P&G studies were seriously flawed by small sample sizes, short time spans, and the other problems noted in Table 35. CSPI also criticized the design of P&G's studies, especially given that the few independent investigations confirmed some of the flaws. For example, studies sponsored by Unilever, a P&G competitor, reported that high doses of olestra caused gastrointestinal problems in 15–30% of recipients and that a dose of just 3 grams—less than the amount in an ounce of potato

TABLE 35. Scientific concerns about the potential physiological effects of olestra and the methods used to study those effects

---

Concerns about potential physiological effects

　Olestra causes gastrointestinal problems (pain, gas, diarrhea, leakage) in some
　　people.

　Olestra reduces absorption of fat-soluble vitamins.

　Olestra reduces absorption of carotenoids and, presumably, other fat-soluble
　　antioxidants and phytochemicals.

　The effects of reduced absorption of fat-soluble nutrients on disease risks are
　　unknown.

　It is not known whether olestra is effective in inducing weight loss or reducing
　　risk factors for chronic diseases.

Concerns about scientific studies conducted by P&G

　The studies were of short duration.

　Doses of olestra were lower than those likely to be consumed.

　The studies involved too few people.

　The statistical power of the studies was too low to produce meaningful
　　results.

　The studies did not pay enough attention to frequent or high users of olestra.

　The studies lacked confirmation by independent investigators.

---

chips—reduced blood levels of fat-soluble vitamins and carotenes by significant amounts.[9] Such findings suggested that olestra might increase risks for heart disease, stroke, cancer, and cataracts. As it turns out, olestra is so efficient at eliminating fat-soluble substances from the intestine that clinicians can use chips fried in olestra to reduce symptoms of dioxin poisoning in patients with toxic levels of this chemical in their bodies.[10]

Despite such findings, and despite the 6,600 anecdotal complaints of gastrointestinal problems that had been filed with FDA by the time of the meeting, the Food Advisory Committee judged P&G's research sufficient and acceptable. Most members were not convinced that any serious harm would result from the losses of fat-soluble vitamins or carotenes. They also believed that the warning notice was sufficient to handle concerns about gastrointestinal distress. Thus both FDA advisory committees recommended approval, although some members sharply dissented.

On January 24, 1996, the FDA announced approval of olestra for use in savory snacks, but with some provisos. P&G would need to formulate olestra to meet certain specifications for composition and stiffness. Manufacturers of products containing olestra would have to fortify them with fat-soluble vitamins A, D, E, and K to compensate for potential losses, and they would also have to include a warning notice on the package label. Recognizing that P&G planned to conduct postmarket surveys of consumer responses to olestra, the FDA also announced that it would review the results of those surveys and any new data in 30 months and would reconsider the approval at that time.

FDA food additive regulations do not demand demonstration of absolute safety, but only "reasonable certainty in the minds of competent scientists that the substance is not harmful under the intended conditions of use."[1] In practice, the rules did not require P&G to demonstrate—nor was the FDA permitted to consider—whether olestra might be *beneficial*. As explained by then FDA Commissioner Dr. David Kessler, questions about whether olestra might make sense or contribute to the nutritional health of the nation were irrelevant to the FDA's approval processes.[11]

The 30-month trial period ended in June 1998, when the FDA asked the Food Advisory Committee to evaluate whether P&G's postmarket studies had raised any significant public health concerns and whether any changes were needed in labeling requirements. The committee reviewed data presented by P&G scientists and P&G-sponsored researchers. Its members also listened to testimony from about 30 people, at least half of them employed by P&G or connected to the company in some other way. The committee heard testimony from consumer advocates and independent scientists about reported and potential adverse effects, but most committee members viewed these concerns as minor. When the committee voted to reaffirm its original approval, it enabled the FDA to conclude a matter that had demanded substantial attention from the agency for 27 years.

Getting Help from Congress

By 1988, P&G's first patent on olestra had expired, and three additional patents were due to lapse in 1994. The FDA's lengthy regulatory review appeared to be threatening the company's nearly $200 million research investment. P&G, which is headquartered in Ohio, induced five of the state's congressmen (four of whom were reported to have received campaign funds from the company) to get their colleagues to revive the original patent and to extend the company's control of the other patents for ten years following the date of FDA approval.[12]

Such an action would establish a precedent. Typically, Congress opposes patent extensions for private companies on the grounds that such favors might inhibit free-market competition. At a hearing on the matter, House members expressed particular concern about recent increases in extension requests. They viewed such requests as troubling, because "the patent system was not designed to guarantee every inventor a financial reward for his efforts . . . uncertainty in the length of the patent term may also have a chilling effect on competitors. . . . a 'Pandora's box' would be opened."[13]

Despite such concerns, both houses introduced legislation for private patent extensions in the 1991–1992 congressional sessions and held three separate Judiciary Committee hearings on the bills. During the Senate hearing, Ed Artzt, P&G's chairman of the board and CEO, emphasized that his company was not blaming the FDA for the years of delay: "The FDA has also had to create . . . completely new regulatory standards during the olestra review . . . [olestra] is a macro-ingredient which will be consumed at much higher levels. To deal with this, the FDA has had to create new safety criteria and then we had to develop testing protocols. . . . So to be clear, we are not faulting the FDA."[14] Nevertheless, in answer to specific questions from the committee, Mr. Artzt did suggest that the FDA was responsible for the problem: "As recently as last year, the FDA established a new set of requirements for the review of olestra. . . . The decision to adopt the drug approval route was primarily dictated by FDA."

Congress immediately ordered the General Accounting Office (GAO), its federal watchdog agency, to investigate why the FDA had taken so long to approve olestra. After a four-month investigation, the GAO agreed that the delay was due in part to the FDA's dithering over lack of regulatory precedents. However, it also judged the delay to be due just as much to P&G's indecisiveness about whether to pursue approval of olestra as a drug or as an additive.[3] In the meantime, six consumer groups publicly opposed the patent extension on the grounds that the bills showed "favoritism" to P&G and would be rewarding the company for its "lack of diligence in developing, testing and applying for approval."[15] A competing firm, Unilever, also opposed the extensions on the grounds of unfair competition.

Because patent laws require requests for extensions to be filed before patents actually expire, the Judiciary Committees did not believe "that there is any justification for reviving the expired patent, or for granting the company's request for an open-ended 10-year extension of the existing patents, to run from the time, if ever, that the FDA approves Procter & Gamble's food additive petition."[16] The committee did find that some relief was appropriate, however. On that basis, both the House and Senate passed amended bills to extend the three remaining patents until the end of 1997, but these bills failed by default when Congress adjourned without taking final action on them.[17]

Congress again introduced similar bills during the 1992–1993 sessions and held three additional hearings. Eventually, these efforts brought P&G at least partial relief. Congress passed a generic law granting limited extensions on patents for any product under lengthy regulatory review. Nowhere in the law is there a mention of P&G or olestra, but its net effect was to extend one P&G patent for two years—until January 25, 1996—a term that could be lengthened by another two years if the FDA agreed to approve olestra by that date. In what hardly seemed a coincidence, the FDA announced its approval of olestra on January 24, 1996, precisely one day before the patent extension was due to expire.[18]

Reasonable people might find patent issues too arcane to be of interest. This one, however, produced remarkable effects. It preoccupied the Judiciary Committees of both houses of Congress for more than two years. It caused Congress to order a GAO investigation of the FDA, and the GAO to spend four months on that project. It led the House and Senate to pass an act of Congress simply to benefit one private company. Not least, it caught the FDA in an apparent conflict of interest. Coincidence or not, the FDA's convenient announcement date gave the appearance of collusion with P&G to get olestra approved.

P&G'S MARKETING CAMPAIGN

Once the FDA had approved olestra, P&G needed to sell it to the public. It did so under the brand name Olean. P&G's promotion of Olean products was unusual only in that the campaign was exceptionally comprehensive, visible, and expensive. P&G spent huge sums on media advertising, much of it suggesting that Olean was nothing more than calorie-free soybean oil. An example of that kind of advertising is shown in Figure 31. The company also employed more subtle forms of promotion, such as educating health professionals, and it used "hardball" tactics to discredit its critics.

Launching the Products

P&G does not make potato chips or other savory snacks, but Frito-Lay (a division of PepsiCo) does. P&G sold exclusive rights to Frito-Lay to make olestra chips in exchange for what was said to be an "eight-figure" investment in a new manufacturing plant. To launch the test-marketing of the new products, P&G worked with numerous public relations people, some of them well connected former advisors to President Clinton.

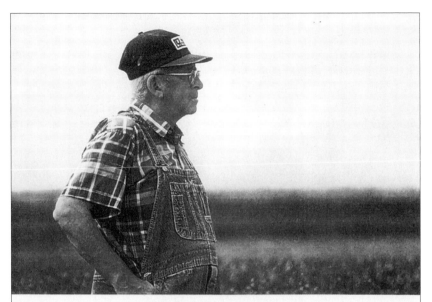

"Doing good starts in your own backyard. Of course, mine is 250 acres of soybeans."

I remember the day I first heard about it. How soybeans like mine were going to be used to make a new kind of cooking oil.

Now usually a day like that wouldn't be so special, except this was something that had never been done before.

Seems the folks who make Crisco® had come up with Olean, an oil that would fry up fat-free snack chips without adding any calories. Make them taste especially good. Yet still be a little healthier to eat than regular snacks.

It only goes to show, good things can start from anywhere. Even your own backyard.

FIGURE 31. Procter & Gamble's advertising campaign emphasized the home-grown origins of olestra.

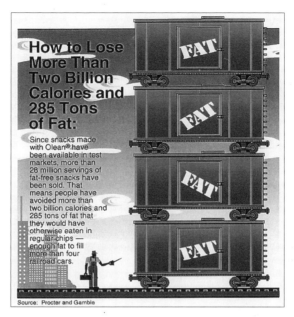

FIGURE 32. In 1998 Procter & Gamble estimated that Americans already had consumed 28 million olestra snacks, thereby saving more than two billion calories and 285 tons of fat—enough to fill four railroad cars.

P&G and Frito-Lay officials personally visited media outlets, and the companies distributed hundreds of thousands of free samples, recruited and trained dietitians, collected testimonials from satisfied customers, ran tour buses, hired cheerleaders, and did Christo-like wrappings of super-markets in Olean banners. They distributed pamphlets to consumers, gave "educational" packets to junior high school and high school students, and donated videotapes. These activities were said to have generated "gobs" of free publicity and sales of 28 million servings by mid-1997.[19] P&G's press materials boasted that enough fat had been saved to fill four railroad cars (see Figure 32).

Defending the Investment

New products are expensive to launch, and companies expect to invest substantial sums in advertising and promotion. P&G's investment in bringing olestra to market, however, seemed unusually large. Although the amount can only be estimated, it appears to be at least $500 million. During the 1993 patent hearings, P&G officials reported expenditures of

$200 million for olestra research and development. Other sources reported estimates of $160 million to $250 million for the olestra processing plant and $5 million to $10 million for the Ohio test-marketing (the costs of the three other test markets were believed to be somewhat lower). In addition, Frito-Lay was reported to have spent $7.4 million, and P&G $22 million, on advertising for olestra products just in the *first quarter* of 1998. To these costs must be added expenditures for the 700,000 acres of land used for growing soybeans and cotton to produce olestra's fatty acids and costs of purchasing sugar raw materials.[20]

Such astronomical expenditures must be understood in context. In 1996 P&G earned $35.3 billion in revenues and spent $3.25 billion to advertise its full line of products, of which $30 million was spent just to advertise pre-olestra Pringles potato chips. That same year, Americans bought 5.5 billion pounds of salty snacks worth $13 billion. Olestra chips would not have to capture a very large share of this market to recoup P&G's investment. Indeed, company officials predicted annual revenues of $400 million to $500 million by 1999. If the FDA could be convinced to approve olestra cooking oil, P&G also could enter the billion-dollar annual markets for fried snack and restaurant foods.[21]

Whether the company would achieve its financial goals seemed questionable, at least in the short term. Although more than 100 million bags of chips were reported sold from the February launch through July 1998, tracking data from one of the early test markets indicated that sales fell markedly as soon as the advertising blitz ended. And although P&G officials maintained that olestra was on track to earn the $400 million that had been expected in the first year, other sources reported that sales had fallen from $41 million to $28 million per month from May to August 1998, meaning that olestra was not turning out to be "the second coming some people thought it would be."[22] From March 1998 to March 1999, Frito-Lay's sales of olestra chips totaled $260 million, far below expectations, a shortfall attributed to olestra's "image" problem. As one business analyst put it, "the consumer has spoken . . . it seemed like people had a negative perception of it right off the bat."[23] When by July 2000 sales of Frito-Lay's olestra chips had fallen another 30% or so, and P&G's post-market surveys showed little evidence of gastrointestinal effects, the companies argued that the label warning was misleading and was being misunderstood by consumers, and they petitioned the FDA to delete the warning label.[24] Late in 2000, in a further effort to improve this market niche, P&G began test-marketing sandwich crackers made with olestra in peanut butter, cheese, and "veggie" cream cheese varieties.[25]

Whether removing the warning statement would improve sales was also questionable. Olestra chips had been introduced at a time when people were eating fewer reduced-fat products, and other snack foods were becoming more competitive. Consumers were disappointed that Olean chips tasted just like ordinary potato chips. I did my own taste comparison and thought they tasted about the same as other commercial chips, though I noted that they were priced a bit higher. My local supermarket shelved bags of olestra chips intermingled with regular chips, and they were difficult to identify except by a small "Olean" in the lower right corner. People also were disappointed that the chips did not help them lose weight. Despite these discouraging observations and predictions of doom, P&G remained optimistic. Company officials noted that "consumers have already enjoyed more than 1.5 billion servings . . . avoiding 140 billion calories and 35 million pounds of fat" and that reports of the demise of olestra were greatly exaggerated.[26]

Co-Opting Health Professionals

P&G garnered support from nutrition and health professionals through efforts targeted at organizations, publications, and individuals. The company gave grants to organizations to develop educational materials and to hold conferences on olestra and related topics. It sponsored focus groups and booths at annual meetings and paid publication costs for special issues of professional journals. For example, a P&G official sits on the board of the International Life Sciences Institute, which sponsored a conference funded in part by the company; proceedings of the conference were published through the New York Academy of Sciences. P&G also is one of many corporate sponsors of professional publications that publish articles on olestra (both pro and con), such as the *American Journal of Clinical Nutrition* and the *Journal of Nutrition*. The company has supported scientists, educators, and practitioners through research grants, travel funds, honoraria, educational materials, samples, and meals. It mailed educational brochures and samples of olestra chips to tens of thousands of physicians, nurses, and dietitians and sent its research summaries and articles to thousands more. P&G officials paid personal visits to professionals perceived as influential, and the company recruited dozens of paid consultants, among them two former secretaries of Health and Human Services and many prominent researchers and clinicians; these people wrote articles, testified, or appeared in commercials supporting olestra.[27]

Such actions raise concerns about potential conflicts of interest, especially when the financial relationships are not disclosed. One former Health and Human Services Department secretary, for example, appears in a promotional videotape but does not reveal his consulting relationship. Other materials also display or quote spokespersons whose connections with the company are not stated. At the very least, disclosure provides a more thorough basis for critical judgment. The American Dietetic Association's fact sheet on olestra, for example, emphasizes benefits, does not mention the warning notice or any of the reasons for it, and dismisses inhibitory effects on absorption of carotenes as insignificant. Because the fact sheet fully discloses P&G sponsorship, readers should not be surprised that it reflects the company's viewpoint. Even so, the association's Web site does not mention P&G's reported $100,000 donation to the organization during the previous decade. Disclosure also might prevent embarrassing situations such as that involving the American Medical Association, which was reported to be negotiating for an $800,000 health education grant from P&G in the same month that it issued a statement supportive of olestra.[28]

Although recipients of corporate funding do not inevitably support corporate interests, such financial connections give the appearance of conflict of interest. Most people who accept P&G funds undoubtedly do so because they believe that olestra is beneficial or that the arrangement is unlikely to influence their critical judgment. In my personal experience, it is virtually impossible for any nutritionist interested in the benefits and risks of olestra to avoid some sort of financial relationship with P&G unless one systematically refuses all speaking invitations, travel reimbursements, honoraria, and meals from outside parties. I consider myself independent of P&G, yet I have had a professional relationship with the company that dates back to 1988 when I spoke at a P&G-sponsored press luncheon announcing release of the *Surgeon General's Report on Nutrition and Health*. I gave a similar talk some months later at a P&G conference on olestra, for which I received meals, travel and hotel expenses, and a $1,000 honorarium. Since then, I have discussed product development at meals hosted by P&G officials and explained my views of olestra to company staff ($500 honorarium), I also co-chaired a session of, and was lead author of a report from, a P&G-sponsored conference on fat-modified foods for which I was paid travel, hotel, meals, and a $4,000 honorarium. Because I make it a policy not to accept honoraria from food companies, I asked P&G to write the checks to my department's scholarship fund—or, in one case, to CSPI—which it did without comment. P&G nutritionists also have been unfailingly gracious in responding to my requests for information or materials. Although P&G officials asked to meet with me shortly after publication of a critical article I had written on olestra for a professional journal, their only comment was that it was "well researched," and their follow-up letter to the journal's editor merely suggested that readers could contact the company for further information.[29] Whether intended to engage us in P&G's mission or not, such courtesy and generosity surely makes recipients feel churlish to attack the company for the quality of its products or its tactics.

P&G, however, has no such compunctions about attacking critics, as illustrated by its reaction to CSPI's interventions. As detailed in several investigative reports, the company does not take CSPI's actions lightly. It hired Washington's "most feared and vilified" private-investigation firm to obtain information that might undermine CSPI's credibility, and it placed media stories critical of CSPI in publications with financial connections to the company. For example, a *Reader's Digest* article characterizing CSPI as the "food police" failed to mention that P&G is the magazine's third-largest advertiser and had spent a million dollars on advertising in that particular issue alone.[30]

DOES OLESTRA WORK?

P&G's campaign to promote olestra distracts attention from what should be the most critical question: Do Olean-branded foods help people reduce their fat intake and lose weight? Not unexpectedly, research studies funded by the company find "healthful changes in dietary fat intake and serum cholesterol concentrations among consumers who chose to consume olestra-containing foods."[31] For several reasons, such findings are unlikely to be reproduced across broad sections of the population. To begin with, olestra addresses just the fat component of an overall dietary pattern. Its use in snacks might help some people reduce their intake of fat and calories—and, perhaps, their body weight and certain chronic disease risk factors—but its effects on absorption of fat-soluble vitamins and phytochemicals might interfere with the health benefits of fruits and vegetables. Furthermore, foods containing olestra may not contain fat, but they do contain calories—and plenty of them; olestra saves just one-third to one-half the calories of natural-fat products. People who eat olestra chips may believe that they can eat such foods with caloric impunity and compensate by eating *more* of them. One user of olestra products told me, "I love olestra. It means I get to eat potato chips—the whole bag," and she was not talking about a one-ounce package. According to other studies sponsored by P&G, early adoption of olestra products tracks with other indicators of good health habits (white ethnicity, higher education, lower fat intake).[32] People who frequently eat chips and other savory snacks, however, generally have diets of rather poor quality. Given this situation, eating olestra chips does not seem a particularly efficient way to improve anyone's overall diet.

Experience with artificial sweeteners also suggests that olestra is unlikely to have much effect on weight or, for that matter, on overall fat intake. In 1970, not long after first introducing artificial sweeteners, manufacturers produced enough of them to replace the equivalent of 5.8 pounds of sugars per person per year. In 1991, the last year for which such figures were available, they produced enough to replace nearly 25 pounds of sugars per capita. From 1970 to 1991, however, the availability of caloric sugars in the food supply *increased* from 122 to 138 pounds per person per year, and it increased further to 154 pounds in 1997.[33] Some individuals who use artificial sweeteners may reduce their sugar intake, but most do not. If olestra indeed reduces inhibitions about eating salty snacks, or encourages deliberate misuse to induce laxative effects (as has been reported),[34] people may well eat more of these products and increase their calorie intake. Given the uncertainties about olestra's long-term effects on vitamin absorption, the lack of evidence for long-term benefits, the overabundance of food produced in the United States, and the pressing need to find ways to feed the world's growing population, P&G's herculean efforts to develop and market olestra might well be viewed as an astonishing waste of human, land, food, and economic resources. Whether these efforts will continue to reward stockholders remains to be determined.

TECHNO-FOODS: IMPLICATIONS

In developing olestra and other techno-foods, manufacturers appeared to be responding to policy recommendations from government health officials and to be doing precisely what they were asked to do to improve the nation's health. In return, they demanded—and won—the ability to make health claims for their products. Health claims drive the design of functional foods; manufacturers have a firm notion of the claims they would like to make for their products before they even start to develop them. Authorized health claims—and, more recently, structure/function claims—have greatly stimulated development of products reduced or substituted in fat or sugar, and of products fortified with nutrients, fiber, or herbals and phytochemicals. P&G's $500 million investment in olestra research and development (and the expected returns on that investment) give some indication of what is at stake in today's functional-foods marketplace.

Some of these foods indeed may be beneficial, especially to the already health-conscious, higher-income consumers most likely to purchase them. Such people already follow recommended health practices and can easily adopt another. Fortification of the food supply certainly raises the overall consumption levels of the nutrients used and improves the nutritional status of people with low intakes of those nutrients. Fiber- and soy-supplemented foods should help reduce blood cholesterol levels among people who eat enough of them *and* who follow low-fat diets. Stanol- and sterol-supplemented margarines also should help lower blood cholesterol levels when they replace other fats in already healthful diets, as should the replacement of high-fat snack foods with those lower in fat or made with olestra.

But no functional foods can ever replace the full range of nutrients and phytochemicals present in fruits, vegetables, and whole grains, nor can they overcome the detrimental effects of diets that are not already healthful. Although it makes sense to foster the development, marketing, and consumption of products that really do provide health benefits, it makes no sense whatsoever to flood the market with "exaggerated claims and products of dubious benefit."[35] Because messages to eat less fat and sugar are so well recognized by the public, potato chips, sugared cereals, and candies can appear to be healthful just because they are low in fat or contain added vitamins or minerals. Low-fat cookies, olestra-fried chips, zinc-fortified breakfast cereals, vitamin-supplemented candies, and stanol-supplemented margarines may lull people into a false sense of dietary security: "Fortified junk foods are still junk. . . . Fruits and vegetables, whole grains, beans, and low-fat milk and yogurt are packed with nutrients or phytochemicals. . . . Chips, candy bars, and cookies—even if they're fat-free, low-salt, and contain no preservatives—can't take the place of foods that come with no label, no advertising, and no gimmicks."[36]

This point is nicely illustrated in Figure 33. From the standpoint of nutrition, techno-foods simply are not necessary. From the standpoint of food traditions, they may not be desirable. The food marketplace already is glutted with an enormous overabundance of calories and products, and

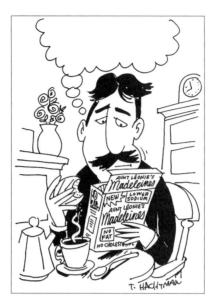

FIGURE 33. To some cultural critics such as the cartoonist Tom Hachtman, techno-foods seem tasteless and uninspiring. Would Proust ever have written a word if his madeleine had been made with olestra? (©The New Yorker Collection 1998. Tom Hachtman from **cartoonbank.com**. All rights reserved.)

it is not difficult to select a health-promoting diet from this supply at quite low cost. The techno-food approach misses the point that the best health outcomes are associated with dietary *patterns* that follow recommendations, not just eating or avoiding one or another single food.

What is particularly disturbing about functional foods is how they change the way people think about dietary patterns. They suggest that foods are medicines, and they convert the pleasures of eating into the perils of drug taking. My esteemed colleague Joan Gussow, who has thought long and deeply about such matters, observes that if we view foods simply as containers of nutrients or curative substances, we encourage manufacturers to think of more ways to invent more new products to meet some perceived health need. She argues that foods should be appreciated for the richness and complexity of their taste and cultural context, as well as for their nutritional aspects. She concludes, "eating healthfully is neither complicated, nor time-consuming, nor punishing. And we don't need any more new products to do it."[37]

As this discussion has demonstrated, the primary beneficiaries of techno-foods are most likely to be the companies that make them. The degree of benefit to the public is much less certain, and the potential for harm—in more frequent and blatant health claims, more products claiming special health benefits, products that actually do damage, increased pressure to "eat more," and greater public confusion about diet and health—is not insignificant and should concern all of us.

CONCLUSION

THE POLITICS OF FOOD CHOICE

WE HAVE SEEN HOW THE FOOD INDUSTRY USES LOBBYING, lawsuits, financial contributions, public relations, advertising, partnerships and alliances, philanthropy, threats, and biased information to convince Congress, federal agencies, nutrition and health professionals, and the public that the science relating diet to health is so confusing that they need not worry about diets: When it comes to diets, anything goes.[1]

Representatives of food companies and their trade associations repeatedly make the following claims:

- The keys to healthful diets are balance, variety, and moderation (especially when their products are included).

- All foods can be part of healthful diets (especially theirs).

- There is no such thing as a good or a bad food (except when their products are considered good).

- Dietary advice changes so often that we need not follow it (unless it favors their products).

- Research on diet and health is so uncertain that it is meaningless (except when it supports the health benefits of their products).

- Only a small percentage of the population would benefit from following population-based dietary advice (if that advice suggests restrictions on intake of their products).

- Diets are a matter of personal responsibility and freedom of choice (especially the freedom to choose their products).

- Advocacy for more healthful food choices is irrational (if it suggests eating less of their products).
- Government intervention in dietary choice is unnecessary, undesirable, and incompatible with democratic institutions (unless it protects and promotes their products).

Dr. Rhona Applebaum of the National Food Processors Association, for example, succinctly expresses such views when she says that diets should conform to "the three principles of sound nutritional advice: balance, variety, and moderation" and that societal measures to support more healthful food choices are unnecessary. Changing the environment of food choice is possible, she maintains, only

> if the federal government, in the role of "Big Brother," mandates what foods can or cannot be produced—which is not the role of government in a free market economy. Controlling, limiting, and outright banning of products deemed "unfit" does not work, and history attests to the failure of such extremist measures. . . . Food consumption is not supply driven, it is demand driven, and consumers are in the driver's seat . . . you cannot force people to comply with the Dietary Guidelines and it is wrong to try. It is an unworkable, totalitarian approach that brings with it all the evils associated with such a philosophy.[2]

With such statements, food industry officials appeal to emotion (in this case, fears of totalitarianism) to argue against something that no nutritionist, private or governmental, advocates. Nutritionists are simply trying to educate the public that some foods *are* better for health than others. The food industry fiercely opposes this idea and uses its substantial resources, political skills, and emotional appeals to discourage attempts to introduce "eat less" messages into public discussion of dietary issues and, instead, to encourage people to eat more.

These tactics on the part of food companies are, in one sense, a routine part of doing business; they are no different from those used by other large commercial interests, such as drug companies, or—as we shall see—tobacco companies. But sellers of food products do not attract the same kind of attention as purveyors of drugs or tobacco. They should, not only because of the health consequences of dietary choices, but also because of the ethical issues raised by industry marketing practices. Food marketing raises ethical dilemmas, but so does attempting to regulate or change people's food choices, deciding how government should protect health within the context of a free market economy, determining what kinds of policy changes might support more healthful food choices, and identifying the role of individual responsibility in making such choices. This concluding chapter explores such dilemmas.

THE ENVIRONMENT OF FOOD CHOICE

We are fortunate to live in a free market economy that gives us an abundant—indeed an overabundant—food supply at low cost. What we choose to make of this supply is, of course, a matter of personal responsibility, as food company officials are quick to argue. But we do not make food choices in a vacuum. We select diets in a marketing environment in which billions of dollars are spent to convince us that nutrition advice is so confusing, and eating healthfully so impossibly difficult, that there is no point in bothering to eat less of one or another food product or category. We may believe that we make informed decisions about food choice, but we cannot do so if we are oblivious of the ways food companies influence our choices. Most of us, if we choose to do so, can recognize how food companies spend money on advertising, but it is far more difficult to know about the industry's behind-the-scenes efforts in Congress, federal agencies, courts, universities, and professional organizations to make diets seem a matter of personal choice rather than of deliberate manipulation. The emphasis on individual choice serves the interests of the food industry for one critical reason: if diet is a matter of individual free will, then the only appropriate remedy for poor diets is education, and nutritionists should be off teaching people to take personal responsibility for their own diet and health—not how to institute societal changes that might make it easier for everyone to do so.

That suggestions to change the social environment of food choice are threatening to industry is evident from the vehemence with which trade associations and the business press attack advice to restrict intake of one or another food group, to get "junk" food out of schools, to label foods more explicitly, or to tax sales of foods to generate funds for nutrition education. Business commentators equate such approaches with nothing less than fascism: "If [President] Bill Clinton really wants ideas for a healthy eating crusade, he must surely look to the only political regime that thoroughly made them part of national policy: Nazi Germany."[3] They could not be more sarcastic about societal approaches to dietary change: "This being America, of course, ordering Biggie Fries instead of the salad bar can't possibly be our own fault. . . . If all this sounds a bit preposterous, it only means you have an underdeveloped sense of victimhood. The parallels between Big Tobacco and Big Fat are too striking to be overlooked. . . . Come on, America. Get off that couch and sue."[4]

Sarcasm aside, if the business press finds parallels between the tobacco and food industries, it is because the parallels are impossible to avoid. Cigarette companies famously argue that smoking is a matter of individual choice and that it is wrong for government to interfere unduly in the private lives of citizens. They use science to sow confusion about the harm that cigarettes can cause. They set the standard in use of public relations, advertising, philanthropy, experts, political funding, alliances, lobbying, intimidation, and lawsuits to protect their sales. In efforts to expand markets, they promote cigarette smoking to children and adolescents; to minorities, women, and the poor; and to people in countries throughout the world, developing as well as industrialized.[5] The similarities between the actions of cigarette companies and food companies are no coincidence. As explained in the Introduction, some cigarette companies own food companies.

No matter who owns them, food companies lobby government and agencies, and they become financially enmeshed with experts on nutrition and health. Although the food industry frames such tactics as promoting individual liberty and free will, its true objective is (not surprisingly) "trade and unrestricted profit."[6] With respect to cigarettes, most Americans by now are thoroughly aware of the marketing practices of tobacco companies; we learned about them through decades of antismoking campaigns. These campaigns succeeded in getting warning labels on cigarette packages, getting smoking-restricted areas in businesses and on airplanes, and even inspiring an attempt by the Food and Drug Administration (FDA) to regulate tobacco as a drug. The parallel practices of food companies, however, have elicited nowhere near this level of protest.

The principal reasons for this difference must surely lie in the complexity of the messages about foods and their health effects. Although cigarettes and diet contribute to comparable levels of illness and death across the population, cigarettes constitute a single entity, in contrast to a food system that currently supplies 320,000 food products.[7] No nutritionist could ever suggest that eating an occasional candy bar or bag of potato chips might cause disease—it truly is the overall dietary pattern that counts, and it counts over a lifetime. Unlike the straightforward "don't smoke" advice, the dietary message can never be "don't eat." Instead, it has to be the more complicated and ambiguous "eat this instead of that," "eat this more often than that," and the overall prescription, "eat less."

The actions of food companies greatly add to the confusion and, in some ways, create it. Companies are in business to make money; that is their job. From the perspective of stockholders, it is irresponsible for companies to make decisions that will *not* lead to increased profits. If companies offer foods of minimal nutritional value and people buy them, companies will continue to make and market them. If fat, sugar, and salt help to sell products, companies will market top-of-the-*Pyramid* products in the name of freedom of choice. If "nutrition"—added vitamins, reduced fat—helps to sell products, the companies will use nutrition as a marketing tool. If the market is not expanding, they will increase the range of their marketing targets to children, urban minorities, and people in developing countries, whether or not the products displace more nutritious foods in the diet or add unnecessary calories. These actions also parallel the tactics of tobacco companies. And in the same way that cigarette companies' promotion of smoking raises ethical issues, so does the food industry's promotion of minimally nutritious products and of overeating in general.

THE ETHICS OF FOOD CHOICE

Ethical issues arise whenever actions that benefit one group harm another. Food choices have economic, political, social, and environmental consequences that place improvements to the health of individuals or populations in conflict with other considerations. Table 36 summarizes some of these conflicts. Underlying the notion of food ethics is the assumption that following *Dietary Guidelines* improves health and well-being. If ethics is viewed as a matter of good conduct versus bad, then choosing a healthful diet—and advising people to do so—would seem to be virtuous actions. As we have seen, food industry representatives question this assumption when they say that *Dietary Guidelines* apply only to a small percentage of the population or claim that they do more harm than good by causing unnecessary deprivation and anxiety. I have heard ethicists call such problems "mass communication risks," meaning, in this case, that education about nutrition out of its dietary context makes people misinterpret advice, whether the advice comes from government, academics, or industry.[8]

Beyond concerns about whether it is appropriate for anyone to tell anyone else what to eat in the name of health, the principal ethical issues related to dietary practices involve the implications of advice to "eat less" for food producers and the food service industry. Some years ago, the nutrition educators Joan Gussow and Kate Clancy began to ask whether it is ethical for food companies to market large numbers of resource-intensive, high-calorie, low-nutrient food products to people who neither need nor can afford them and, in the case of children, do not understand the difference between advertising and education. They questioned the ethical implications of promoting a "seasonless, regionless" diet in which an average food travels thousands of miles before it is eaten—a practice that wastes natural resources; requires extensive use of pesticides, energy-intensive fertilizers, antibiotics, and hormones; and causes people in developing countries to produce food for export rather than for themselves.[9] In their view, the overriding ethical dilemma associated with *Dietary Guidelines* is the conflict between following the advice (and eating more plant foods but less meat, dairy, and processed foods) and the effects of doing so on food producers: "These economic realities are a problem worth worrying over. We all need to be concerned—if people start to eat less beef and sugar and Pringles—about the cattle growers, the cane raisers and the Pringle makers. . . . but we must also recognize that consumers need help choosing foods, and there is no way we can help them select better diets without causing economic disruption to some sectors of the food industry."[10]

That "virtuous" dietary choices can result in economic harm to food producers is evident from U.S. Department of Agriculture (USDA) studies. USDA economists estimate that eating more fruit and vegetables and fewer foods of animal origin would upset the existing "volume, mix, production, and marketing of agricultural commodities" and would require large "adjustments" in international food trade, nonfood uses of basic commodities, and food prices.[11] Some agricultural sectors (fruits, vegetables) would benefit if people followed dietary guidelines, but others (beef, corn, sugar) would suffer. What might seem a virtue to some people might seem a vice to others—hence, ethical and policy dilemmas.

Ethical or not, a message to eat less meat, dairy, and processed foods is not going to be popular among the producers of such foods. It will have only limited popularity with producers of fruits and vegetables because their scale of production is limited and they cannot easily add value to their products. The message will not be popular with cattle ranchers, meat packers, dairy producers, or milk bottlers; oil seed growers, processors, or transporters; grain producers (most grain is used to feed cattle); makers of soft drinks, candy bars, and snack foods; owners of fast-food outlets and franchise restaurants; media corporations and advertising agencies; manufacturers and marketers of television sets and computers (where advertising takes place); and, eventually, drug and health care industries likely to lose business if people stay healthier longer. The range

TABLE 36. Ethical dilemmas that arise in applying the 2000 *Dietary Guidelines for Americans* to food choices

Dietary Guidelines	Ethical and Policy Dilemmas
Aim for fitness	
Aim for a healthy weight.	Eat less, *and cause economic harm to food producers.*
	Revise government agricultural support, advertising, tax, and other policies to promote "eat less," *and cause economic harm to some corporations and individuals.*
	In developing countries, establish policies to increase food intake, *and increase the risk of obesity.*
Be physically active each day.	Institute taxes and other policies to promote more active lifestyles, *and increase costs to consumers.*
Build a healthy base	
Let the *Pyramid* guide your food choices.	State "eat less" messages explicitly, *and provoke political opposition,* or say that there are no good or bad foods, *and confuse the public.*
	Insist that dietary advice be issued by independent agencies, *and incur political consequences,* or accept euphemistic dietary guidelines from agencies with conflicting missions, *and confuse the public.*
Eat a variety of grains daily, especially whole grains.	Recommend unprocessed grain products low in added fat, sugar, and salt, *and risk opposition and higher costs*, or advise "no good foods, no bad foods," *and add to public confusion.*
Eat a variety of fruits and vegetables daily.	Insist that fruits and vegetables be grown under conditions that conserve resources, limit pesticides and herbicides, and support farm workers adequately, *and pay more for food.*

of economic sectors that would be affected if people changed their diets, avoided obesity, and prevented chronic diseases surely rivals the range of industries that would be affected if people stopped smoking cigarettes.

Perhaps for this reason, USDA officials believe that really encouraging people to follow dietary guidelines would be so expensive and disruptive to the agricultural economy as to create impossible political barriers. Rather than accepting the challenge and organizing a concerted national campaign to encourage more healthful eating patterns, they propose a more politically expedient solution: the industry should work to improve the food supply through nutrient fortification and the development of

TABLE 36. *(continued)*

Dietary Guidelines	Ethical and Policy Dilemmas
Keep foods safe to eat.	Require food companies to produce safe food and test for pathogens, *and risk political opposition and higher costs*, or focus safety efforts on consumer education, use of irradiation, or other postmarket methods, *and ignore basic causes of safety problems.*
Choose sensibly	
Choose a diet that is low in cholesterol and moderate in total fat.	Eat less meat, dairy, and eggs, *and cause economic harm to food and feed producers as well as inducing higher food costs.*
Choose beverages and foods to moderate intake of sugars.	Eat less of high-sugar foods, *and cause economic harm to sugar producers, product producers, and workers in those industries.*
	Remove price supports from sugar production, *and risk the companies' closing and moving elsewhere.*
	Regulate marketing of soft drinks and other high-sugar foods to children, especially in school, *and cause economic harm to soft-drink companies and to schools.*
Choose and prepare foods with less salt.	Eat less of high-salt foods, *and cause economic harm to their producers and to workers in those industries.*
	Advise salt restriction as a means of preventing hypertension, *and inconvenience people who do not need such advice.*
If you drink alcoholic beverages, do so in moderation.	Drink less alcohol to reduce social and health problems, *and eliminate a means of reducing heart-disease risk in certain population segments.*

functional foods with added nutritional value.[12] Such proposals raise ethical dilemmas of their own. These foods are not necessarily "healthier," and they encourage people to eat more, not less.

TAKING ACTION: IMPROVING PUBLIC AND CORPORATE POLICIES

Given the ethical and political implications just discussed, we must now ask two questions: What should health professionals and concerned citizens do to improve the social and political environment in which people make food choices? And how can we make sure that the actions we take are both responsible and effective? Once again, the parallel with tobacco is instructive. In the 30 years or so since publication of the surgeon general's first report on smoking and health, cigarettes have become socially unacceptable—on health grounds—among many groups and in many locations. Many of the lessons learned from the "tobacco wars" apply just as well to food, especially the lesson that the industry will relentlessly counter even the slightest suggestion to use less of its products. That actions typical of antismoking campaigns are only rarely applied to nutrition issues is a tribute to how well the food industry has sown confusion about the research linking diet to health, about advice based on that research, and about dietary choices based on that advice. The result is the widely held idea that "eat less" need not apply to categories of foods, to specific food products, or to food in general.

In this regard also, we have much to learn from the tobacco wars. Successful antismoking campaigns are based on four elements: a firm research base, a clear message, well-defined targets for intervention, and strategies that address the societal environment as well as the education of individual smokers. The research basis of antismoking messages is firmly established: Cigarettes cause lung cancer. The message is simple: don't smoke. The targets are well defined: antismoking efforts focus not only on individuals who smoke but also on the companies that produce cigarettes. The strategies include education but also encompass environmental measures, such as age thresholds for buying cigarettes, cigarette taxes, and bans on smoking in airplanes, restaurants, and workplaces.[5]

Could the four principal elements of antismoking campaign strategies—research, message, target, and tactics—be applied to dietary change? With regard to research, the evidence for the health benefits of hierarchical dietary patterns that emphasize fruits, vegetables, and grains is strong, consistent, and associated with prevention of as much illness as cessation of smoking. The message to follow *Pyramid*-like dietary patterns is more complicated than "don't smoke" but not impossible to understand. Just as "don't smoke" applies to everyone, so does the dietary message; everyone benefits from following a dietary pattern that contributes to prevention of so many diseases. Perhaps the most important lesson of all concerns tactics: antismoking campaigns succeeded when they began to focus on *environmental* issues rather than on the education of individuals. If we want to encourage people to eat better diets, we need to target societal means to counter food industry lobbying and marketing practices as well as the education of individuals.

TABLE 37. Modifications of public policies that would promote better food choices and more active lifestyles

Education
> Mount a major, national campaign to promote "eat less, move more."
> Teach teachers about nutrition and weight management.
> In schools, ban commercials for foods of minimal nutritional value and teaching materials with corporate logos.
> End the sale in schools of soft drinks, candy bars, and other foods of minimal nutritional value.
> Require school meals to be consistent with *Dietary Guidelines.*
> Require daily opportunities for physical education and sports in schools.

Food labeling and advertising
> Require fast-food restaurants to provide nutrition information on packages and wrappers.
> Require containers for soft drinks and snacks to carry information about calorie, fat, or sugar content.
> Restrict television advertising of foods of minimal nutritional value; provide equal time for messages promoting "eat less, move more."
> Require print food advertisements to disclose calories.
> Prohibit misleading health claims in advertising and on package labels.

Health care and training
> Require health care training programs to teach nutrition and methods for counseling patients about diet, activity, and health.
> Sponsor research on environmental determinants of food choice.

Transportation and urban development
> Provide incentives for communities to develop parks and other venues for physical activity.
> Modify zoning requirements to encourage creation of sidewalks, pedestrian malls, and bicycle paths.

Taxes
> Levy city, state, or federal taxes on soft drinks and other "junk" foods to fund "eat less, move more" campaigns.
> Subsidize the costs of fruits and vegetables, perhaps by raising the costs of selected foods of minimal nutritional value.

Table 37 provides suggestions for actions that might improve the social environment of food choice in order to make it easier for people to eat better diets and be more active. Some of these suggestions involve government action—new policies as well as tweakings of existing policies. The government, of course, represents all constituencies and must balance a cacophony of diverse interests. In all too many instances, as we have seen, the government serves business interests at the expense of public health. Achieving a more equitable balance necessarily starts with

Congress and, therefore, with the reform of laws governing campaign contributions and lobbying. History, however, suggests little basis for optimism that such reforms can occur soon without much more forceful advocacy of consumer perspectives.

A related reform would be to erect a higher and stronger "firewall" between Congress and regulatory agencies. This kind of reform might benefit industry as well as the public, because it would allow companies to compete from the same starting point. To achieve this firewall, Congress would need to reconsider the provisions of laws affecting FDA functions—especially the Dietary Supplement Health and Education Act of 1994 (DSHEA) and the FDA Modernization Act of 1997 (FDAMA)—that so handicap the agency's ability to regulate the food and supplement supply. Congress needs to allocate more funding for the agency's regulatory missions—not less as has been its recent practice. In strengthening the FDA, Congress will need to address the long-standing historical anomaly that its appropriations for the FDA are negotiated through congressional *agriculture*—not health—committees. This anomaly derives from the original assignment of the FDA to the USDA in 1906. The FDA was transferred to a health agency (the Department of Health, Education and Welfare) in 1953 and has been a unit of the Department of Health and Human Services since that department's creation in 1979. Nevertheless, congressional decisions about which of the FDA's functions are funded, and at what level, depend more on how they might affect agriculture than on how they might affect the health of Americans. To select just one example: Public health might be better served if the FDA could sponsor research by independent investigators to further its regulatory decisions, yet congressional agriculture committees consistently deny requests for such funding.

The regulatory agencies themselves also could help create a more independent environment for their work. They could institute greater restrictions on the ability of officials to take jobs with industry and could insist on full disclosure of conflicts of interest by members of advisory committees. The FDA and USDA could be more sensitive to the need to avoid even the appearance of working hand in glove with the industries they regulate. As we have seen, the USDA's conflicting missions—to promote agribusiness and to advise the public about diet and health—cause no end of trouble; such problems are unlikely to be resolved until the USDA's education functions are transferred to an agency less intimately tied to industry interests. Advocates have proposed instituting a single food agency as a way to settle coordination conflicts among the various federal agencies that deal with food safety, and nutrition education might well flourish in such a venue. In this instance also, history suggests that it will be politically inexpedient—if not downright impossible—to accomplish such restructuring.

More realistic are shorter-term actions that community and state governments could take to help people make more healthful dietary choices. The current epidemic of obesity is reason enough to demand action, and the associated health care costs are sufficient grounds for believing that at least some of the actions listed in Table 37 might be politically feasible. Today, numerous government policies support the present food system; these policies could be revised to promote more healthful diets rather than the economic interests of the food industry.[13]

Efforts to promote better food choices begin with education; simply put, an educated public is a healthier public. At issue is how to raise the "dietary literacy" of the general public. Although government agencies create *Dietary Guidelines* and food guides, they in effect delegate the responsibility for promoting this advice to industry. Industry, as we have seen, is unlikely to promote any message to eat less. Therefore, the fact that people do not follow dietary advice cannot be considered evidence that this advice—or nutrition education in general—is ineffective. For reasons of politics as well as finances, the government is unlikely to fund a nationwide campaign to educate people to eat less. Federal agencies do not even support the least controversial of nutrition education campaigns—eat more fruit and vegetables—with anything approaching an adequate budget. As discussed in Chapter 5, the annual budget for the educational component of the National Cancer Institute's 5 A Day partnership with industry (to promote consumption of five servings of fruits and vegetables each day) is less than the amount spent to advertise a single candy bar or soft drink—and by a factor of 50 to 100.

Despite demonstrations that advertising can be extraordinarily effective in promoting desirable dietary changes (such as a switch from whole to lower-fat milk), and at a cost of less than one dollar for every person reached,[14] no government agency can possibly spend that kind of money to reach everyone in the population without a substantial change in tax allocations. USDA economists tell us that rising incomes, time constraints, and low food prices outweigh nutrition education as factors influencing dietary choices and that as incomes rise, people eat more, become less active, and gain weight. As incomes rise further, however, health goals become more important. This last observation suggests that a burgeoning economy creates a stronger base of advocacy for dietary change.[15]

One place to begin is with children. If the roots of obesity are in childhood, then marketing of foods to children deserves substantial public opposition. Banning commercials for foods of minimal nutritional value from children's television programs and from schools, and preventing such foods from replacing more nutritious foods in school lunches, are actions ripe for advocacy—school by school, district by district, state by state.

Tax and price policies are another option. Sales of soft drinks, candy, chewing gum, and snack foods already are taxed in at least 18 states and one major city, and these taxes generate more than $1 billion annually. Some advocates propose that state and local governments tax such products at levels too small to affect sales (less than a penny per soda, for example) and use the accumulated funds to support health promotion campaigns.[16] Price changes clearly influence buying decisions and can be manipulated to improve dietary intake. For example, reducing the prices of low-fat snacks in vending machines, and of fruits and vegetables in school cafeterias, increases sales of these items.[17] The prices of fruits and vegetables also could be subsidized to compensate in part for the low economic added value of these foods—just as is already done through price supports for dairy foods and sugar. These and other fiscal measures to fund health promotion programs are certain to encounter opposition, and USDA officials characterize such proposals as unrealistic and unfriendly to consumers.[12] Nevertheless, judging from experience with the states that have passed such taxes, it appears that the public is willing to vote for them, especially if they are not unduly burdensome and are targeted to desirable social goals such as health promotion.

Given the environment in which food corporations operate, it is worth considering how companies might continue to please stockholders yet market their products more ethically. As a starting point, companies could stop attacking and undermining regulatory agencies. They could stop marketing directly to children. They could stop touting misleading health benefits for their products, invoking individuality and free will, and complaining about Big Brother government. They could bring reality in line with their rhetoric; if food companies really do have the public interest at heart, they could act accordingly. Charles Piller, the technology columnist for the *Los Angeles Times*, urges companies to provide explicit help to the communities in which they operate (and from which they receive substantial subsidies) by committing 1% of annual profits to support local public schools—and not just by giving them computers.[18] This excellent idea is well worth the attention of officials concerned about the quality of their companies' future work force, if nothing else.

In considering ways to improve the environment of food choice, we need to examine the role of health experts. In this context, let me speak directly to my professional colleagues. We nutritionists are not trained to be extremists or revolutionaries, and few us of would want to turn nutrition into a moral issue. Most of us think that food is delightful to eat (as well as to study), and that it should be enjoyed for the pleasures it gives as well as for its health benefits. Even those of us who are concerned about the practices of food companies are not trying to shut down the food industry; foods, after all, are not cigarettes. Nevertheless, it is difficult to avoid noticing that food companies work just like tobacco companies to sell their products. In forging alliances with food companies, we lose sight of this resemblance and of the influence of food-marketing practices on public health. Many of us find it easier to take the "innocuous" *balance–variety–moderation* approach to dietary advice than to face the consequences of saying, "choose this over that" or just "eat less."

On the basis of the examples given in this book, it seems difficult (if not impossible) for food and nutrition professionals to maintain independence—or to be perceived as independent—when we enter into partnerships and alliances with food companies. We may view alliances with industry as a logical way to reach the public with dietary messages or to fund our research, but such alliances inevitably raise questions of conflict of interest. All of us who are educators, practitioners, or researchers—as well as the professional societies that represent us—need to be better aware of the potential compromises inherent in accepting industry funding and to think about how we might take precautions to maintain our independence and integrity. If it is any consolation, we are not alone in needing to worry about such concerns. In the comparatively benign context of corporate sponsorship of science museum exhibits, for example, the eminent scientist Stephen Jay Gould explains that he is "neither an idealist nor a Luddite in this matter. I just feel that the world of commerce and the world of intellect, by their intrinsic natures, must pursue different values and priorities—the commercial world looms so much larger than our domain that we can only be engulfed and destroyed if we make a devil's bargain of fusion for short-term gain."[19]

If we are going to make real progress in helping the public improve diet and health, we are going to have to face the political issues head on, say what we really mean, and be willing to take the consequences of substantial opposition from many sectors of society. At stake are credibility, integrity, and ethics. One suggestion about how to do this comes from Sir Joseph Rotblat, the 1995 Nobel laureate for peace. He thinks that all

TABLE 38. Ethical questions related to food choice

Production methods
Do they protect and preserve natural resources?
Do they avoid pollution of air, land, and water?
Do they adequately reward producers of basic farm commodities?
Do they ensure food safety?
Do they ensure worker safety and economic benefits?
Do they promote nutritional quality?

Marketing methods
Do they avoid inappropriate targeting of children?
Do they emphasize products of high nutritional quality?
Do they disclose the contents of products?
Do they avoid making inappropriate or misleading health claims?
Do they avoid exerting inappropriate pressure on officials in legislative, judiciary, and executive branches of government?
Do they avoid exerting inappropriate pressure on journalists or their employers?
Do they avoid exerting pressure on nutrition and food professionals to engage in activities that give rise to conflicts of interest?

Advising methods
Do they consider the balance between risks and benefits whenever possible?
Do they take ethical issues into consideration?
Do they promote ethical choices whenever possible?

scientists should take an ethics oath that includes this precept, among others: "Throughout my career, I will consider the ethical implications of my work before I take action."[20] This seems like a reasonable first step. In Table 38, I suggest a range of questions that we might consider as we engage in our professional work.

TAKING ACTION: VOTING WITH FORKS

I have argued that one of the most important lessons of antismoking campaigns is that efforts to improve eating habits must be environmental as well as personal, societal as well as individual. A focus on societal determinants does not in any way deny the importance of individual responsibility for food choices. Indeed, there is much that people can do to deal with and counter the lobbying, marketing, and public relations practices of the food industry.

Our overabundant food system, a result as well as a cause of our flourishing economy, gives most of us the opportunity to make a political statement every time we eat—and to make a difference. The questions in

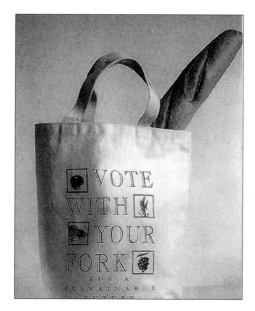

FIGURE 34. An early 1990s souvenir of the Oldways Preservation & Exchange Trust (Boston, Massachusetts) Chefs Collaborative campaign to encourage chefs to forge alliances with local growers of organic foods. Its slogan: "Vote with your fork for a sustainable future." (Photo by Shimon and Tammar Rothstein, 2000)

Table 38 suggest guidelines for making such decisions. For example, buying locally produced, organically grown food not only improves the taste and nutritional quality of the diet (if for no other reason than that the foods have not traveled so far or been stored so long) but also supports local farmers, promotes the viability of rural communities, and creates greater diversity in agricultural production. In the early 1990s, Oldways Preservation & Exchange Trust (a Boston-based group devoted to incorporating traditional foodways into current dietary choices) recognized the political implications of food choice when it urged chefs and restaurateurs to forge alliances with local food producers and "vote with your fork!" (see Figure 34).

The value of such alliances is vividly illustrated by the purchasing practices of a small (65-seat) vegan restaurant, Angelica's Kitchen, in New York City's East Village neighborhood. Among many other products, the restaurant buys 830 pounds of parsley, 2,100 pounds of greens (collards, kale), 3,400 pounds of squash, and 7,800 pounds of carrots every *month*, all of it organically grown and much of it from local suppliers.[21] Another example: The celebrity chef Eberhard Müller and the food consultant Paulette Satur run an organic farm on Long Island that produces 3,000 pounds of organic lettuce every week while the season lasts; they distribute the farm's produce to more than 50 New York restaurants.[22] Such alliances between restaurant owners, chefs, cooks, and farmers hold the promise of economic viability for everyone concerned.

In his book *The McDonaldization of Society*, George Ritzer advocates "subverting the process" by making what he calls "personal irrational choices": Never buy artificial (processed) food products, buy organic, avert your eyes during television commercials, and don't take children to fast-food restaurants.[23] Michael Jacobson and Laurie Ann Mazur argue for downsizing commercialism to a more appropriate role in society. Their advice: Pay attention (count advertisements), declare yourself a personal ad-free zone (don't wear corporate logos), boycott products, turn off the television, get television commercials and soft drinks out of schools, and teach critical media skills so everyone can tell the difference between advertisements and program content.[24] The manifesto of the international Slow Food Movement (its logo is a snail) says, "Our defense should begin at the table with Slow Food. Let us rediscover the flavors and savors of regional cooking and banish the degrading effects of Fast Food."[25]

Adopting such actions is one way to apply ethical principles, but the higher cost and inconvenience of doing so are certain to preclude those choices for many (if not most) people. Unless we are willing to pay more for food, relinquish out-of-season produce, and rarely buy anything that comes in a package or is advertised on television, we support the current food system every time we eat a meal. That is why voting with our forks must extend beyond the food choices of individuals to larger political arenas. Countless community, state, and national organizations deal with food issues, and it is not difficult to find one to suit any political viewpoint or taste. As has been demonstrated by the support for creating federal standards for organic food, such groups can join together quickly and effectively when an issue of mutual interest emerges. This ability to exercise democratic power holds much hope for achieving a more equitable balance of interests in matters pertaining to food and health.

ISSUES IN NUTRITION
AND NUTRITION RESEARCH

TO EVALUATE THE QUESTIONS AND ARGUMENTS EXPLORED IN THIS book, some background information about nutrition may be helpful. This Appendix provides a brief, nontechnical overview of basic principles of nutrition, as well as a discussion of some fundamental issues that affect our ability to interpret research studies that examine the ways in which specific dietary components—or overall dietary patterns—affect health.[1]

NUTRITION BASICS

The importance of nutrition to health is self-evident: People must eat to live. Humans require a continuous supply of energy, nutrients, other food components, and water to maintain life, grow, and reproduce. By definition, *essential nutrients* are those that cannot be synthesized in adequate amounts by the human body through normal metabolic processes and, therefore, must be obtained from food plants and animals.[2]

The list of nutrients that are essential or otherwise useful to human physiology is long, is complicated by conditions, restrictions, and ambiguities, and is almost certainly incomplete. It includes the nearly 70 distinct substances listed in italics in Table 39 and its footnotes. These are categorized as sources of energy (carbohydrate, fat, protein, alcohol); essential amino acids, fatty acids, vitamins, minerals, and trace elements; fiber; and water. Other nutrients also may be required under certain conditions. In addition, "phytochemical" substances in plant foods, although they are not considered essential (because people can live without them), may nevertheless protect the body against cancer and other diseases. A great deal of attention is focused on dietary fat, and Table 40 explains the different types.

Because plants can extract minerals from soil and use solar energy to synthesize vitamins and other essential nutrients, and because animals eat plants and

TABLE 39. Dietary components generally considered essential or beneficial to human health

Category	Definition: *Examples*
Calorie sources	Large molecules that are broken down by digestive enzymes, absorbed, and metabolized or used to construct body molecules: *carbohydrate, fat, protein, alcohol.*[a]
Essential amino acids	Building blocks of protein; those that are not made in the body and must be provided in the diet are: *isoleucine, leucine, lysine, methionine, phenylalanine, threonine, tryptophan, valine, histidine.*[b]
Essential fatty acids	Building blocks of fat, of which two must be provided in the diet: *linoleic acid, linolenic acid.*[c]
Vitamins	Carbon-based compounds that catalyze or participate in the synthesis of body molecules or metabolic reactions.
Water-soluble	The vitamins in this group dissolve in water, are excreted in urine, and are rarely toxic: *ascorbic acid (vitamin C), biotin,*[d] *cobalamin (vitamin B_{12}), folic acid, niacin, pantothenic acid, pyridoxine (vitamin B_6), riboflavin, thiamin (vitamin B_1), choline.*[e]
Fat-soluble	These vitamins are absorbed, transported, and stored along with fat; excessive amounts can accumulate to toxic levels: *vitamin A,*[f] *vitamin D,*[g] *vitamin E, and vitamin K.*[d]
Minerals	Required from food or water in amounts greater than 100 mg per day: *calcium, chloride, magnesium, phosphate, potassium, sodium.*

incorporate the nutrients into their own tissues, we can obtain the nutrients we need by eating food plants and animals. Any plant or animal food that has not yet been processed contains many essential nutrients, although in varied proportions. Green peppers are especially high in beta-carotene and vitamin C, for example, and dairy products are especially high in calcium. Some nutrients are found only in certain food groups: Vitamin C derives only from foods of plant origin, and vitamin B_{12} derives only from foods of animal origin (this vitamin is synthesized by common bacteria present in foods consumed by animals). For these reasons alone, the human diet should contain sufficient amounts of a wide variety of foods to provide the full range of needed nutrients. Throughout human history, population groups have found many ways to meet nutrient requirements through consumption of available plants and animals. No one food (other than breast milk) is either perfect or absolutely necessary. To create healthful diets, foods can be mixed and matched to suit any taste and any cultural, ethnic, or religious preference.

TABLE 39. *(continued)*

Category	Definition: *Examples*
Trace elements	Required in microgram or milligram amounts: *chromium, cobalt,[b] copper, fluoride, iodine, iron, manganese, molybdenum, selenium, zinc.[i]*
Fiber	Carbohydrate molecules in plant foods that cannot be broken down by human digestive enzymes and are only minimally absorbed and metabolized.[j]
Phytochemicals	Plant chemicals that appear protective against disease, perhaps because they stimulate detoxifying enzyme systems: *carotenes, lutein, lycopene, allium, sulforaphane, flavonoids, others.[k]*
Water	

[a]Carbohydrates (starches and sugars) contribute about 4 calories per gram (20 calories per teaspoon); proteins, fats, and alcohol contribute about 4, 9, and 7 calories per gram, respectively. Fat is fattening because it is so high in calories.

[b]Histidine is essential for infants; its adult requirement is uncertain. The amino acids *arginine, cystine, glycine, glutamine, proline,* and *tyrosine* are considered to be "conditionally essential"; they may be required under certain conditions, genetic and otherwise. The protein metabolites *carnitine, ornithine,* and *taurine* also may be conditionally essential.

[c]Other fatty acids in the omega-3 series also may have essential functions.

[d]Synthesized by intestinal microorganisms; dietary requirement uncertain.

[e]Choline is synthesized by the body to some extent; the dietary requirement is uncertain.

[f]Includes *beta-carotene,* a precursor of vitamin A in plant foods.

[g]Most vitamin D is synthesized from the action of sunlight on precursors of the vitamin in skin.

[h]Cobalt is an essential component of vitamin B_{12}.

[i]*Arsenic, boron, nickel, silicon, tin,* and *vanadium* are required by certain animal species, but human requirements are not well defined.

[j]Evidence supports the health benefits of fiber, particularly of diets that contain 20–35 grams per day, but no specific requirement has been established.

[k]These compounds in fruits and vegetables appear protective against cancer and other diseases; their mechanisms of action are under active investigation.

Standards of Nutrient Intake: DRIs and RDAs

In the United States, standards of nutrient intake for populations are developed by the Food and Nutrition Board (FNB) of the Institute of Medicine. From the early 1940s until the late 1990s, the standards were the Recommended Dietary Allowances (RDAs). Beginning in 1997, the Food and Nutrition Board incorporated the RDAs into a more complicated set of standards, now called Dietary Reference Intakes (DRIs). By 2001, DRIs had been established for 32 nutrients, with more to come.[3] The DRIs encompass four categories of standards—one of them RDAs—that depend on the extent and quality of the available research. RDAs are established for nutrients for which the most research is available (we do not need to be concerned with the other three categories here). Under the new DRI system, RDAs are defined as they always have been: the dietary intake level of specific nutrients that meets the requirements of most—about 97%—of the individuals in a population. The RDAs are used to assess dietary adequacy, interpret food consumption records, establish levels of food assistance, evaluate the nutritional

TABLE 40. Dietary fats[a]

Fatty acids

Saturated	All carbon binding sites filled with hydrogen atoms (most characteristic of animal fats). Raises blood cholesterol levels.
Unsaturated	All binding sites except one filled with hydrogen atoms (most characteristic of the fats in olives, nuts, and avocados). Relatively neutral with respect to cholesterol raising.
Polyunsaturated	Two or more binding sites not filled with hydrogen atoms (most characteristic of vegetable seed fats). The essential fatty acids are in this category. Lowers blood cholesterol.
Omega-3	A form of polyunsaturated fatty acid especially common in fish and certain plants in which the first unsaturated binding site occurs on the third carbon from one end of the chain (rather than on the sixth or ninth). Appears to reduce risks for coronary heart disease and stroke.
Hydrogenated	Artificially saturated fats made by adding hydrogen to poly-unsaturated fat, as in certain margarines and oils.
Trans-saturated	Saturated fats in which some of the hydrogens are placed unnaturally, making the fat "stiffer," as in hydrogenation. Raises risk for coronary heart disease.
Cholesterol	A fatty (but not fatty acid) precursor of vitamins and sex hormones derived *only* from foods of animal origin— meat, dairy, eggs. Its metabolism does not yield calories. Raises blood cholesterol levels, but by not nearly so much as saturated fat.

---

[a]Food fats are concentrated sources of energy (9 calories per gram, compared to 4 calories per gram for protein or carbohydrate). They usually are composed of three *fatty acids* attached like the letter "E" to a backbone of a small sugar, glycerol. Fatty acids are hydrocarbons: chains of carbon atoms to which hydrogen atoms are attached. Their properties depend on the degree of saturation (whether every place where a hydrogen atom can attach to a carbon actually has one attached) and on the chain length (number of carbons). All fats contain a *mixture* of fatty acids, but some contain more of one kind than of another. As a general rule, animal fats contain more saturated fatty acids than vegetable fats, and vegetable fats contain more polyunsaturated fatty acids than animal fats (but there are exceptions).

status of individuals and populations, establish a basis for evaluating the nutrient content of food on package labels, and develop guidelines for nutrition education and dietary counseling. Because of the obvious importance of these functions, the limitations of RDAs require careful attention. To begin with, they are standards for the entire population, not necessarily for any one individual within that population. They are set at levels that meet the needs of nearly everyone in a population within certain age ranges. Most people (those with average or below-average requirements) meet their nutritional needs at lower levels of intake and are not at risk of deficiency if their intake falls below the RDA standard. For just 3% or less of the healthy population, the RDAs may be too low. For the 97% of the population, the RDA is adequate or more than adequate. What this means is that even if a person's diet does not meet the RDAs, we cannot conclude that the diet is deficient without further information.

Malnutrition: Deficiencies, Excesses, Imbalances

The term *malnutrition* refers to excessive and unbalanced intake of food components as well as to inadequate intake. Fat-soluble vitamins and virtually all of the mineral elements cause disease symptoms when they are consumed or absorbed in excess. Overconsumption of calories, fat, cholesterol, sodium, sugar, alcohol also produces adverse effects on health. For each nutrient or component, a certain range of intake meets physiologic requirements but does not induce harmful symptoms. To date, however, the optimal ranges of intake of specific nutrients can be estimated only for *populations*. Optimal intakes for *individuals* are difficult to define; people vary in nutrient requirements for genetic reasons, and also because diet interacts with other factors that affect the use of nutrients, such as smoking cigarettes, taking medications, and being physically active.

Nutritional Deficiencies   A deficiency of an essential nutrient causes recognizable symptoms. When the deficient nutrient is replaced, the symptoms disappear. Inadequate dietary intake is only one cause of nutrient deficiency, however. Deficiency symptoms also result from conditions that impair nutrient digestion, absorption, or metabolism (such as intestinal infections), interfere with nutrient transport or use (genetic defects in crucial enzymes), or substantially increase nutrient requirements or losses (severe illness, burns). Nutritional deficiencies may appear as starvation, as various forms of protein-energy malnutrition, as syndromes of deficiency of single nutrients, or as a wide range of less specific symptoms that can be diagnosed only with laboratory tests. Deficiencies usually are expressed as digestive, neurological, blood, or skin disorders. For deficiencies of some nutrients, the constellation of symptoms is given a name, such as *scurvy* for vitamin C deficiency, *beriberi* for thiamin deficiency, and *pellagra* for deficiency of niacin. Such conditions were quite common in the United States in the early years of the twentieth century, but they gradually disappeared with economic and public health improvements following World War II. Today iron-deficiency anemia, which affects up to 20% of low-income children, women, and the elderly, is the most prevalent nutritional deficiency disorder observed in this country.

The number of people throughout the world who suffer from nutritional deficiencies, however, is surely in the hundreds of millions. Widespread nutritional deficiencies are observed among populations in developing countries where income, education, housing, and sanitation are inadequate, and where the water supplies are contaminated with infectious organisms and parasites that can induce diarrhea and losses of fluids and blood. These problems are a direct result of poverty. In the United States, as well as in most developing countries, food production is sufficient to meet the energy requirements of the population, but many people are too poor to afford an adequate diet.

In industrialized countries, overt symptoms of dietary deficiencies are less prevalent even in the presence of poor dietary intake. "Hunger"—as defined by inadequate ability to purchase food—affects 20 million children and adults in the United States and numerous surveys have identified nutrient intakes below RDA levels among groups living in poverty. Such findings, however, are only rarely accompanied by clinical signs of nutrient deficiencies. When clinical signs do occur, they are usually associated with the additional nutritional requirements of pregnancy, infancy, and early childhood; with illness, injury, or hospitalization; with aging; or with the toxic effects of alcohol or drug abuse.

Regardless of its cause, inadequate dietary intake profoundly affects body functions. It induces rapid and severe losses of body weight, decreases blood pressure and metabolic rate, causes abnormalities in heart function and losses in muscle strength and stamina, and induces undesirable changes in gastrointestinal function and behavior. The result is a generalized lack of vitality that reduces productivity and impairs people's ability to escape the consequences of poverty. Of special concern is the loss of immune function that accompanies starvation. Malnourished individuals demonstrate poor resistance to infectious disease. Infections, in turn, increase nutrient losses and requirements and, in the absence of adequate nutrient intake, induce further malnutrition. This cycle is the principal cause of death among young children in developing countries and an important cause of illness in malnourished adults. Protein-calorie (or protein-energy) malnutrition is the collective term for the clinical effects of this cycle on young children. Survivors display typical effects of starvation: depression, apathy, irritability, and growth retardation.

Given the political will to do so, it is not difficult to prevent poverty-associated malnutrition in adults and children, and numerous methods have been demonstrated to be effective in developing countries. Among them are programs that redistribute income, subsidize food prices, promote agricultural production, provide food supplements, and provide education. Improvements in sanitation and in primary health care are also essential components of programs to reduce nutritional deficiencies.[4]

Nutritional Excesses and Imbalances   As nutritional deficiencies decline in prevalence in industrialized—as well as developing—countries, they are replaced by chronic conditions of dietary excess and imbalance. In today's rapidly changing socioeconomic environment, populations throughout the world exhibit rising rates of chronic diseases superimposed on classic patterns of malnutrition.[5] In the United States, four of the ten leading causes of death—coronary heart disease, cancer, stroke, and diabetes—are chronic diseases related in part to diets providing excessive energy, fat, cholesterol, or salt. Chronic liver disease and cirrhosis are associated with excessive intake of alcohol. Table 41 lists dietary factors associated with the principal diet-related chronic diseases that affect Americans. These dietary components also are associated with hypertension, obesity, dental diseases, osteoporosis, and kidney disease. The proportion of the burden of illness that can be attributed to dietary factors alone, however, is uncertain. Most estimates are that about one-third of cancers and heart disease cases are attributable at least in part to the combination of poor diet, inadequate activity, and excessive alcohol use, and that diseases caused by inappropriate diets are responsible for $200 billion annually in medical care and lost productivity in this country alone.[6]

TABLE 41. Dietary components associated directly or indirectly with some increase in risk of chronic disease[a]

Disease	Excess Calories	Excess Fat[b]	Inadequate Fiber	Excess Salt	Excess Alcohol
Coronary heart disease	×	×	×	×	×
Cancer	×	×	×	×[c]	×
Stroke	×	×		×	×
Diabetes (type 2)	×	×	×		×
Liver cirrhosis					×
Digestive diseases	×	×	×		×

[a]Diet affects disease indirectly by raising levels of risk factors: obesity, high blood pressure, and high blood cholesterol. The evidence for these associations varies in quality and strength from very strong (alcohol and liver cirrhosis) to rather weak (salt and cancer).

[b]It is difficult to distinguish the effects of *total fat* on disease risk from the effects of the "good" polyunsaturated, monounsaturated, and omega-3 fats, or of the "bad" saturated and *trans*-saturated fats, or of the calories contributed by fat. Current evidence suggests that total fat is unlikely to raise heart disease risk unless it is high in saturated or *trans*-saturated fatty acids.

[c]Some evidence connects consumption of very large amounts of salt-cured foods with an increased risk of stomach and certain other cancers.

ISSUES IN NUTRITION RESEARCH

The uncertainties in estimates of the burden of illness attributed to diet are due in part to difficulties in the design, conduct, and interpretation of research on nutritional factors and disease. Nutrition research is complicated by genetic variations in individual nutritional requirements, by the complexity of dietary intake, and by interactions among dietary and other behavioral and lifestyle factors. It is also complicated, as discussed below, by limitations in the ability to obtain accurate information about the dietary intake of individuals or populations. Proof of dietary causality is difficult to demonstrate for diseases that are also influenced by so many other genetic, environmental, and behavioral factors.

No Method Is Perfect; Association Is Not Proof

An association between a dietary component and a particular disease is derived from studies of laboratory animals and from biochemical (test tube), epidemiological (population), and clinical (medical) investigations in humans. Each of these types of studies has limitations. Biochemical studies may not be closely related to "real-life" situations. Epidemiological studies usually describe correlations between a dietary factor and a disease across many different populations or within the same population; the results describe *associations* between a dietary factor and a disease and generate testable hypothesis about causality, but they never *prove* that a dietary factor causes a disease.[7] The high cost of clinical investigations, in which the effects of a dietary factor on a disease are followed over time, limits the size of the population studied. A host of other factors (drinking, smoking, medications, exercise) also can affect the results. Thus, whereas it is relatively easy to demonstrate that iron or any other single nutrient can prevent or treat symptoms of its deficiency, it is not so easy to demonstrate that single nutritional factors affect heart disease, cancer, or other such conditions.

Assessing the effects of nutritional supplements illustrates this problem. People who take supplements are demonstrably healthier than those who do not, but their good health may have less to do with the supplements than with their being white rather than members of minority groups (an index, however imperfect, of social class), or wealthier, or better educated, or smokers of fewer cigarettes, or drinkers of less alcohol. As a group, people who take supplements also exercise more and care more about health. Placebo effects introduce a further complication (see the next section). The most scientifically convincing evidence that a dietary factor affects a disease is a "double-blind, clinically controlled, prospective study" in which neither the investigators nor the participants know whether the study subjects are taking a nutrient or a placebo—a pill with no physiologic effects—during the many years that it takes for diseases to develop. Such studies find it difficult to recruit and retain participants, cost many millions of dollars, and rarely produce results that can be interpreted unambiguously, not least because they examine the effects of single nutrients in isolation from the overall dietary context. Because of such limitations, diet–disease associations are usually inferred from the totality of available evidence and are considered most compelling when data from all sources are consistent, strongly correlated, highly specific, related to the dose used, and biologically plausible.

Despite research uncertainties, nearly every expert committee that has ever examined the evidence linking diet to disease finds support for the associations listed in Table 41. They consider most compelling the evidence for saturated fat as a causative factor and that for fruits and vegetables as protective factors; the evidence for the other associations appears strongly suggestive, if not utterly convincing.

Placebo Effects Are Powerful

A critical difficulty encountered in research studies that examine the effects of taking one or another nutrient is the need to distinguish true effects from placebo (or other self-healing) effects. Because taking *anything* often makes people feel better, rigorous standards of scientific proof require the same kinds of evidence for dietary components as they do for drugs; the component must be shown to produce health benefits greater than those that can be obtained with placebos as well as with no treatment at all. Whether or not placebo effects are "real" or just the result of diseases getting better by themselves, about 30% of people are "responders," which means that whenever they take something—anything—their colds, aches and pains, feelings of tension or anxiety, and other such minor problems appear to go away or become less severe.

The power of placebo effects in nutrition is illustrated by a now classic study of the effects of vitamin C on cold symptoms conducted by the National Institutes of Health (NIH) in the early 1970s. Having heard Dr. Linus Pauling, twice winner of the Nobel Prize, extol the benefits of vitamin C as a preventive measure and cure for the common cold,[8] the investigators wanted to see whether the vitamin would be effective against colds if tested against a placebo. They recruited about 300 NIH employees to take either vitamin C or a placebo (not knowing which was which) and asked the volunteers to report whenever they caught a cold and how long it lasted. The initial results: People who were taking vitamin C reported fewer colds and milder symptoms than people who were taking placebos.

During the study, however, an unusually high rate of people withdrew from participation. The investigators realized something was amiss and asked why. They soon discovered that the dropouts had tasted the pills, had figured out (or thought they had figured out) what they were taking, and had given up on the study. The investigators then reanalyzed the data according to whether the study participants really knew what they were taking or only thought they did. This analysis produced quite different results: People who *thought* they were taking vitamin C reported fewer colds and milder symptoms, whether they really were taking vitamin C or were actually taking the placebo. Those who *thought* they were taking vitamin C felt better.[9] This example suggests the benefits of placebos in such situations, and also reveals the reasons why it is so important to control for placebo or other self-healing effects when designing dietary studies.[10]

Dietary Intake Is Difficult to Assess

All research on diet and health depends on the investigators' ability to find out what people are eating, but doing so with any reasonable degree of accuracy is remarkably difficult. Indeed, the most intellectually demanding challenge in the field of nutrition is to determine dietary intake. As we shall see, just asking people what they eat biases their answers. The most frequently used methods for directly determining dietary intake ask people to

- Report what they ate or drank in the previous day (24-hour diet survey, reported retrospectively).
- Keep a record of what they eat for a day or more (diet record, recorded at time of consumption).
- Mark off on a list of foods the ones eaten within the last day, week, month, or year (food frequency questionnaire, recorded retrospectively).

The difficulties inherent in these methods cannot be overestimated. People do not easily remember what they eat, and they may be uncomfortable reporting late night snacks, alcohol, or the amounts of foods they consume. As a result, most people underestimate their caloric intake, the sizes of their food portions, and the consumption of foods they think are bad for them; they also tend to overestimate their intake of "good" foods.[11] Furthermore, researchers have not yet resolved questions related to whether one method is better than another, whether collecting information on portion sizes is useful or necessary, or indeed whether *any* method can capture the complexities of diets that vary so much from person to person and from day to day.

A second source of information on dietary intake is indirect; it comes from data on the availability of commodities in the food supply. Food supply data express the amounts of foods produced annually in the United States, plus the amounts imported, less the amounts exported. These amounts are divided by the number of people in the population at midyear, and then presented as the amount available annually for every person in the population, regardless of age. The U.S. Department of Agriculture (USDA) has been collecting and producing this information since 1909. Food supply data have their own kinds of reliability problems (imagine what it would take to count the number of pounds of corn or gallons of milk produced in this country, let alone the amounts imported or exported), but to the extent that collection methods remain the same from year to year, they yield useful information on trends in the U.S. food supply. Another point is that food supply data indicate the amounts of foods *available* for consumption, not necessarily the amounts actually eaten. Some food is wasted, although how much can only be estimated. Similarly, it is difficult to know how much food is produced in home gardens (which would increase the per capita availability) or fed to pets (which would decrease it). Overall, food supply figures are most likely to overestimate actual food consumption.[12]

If dietary intake data underestimate nutrient consumption and food supply data overestimate nutrient consumption, the truth probably lies someplace in between. Given this situation, reports on what Americans are eating require careful interpretation. Trends seem most believable when the data from all sources point in the same direction. For example, the food supply figure for calories is 3,800 per day per capita (this means the figure applies to infants and children as well as to adults of all ages), but dietary intake surveys indicate that *adults* consume about 2,000 calories per day. Wastage accounts for some of the discrepancy, but not all, and the lower figure hardly seems sufficient to account for rising rates of overweight and obesity.[13] A more probable explanation for the lower figure is underreporting of food intake on dietary surveys. Actual average caloric intake probably lies between 2,000 and 3,800 calories per person per day, but closer to the lower than to the higher figure.

A further problem is translating intake of *foods* into calories and nutrients. Doing so requires reference to tables of food composition in a database managed by the USDA. Every study of diet and health depends on the accuracy and reliability of this database. To determine whether calcium protects against osteoporosis, for example, we need to know how much calcium people are eating. This requires knowing how much calcium we would get if we ate a carrot, for example (yes, carrots do contain calcium). But is the calcium content of carrots grown in California the same as that of carrots grown in Arkansas or Massachusetts? Does carrot variety X contain the same amount as variety Y? Does it matter whether the carrot was grown organically? Such questions raise issues of sampling techniques and sample numbers, not to mention the reliability of the laboratory tests for the calcium content of food. Finally, composition determinations are expensive and time-consuming, and the USDA has only a limited budget for such studies. Instead, it must rely on composition information provided by food companies for the hundreds of thousands of packaged foods on the market. In many instances, companies are reluctant to provide nutrient-content information that they consider proprietary.[14] Taken together, these problems mean not that dietary intake information is necessarily false but, rather, that it requires careful interpretation laced with a good deal of common sense.

Nutrition Research Must Be Interpreted Critically, in Context

Nutrition is a thinking person's field, requiring critical analysis at every step of learning and interpretation, as well as an unusually high tolerance for ambiguity and uncertainty. The difficulties in interpretation discussed here—and the emphasis in research and food advertising on single nutrients rather than dietary patterns—create ample opportunity for controversy. The contradiction between the seemingly endless debates about the meaning of nutrition research, and the equally endless similarity of dietary guidelines can best be explained by experts' use of context and judgment. Every committee examining the available research on diet and disease risk has been impressed by the health benefits of consuming largely plant-based diets, balancing energy intake with energy expenditure, and limiting intake of animal fats, alcohol, and processed foods high in fat, sugar, and salt. Such committees place new research findings in context and accept them when they are reasonably consistent with other sources of information and make biological sense, as I also have tried to do in this book.

NOTES

This section contains reference citations along with occasional notes. Citations follow the spare, unpunctuated "Vancouver" style used by most biological science journals as described in JAMA 1993;269:2282–2286 (*Journal of the American Medical Association,* 1993, volume 269, pages 2282–2286). Issue numbers sometimes follow the volume in parentheses; thus *Food Technology* 1989;43(4): 144–150 refers to a paper published in the April issue. As is customary in Vancouver style, text citations to references sometimes appear out of numerical order; these are cross-references to material cited earlier *in the same chapter.* To save space, references to most U.S. government reports omit their publisher, the U.S. Government Printing Office, and citations to articles in professional journals with more than four authors list only the first three (followed by et al.). For clarity, most references give the full name of the author and the full title of the journal, but the following standard abbreviations are used:

Am	American
Am J Clin Nutr	American Journal of Clinical Nutrition
DHHS	U.S. Department of Health and Human Services
FDA	U.S. Food and Drug Administration
J	Journal, Journal of, Journal of the
J Am Diet Assoc	Journal of the American Dietetic Association
JAMA	Journal of the American Medical Association
N Engl J Med	New England Journal of Medicine
Suppl	Supplement
USDA	U.S. Department of Agriculture

INTRODUCTION: THE FOOD INDUSTRY AND "EAT MORE"

1. Kluger R. Ashes to Ashes: America's Hundred-Year Cigarette War, the Public Health, and the Unabashed Triumph of Philip Morris. New York, NY: Alfred A. Knopf, 1996.

2. DHHS. The Surgeon General's Report on Nutrition and Health. Washington, DC, 1988.

3. Calories measure the energy value of food. Food package labels—and this book—use the erroneous but commonly understood "calories" instead of the correct unit, kilocalories (kcal). A kilocalorie (in this book, calorie) is the amount of energy required to raise the temperature of a liter of water 1° centigrade. In the metric system, energy is measured in joules; 1 kcal = 4.2 kilojoules (kJ).

4. Food and Nutrition Board. Diet and Health: Implications for Reducing Chronic Disease Risk. Washington, DC: National Academy Press, 1989. James WPT. Healthy Nutrition: Preventing Nutrition-Related Diseases in Europe. Copenhagen: World Health Organization, 1988. World Cancer Research Fund. Food, Nutrition and the Prevention of Cancer: A Global Perspective. Washington, DC: American Institute for Cancer Research, 1997.

5. McGinnis JM, Foege WH. Actual causes of death in the United States. JAMA 1993;270:2207–2212. Stampfer MJ, Hu FB, Manson JE, et al. Primary prevention of coronary heart disease in women through diet and lifestyle. N Engl J Med 2000;343:16–22. Frazão E. High costs of poor eating patterns in the United States. In: Frazão E, ed. America's Eating Habits: Changes & Consequences. Washington, DC: USDA, 1999:5–32.

6. Troiano RP, Flegal KM, Kuczmarski RJ, et al. Overweight prevalence and trends for children and adolescents. Archives of Pediatric and Adolescent Medicine 1995;149:1085–1091. Mokdad AH, Serdula MK, Dietz WH, et al. The spread of the obesity epidemic in the United States, 1991–1998. JAMA 1999; 282:1519–1522. Must A, Spadano J, Coakley EH, et al. The disease burden associated with overweight and obesity. JAMA 1999;282:1523–1529. Overweight and obesity are defined in relation to the Body Mass Index (BMI): body weight in kilograms divided by height in meters squared (kg/m^2). Overweight is defined as a BMI at or above the 85th percentile in a national survey conducted in 1976–1980, or a BMI of 25 or above. Obesity is defined as a BMI of 30 or above.

7. Physical activity trends—United States, 1990–1998. JAMA 2001;285: 1835. Anderson RE, Crespo CJ, Bartlett SJ, et al. Relationship of physical activity and television watching with body weight and level of fatness among children. JAMA 1998;279:938–942.

8. Putnam JJ, Allshouse JE. Food Consumption, Prices, and Expenditures, 1970–1997. Washington, DC: USDA, 1999. USDA. Data Tables: Results from USDA's 1994–1996 Continuing Survey of Food Intakes by Individuals and 1994–1996 Diet and Health Knowledge Survey, 1997. Online: http://www.barc.usda.gov/bhnrc/foodsurvey/. Accessed May 23, 2001.

9. Lin B-H, Guthrie J, Frazão E. Nutrient contribution of food away from home. In: Frazão E, ed. America's Eating Habits: Changes & Consequences. Washington, DC: USDA, 1999:71–95.

10. Food Surveys Research Group. Pyramid Servings Data: Results from USDA's 1995 and 1996 Continuing Survey of Food Intakes by Individuals. Beltsville, MD: USDA Agricultural Research Service, 1997.

11. Kantor LS. A dietary assessment of the U.S. food supply. Family Economics and Nutrition Review 1999;12:51–54.

12. Lipton KL, Edmondson W, Manchester A. The Food and Fiber System: Contributing to the U.S. and World Economies. Washington, DC: USDA Economic Research Service, 1998. Gallo AE. The Food Marketing System in 1996. Washington, DC: USDA Economic Research Service, 1998.

13. Beale CL. A century of population growth and change. FoodReview 2000;23(1):16–22. Sommer JE, Hoppe RA, Green RC, Korb PJ. Structural and Financial Characteristics of U.S. Farms, 1995: 20th Annual Family Farm Report to Congress. Washington, DC: USDA, 1998. Online: **http://www.ers. usda.gov/publications**. Accessed May 23, 2001.

14. Nestle M, Wing R, Birch L, et al. Behavioral and social influences on food choice. Nutrition Reviews 1998;56:s50–s74. Nestle M, ed. Mediterranean diets: science and policy implications. Am J Clin Nutr 1995;61(suppl): 1313s–1427s.

15. Popkin BM. The nutrition transition and its health implications in lower-income countries. Public Health Nutrition 1998;1(1):5–21. Gardner G, Halwell B. Underfed and Overfed: The Global Epidemic of Malnutrition. Washington, DC: Worldwatch Institute, 2000. See: http://apps.fao.org.

16. Glanz K, Basil M, Maibach E, et al. Why Americans eat what they do: taste, nutrition cost, convenience, and weight. J Am Diet Assoc 1998;98: 1118–1126.

17. Dunham D. Food Costs . . . From Farm to Retail in 1993. Washington, DC: USDA Economic Research Service, 1994.

18. Meade B, Rosen S. Income and diet differences greatly affect food spending around the globe. FoodReview 1996;19(3):39–44. Huang KS. Prices and incomes affect nutrients consumed. FoodReview 1998:21(2):11–15.

19. Egan T. Failing farmers learn to profit from federal aid. New York Times December 24, 2000:A1,A20.

20. Zizza C, Siega-Riz AM, Popkin BM. Significant increase in young adults' snacking between 1977–1978 and 1994–1996 represents a cause for concern! Preventive Medicine 2001;32:303–310. Bowers DE. Cooking trends echo changing roles of women. FoodReview 2000;23(1):23–29.

21. Shim Y, Variyam JN, Blaylock J. Many Americans falsely optimistic about their diets. FoodReview 2000;23(1):44–50. Hackman EM, Moe GL. Evaluation of newspaper reports of nutrition-related research. J Am Diet Assoc 1999;99:1564–1566.

22. Endicott RC. Top 100 megabrands. Advertising Age July 17, 2000: s1–s18.

23. Gallo AE. Food advertising in the United States. In: Frazão E, ed. America's Eating Habits: Changes & Consequences. Washington, DC: USDA, 1999: 173–180.

24. Novelli WD. Applying social marketing to health promotion and disease prevention. In: Glanz K, Lewis FM, Rimer BK, eds. Health Behavior and Health Education: Theory, Research, and Practice. San Francisco: Jossey-Bass, 1990:342–369. Blisard N. Advertising and what we eat: the case of dairy products. In: Frazão E, ed. America's Eating Habits: Changes & Consequences. Washington, DC: USDA, 1999:181–188. Enyinda CI, Ogbuehi AO. An empirical analysis of retail pricing and multimedia advertising effects on sales performance. J Food Products Marketing 1997;4:3–16.

25. Young LR, Nestle M. Portion sizes in dietary assessment: issues and policy implications. Nutrition Reviews 1995;53:149–158. Hogbin MB, Hess MA. Public confusion over food portions and servings. J Am Diet Assoc 1999;99: 1209–1211.

26. Levenstein H. Paradox of Plenty: A Social History of Eating in Modern America. Oxford: Oxford University Press, 1993.

27. Wilde PE, McNamara PE, Ranney CK. The effect of income and food programs on dietary quality: a seemingly unrelated regression analysis with error components. Am J Agricultural Economics 1999;81:959–971. Alaniz ML, Wilkes C. Pro-drinking messages and message environments for young adults: the case of alcohol industry advertising in African American, Latino, and Native American communities. J Public Health Policy 1998;19:447–472.

28. Salter L. Mandated Science: Science and Scientists in the Making of Standards. Dordrecht: Kluwer Academic Publishers, 1988. Irwin A, Wynne B. Introduction. In: Irwin A, Wynne B, eds. Misunderstanding Science? The Public Reconstruction of Science and Technology. Cambridge: England: Cambridge University Press, 1996:1–18.

PART I. UNDERMINING DIETARY ADVICE

Some of the material in Part I draws on previously published work: Nestle M, Porter DV. Evolution of federal dietary guidance policy: from food adequacy to chronic disease prevention. *Caduceus* 1990;6(2):43–67. Nestle M. Dietary advice for the 1990s: the political history of the food guide pyramid. *Caduceus* 1993: 9:136–153 (with permission, Southern Illinois University School of Medicine and the Department of Medical Humanities); Alcohol guidelines for chronic disease prevention: from prohibition to moderation. *Social History of Alcohol Review* 1996;32/33:1–15 (with permission) and *Nutrition Today* 1997;32(2):86–92. In defense of the USDA food guide pyramid. *Nutrition Today*, 1998;33(5):189–197 (with permission, Lippincott Williams & Wilkins); Commentary. *Food Policy* 1999;24:307–310 (with permission, Elsevier Science).

CHAPTER 1: FROM "EAT MORE" TO "EAT LESS," 1900-1999

1. DHHS and USDA. Nutrition Monitoring in the United States: A Progress Report from the Joint Nutrition Monitoring Evaluation Committee. Washington, DC, 1986.

2. Department of Agriculture Organic Act, 12 Stat. 317, May 15, 1962. USDA. Some Landmarks in the History of the Department of Agriculture. Washington, DC: USDA Bureau of Agricultural Economics, 1951.

3. Atwater WO. Foods: Nutritive Value and Cost. Washington, DC: USDA, 1894:25.

4. Hunt CL, Atwater HW. How to Select Foods. I. What the Body Needs. Washington, DC: USDA, 1917.

5. Hunt CL. Good Proportions in the Diet. Washington, DC: USDA, 1923:1.

6. Stiebling HK, Ward MM. Diets at Four Levels of Nutritive Content and Cost. Washington, DC: USDA, 1933.

7. Roberts LJ. Beginnings of the Recommended Dietary Allowances. J Am Diet Assoc 1958;34:903–908. Harper AE. Origins of Recommended Dietary Allowances—a historic overview. Am J Clin Nutr 1985;41:140–148.

8. Office of Defense Health and Welfare Services. U.S. Needs Us Strong. Washington, DC, 1942. Bureau of Home Economics. When You Eat Out: Food for Freedom. Washington, DC, 1942.

9. War Food Administration. National Wartime Nutrition Guide. Washington, DC: USDA, 1943.

10. Bureau of Human Nutrition and Home Economics. National Food Guide. Washington DC: USDA, 1946.

11. Bureau of Human Nutrition and Home Economics. Food for Growth: Food for Freedom. Washington, DC: USDA, 1946.

12. Hill MM, Cleveland LE. Food guides—their development and use. Nutrition Program News. Washington, DC: USDA, 1970.

13. Citizens' Board of Inquiry into Hunger and Malnutrition in the United States. Hunger U.S.A. Revisited. New York: Field Foundation, 1972:4.

14. George McGovern. Letter of transmittal. In: U.S. Senate Final Report of the Select Committee on Nutrition and Human Needs. Washington, DC, December 1977:1.

15. White House Conference on Food, Nutrition, and Health. Final Report. Washington, DC, 1970.

16. Austin JE, Hitt C. Nutrition Intervention in the United States: Cases and Concepts. Cambridge, MA: Ballinger, 1979:331.

17. U.S. Senate. Final Report of the Select Committee on Nutrition and Human Needs. Washington, DC, December 1977:17–20.

18. U.S. Senate Select Committee on Nutrition and Human Needs. Diet Related to Killer Diseases, III. Hearings in Response to Dietary Goals for the United States: Re Meat. Washington, DC, March 24, 1977.

19. Mottern, N. Dietary goals. Food Monitor March/April, 1978:8–10.

20. Truswell AS. Evolution of dietary recommendations, goals, and guidelines. Am J Clin Nutr 1987;45:1060–1072. Also see: Harper AE. Dietary goals—a skeptical view. Am J Clin Nutr 1978,31:310–321.

21. U.S. Senate Select Committee on Nutrition and Human Needs. Dietary Goals for the United States—Supplemental Views. Washington, DC, November 1977:677.

22. Putman JJ, Allshouse JE. Food Consumption, Prices, and Expenditures, 1970–1997. Washington, DC: USDA, 1999:83.

23. U. S. Senate Select Committee on Nutrition and Human Needs. Dietary Goals for the United States, 2nd ed. Washington, DC, December 1977:4.

24. Broad WJ. NIH deals gingerly with diet–disease link. Science 1979;204: 1175–1178.

25. Report of the task force on the evidence relating six dietary factors to the nation's health. Am J Clin Nutr 1979;32:2627–2748.

26. American Heart Association Committee on Nutrition. Diet and coronary heart disease. Circulation 1978;58:762A–765A. Upton AC. Statement on Diet, Nutrition, and Cancer. Hearings of the Subcommittee on Nutrition, Senate Committee on Agriculture, Nutrition, and Forestry, October 2, 1979. Washington, DC, 1979.

27. U.S. Department of Health, Education, and Welfare. Healthy People: the Surgeon General's Report on Health Promotion and Disease Prevention. Washington, DC, 1979:vii. The first public health revolution was the fight against infectious diseases.

28. Monte T. The U.S. finally takes a stand on diet. Nutrition Action September 1979:4.

29. USDA and HEW unveil guidelines for healthy eating. CNI Weekly Report 1980;10(6): 1–2. CNI is the Community Nutrition Institute.

30. Wolf ID, Peterkin BB. Dietary Guidelines: the USDA perspective. Food Technology 1984;38(7):80–86.

31. Science and Education Administration. Food: The Hassle-Free Guide to a Better Diet. Washington, DC: USDA, 1979:3.

32. Foreman CT. Remarks prepared for a press briefing on the release of Ideas for Better Eating Washington, DC: USDA, January 8, 1981. Ms. Foreman, then in her last month in office, stated that USDA had distributed more than 950,000 copies of Food and that another 490,000 had been requested.

33. Food 2: A Dieter's Guide, and Food 3: Eating the Moderate Fat & Cholesterol Way. Chicago: American Dietetic Association, 1982.

34. Greenberg DS. Nutrition: a long wait for a little advice. Science 1980;302: 535–536.

35. USDA and DHHS. Nutrition and Your Health: Dietary Guidelines for Americans. Washington, DC, 1980.

36. Miller SA, Stephenson MG. Scientific and public health rationale for the dietary guidelines for Americans. Am J Clin Nutr 1985;42:739–745.

37. Food and Nutrition Board. Toward Healthful Diets. Washington, DC: National Academy of Sciences, 1980. Brody JE. Experts assail report declaring curb on cholesterol isn't needed. New York Times June 1, 1980:A1. Wade N. Food board's fat report hits fire. Science 1980;209:248–250.

38. Food and Nutrition Board. Diet, Nutrition, and Cancer. Washington, DC: National Academy Press, 1982. U.S. General Accounting Office. National Academy of Sciences' Reports on Diet and Health—Are They Credible and Consistent? Washington, DC, 1984.

39. Mendeloff AI. Appraisal of "Diet, Nutrition, and Cancer." Am J Clin Nutr 1983;37:495–498. Pariza MW. A perspective on diet, nutrition, and cancer. JAMA 1984;251:1455–1458.

40. Maugh TM. Cancer is not inevitable. Science 1982;217:36–37. USDA, HHS disagree on diet-cancer report. CNI Weekly Report 1983;13(22):1.

41. Schwartz R. The big fuss over good food. New York Times April 24, 1983:C15. USDA readies to carve up the Dietary Guidelines. Nutrition Action 1983;10:3–4.

42. USDA and DHHS. Nutrition and Your Health: Dietary Guidelines for Americans, 2nd ed. Washington, DC, 1985.

43. Reagan administration OK's dietary guidelines. CNI Weekly Report September 26, 1985:2.

44. Board on Agriculture. Designing Foods: Animal Product Options in the Marketplace. Washington, DC: National Academy Press, 1988. DHHS. The Surgeon General's Report on Nutrition and Health. Washington, DC, 1988. Food and Nutrition Board. Diet and Health: Implications for Reducing Chronic Disease Risk. Washington, DC: National Academy Press, 1989. James WPT. Healthy Nutrition: Preventing Nutrition-Related Diseases in Europe. Copenhagen: World Health Organization, 1988.

45. USDA and DHHS. Nutrition and Your Health: Dietary Guidelines for Americans, 3rd ed. Washington, DC, 1990.

46. Surgeon General's dietary recommendations support need for health messages on foods (press release). Washington, DC: The National Food Processors Association, July 27, 1988.

47. McGinnis JM, Nestle M. The Surgeon General's Report on Nutrition and Health: policy implications and implementation strategies. Am J Clin Nutr 1989; 49:23–28.

CHAPTER 2. POLITICS VERSUS SCIENCE: OPPOSING THE FOOD PYRAMID, 1991–1992

1. Human Nutrition Information Service. USDA's Eating Right Pyramid. Washington, DC: USDA, March 1991. This version was never released but reporters had been sent prepublication copies of the graphic design and unofficial photocopies of the text page boards.

2. Sugarman C, Gladwell M. U.S. drops new food chart. Washington Post, April 27, 1991: A1,A10.

3. Burros M. U.S. delays issuing nutrition chart. New York Times April 27, 1991:9.

4. Sugarman C. The $855,000 pyramid: revised U.S. food-group chart is released. New York Times April 28, 1992:A1,A4.

5. Broad WJ. Jump in funding feeds research on nutrition. Science 1979;204: 1060.

6. U.S. House of Representatives. Rural Development, Agriculture, and Related Agencies Appropriations Bill, 1989 (Report No. 100-690A). Washington, DC: June 19, 1988:107.

7. Welsh S, Davis C, Shaw A. Development of the food guide pyramid. Nutrition Today 1992;27(6):12. This is the official account by USDA/HNIS staff nutritionists.

8. Zuckerman S. Killing it softly. Nutrition Action January-February, 1984:10.

9. Human Nutrition Information Service. Dietary guidelines for Americans (Home and Garden Bulletins 232-1 to 232-7). Washington, DC, April 1986.

10. Cronin FJ, Shaw AM, Krebs-Smith SM, et al. Developing a food guidance system to implement the Dietary Guidelines. J Nutrition Education 1987;19: 281–302.

11. The source is an unpublished USDA staff memorandum, dated April 16, 1991, which summarizes the history of the Pyramid's development.

12. Burros M. Rethink 4 food groups, doctors tell U.S. New York Times April 10,1991:C1,C4.

13. Todd JS. Keep meat and dairy products in diet. New York Times May 8, 1991:A22. The author is identified as Executive Vice President of the American Medical Association.

14. Crea J. USDA creates pyramid to make nutrition point. Orange County Register April 11, 1991:1,26.

15. Gladwell M. U.S. rethinks, redraws the food groups. Washington Post April 13, 1991:A1. Mr. Gladwell explained the origin of his story to me in a 1993 telephone conversation.

16. A Pyramid topples at the USDA. Consumer Reports October 1991: 663–666.

17. Combs GF. What's Happening at USDA. AIN [American Institute of Nutrition] Nutrition Notes September 1991:6.

18. Burros M. Are cattlemen now guarding the henhouse? New York Times May 8, 1991:C6. Copies of the American Meat Institute letter were circulated widely by fax.

19. FASEB Office of Public Affairs. House hearings on the USDA. AIN [American Institute of Nutrition] Nutrition Notes December 1991:4–5.

20. Toufexis A. Playing politics with our food. Time July 15, 1991:57.

21. Snider M. Kids draw up their own nutrition blueprints. USA Today June 12, 1991:D1,D4.

22. Burros M. Plain talk about eating right. New York Times Magazine Good Health, October 6, 1991:12.

23. Agriculture food chart's ups and downs. New York Times May 15, 1991: A26.

24. Madigan E. Letter to the editor. Time August 5, 1991: 8.

25. Madigan E. Why was debut of Pyramid put off? Roll Call September 12, 1991:16.

26. Burros M. Testing of food Pyramid comes full circle. New York Times March 12, 1992:C1,C4.

27. Bell Associates, Inc. An Evaluation of Dietary Guidance Graphic Alternatives: Draft Final Report. Cambridge, MA: January 6, 1992. Another Draft Final Report is dated March 13, 1992; the Final Report appeared in April 1992.

28. Pyramid decision due; two options remaining. CNI Nutrition Week January 3, 1992:3.

29. Madigan ER. Statement prepared for Washington, DC, press conference on release of the Pyramid. Washington, DC: USDA Office of Public Affairs, April 28, 1992. The $855,000 figure did not include printing costs.

30. Pyramid survives delay; new graphic to become symbol of healthy diet. CNI Nutrition Week May 1, 1992:4.

31. Burros M. U.S. reorganizes nutrition advice: food educators win battle to depict 5 basic groups in a Pyramid design. New York Times April 28, 1992:A14.

32. Human Nutrition Information Service. The Food Guide Pyramid (Home and Garden Bulletin No. 252, Supersedes HG-249). Washington, DC: USDA, August 1992.

33. American Dietetic Association. Nutrition trends survey 1997. Chicago, IL: American Dietetic Association, 1997. Guthrie JF, Derby BM, Levy AS. What people know and do not know about nutrition. In: Frazão E, ed. America's Eating Habits: Changes & Consequences. Washington, DC: USDA, 1999:243–280.

34. Bruce Ingersoll. U.S. picks pyramid to show how to eat. Wall Street J April 28, 1992:B1.

CHAPTER 3. "DECONSTRUCTING" DIETARY ADVICE

1. Willett WC. Eat, Drink, and Be Healthy. New York: Simon & Schuster Source, 2001.

2. Dixon LB, Cronin FJ, Krebs-Smith SM. Let the pyramid guide your food choices: capturing the total diet concept. J Nutrition 2001;131:461s–472s. This paper appears in Krebs-Smith SM, ed. The Dietary Guidelines: Surveillance Issues and Research Needs. J Nutrition 2001;131:437s–562s.

3. Southamstar Network. Industry forced changes to food guide, papers show. Toronto Star (Canada) January 15, 1993:A2.

4. Clay WD. Preparation and use of food-based dietary guidelines. Food Nutrition and Agriculture 1997:19:42–45.

5. National Nutrition Monitoring and Related Research Act of 1990 (Public Law 101-445). Title III—Dietary Guidance October 22, 1990. This law expired at the end of 2000, leaving uncertain the future of five-year reviews of the Dietary Guidelines.

6. Glanz K. Letter to Karil Bialostosky, Dietary Guidelines Executive Secretariat, Re: impact of change in the format of Dietary Guidelines for Americans. Honolulu: University of Hawai'i at Mānoa, March 1, 1995.

7. USDA and DHHS. Nutrition and Your Health: Dietary Guidelines for Americans, 4th ed. Washington, DC, 1995.

8. Dietary guidelines group debates changes for 2000. CNI Nutrition Week October 9, 1998:8,6.

9. France D. Groups debate role of milk in building a better pyramid. New York Times June 29, 1999:F7. The headline writer confused the Pyramid with the Dietary Guidelines.

10. Bertron P, Barnard ND, Mills M. Racial bias in federal nutrition policy, Part I: the public health implications of variations in lactase persistence. Part II: weak guidelines take a disproportionate toll. J National Medical Association 1999;91:151–157, 201–208. The authors review evidence that lactose intolerance is *normal* and that drinking milk does not prevent osteoporosis.

11. Burros M. Diet panel mixes politics and chicken fat. New York Times January 25, 2000:F7.

12. USDA Center for Nutrition Policy and Promotion. Notice of availability of the final report, public meeting, and public comment period. Federal Register 65, February 18, 2000:8333–8334. The 129-page (plus appendices) document could be downloaded from the USDA Web site: **http://www.ars.usda.gov/dgac**. Accessed June 4, 2001. For a later analysis, see: Krebs-Smith SM, ed. The Dietary Guidelines: Surveillance Issues and Research Needs. J Nutrition 2001;131: 437s–562s.

13. Glickman D. Remarks prepared for delivery at the National Nutrition Summit (news release). Washington, DC: USDA, May 30, 2000.

14. Shalala DE. Statement at the National Nutrition Summit (press release). Washington, DC: DHHS, May 30, 2000.

15. Beef provides essential nutrients in healthful diets (press release). Washington, DC: National Cattlemen's Beef Association, May 30, 2000.

16. Sugars' provisions in draft dietary guidelines are wrong: GMA. Food Regulation Weekly March 27, 2000:12–13.

17. Havala S. Deciphering those dietary recommendations—how do you define moderation? Vegetarian J July/August 1992:8–13. The author asked leading nutritionists, journalists, users of dietary guidelines, and consumers what they thought *moderation* meant. Most said something like "reasonable limits" or "avoidance of extremes," but some viewed it as a "smokescreen to make people think that whatever they're eating is OK."

18. Putnam JJ, Allshouse JE. Food Consumption, Prices, and Expenditures, 1970–1997. Washington, DC: USDA, April 1999:83.

19. Scrimshaw NS, Murray EB. The acceptability of milk and milk products in populations with a high prevalence of lactose intolerance. Am J Clin Nutr 1988;48 (suppl):1083–1159. The level of indigestion caused by lactose is controversial. Studies, often funded by the National Dairy Council, show that perceived symptoms do not always correlate with physiological measurements of lactose malabsorption. See Suarez FL, Savaiano D, Arbisi P, Levitt MD. Tolerance to the daily ingestion of two cups of milk by individuals claiming lactose intolerance. Am J Clin Nutr 1997;65:1502–1506.

20. Kushi LH, Lenart EB, Willett WC. Health implications of Mediterranean diets in light of contemporary knowledge. 1. Plant foods and dairy products. Am J Clin Nutr 1995;61:1407s–1415s.

21. Cohen R. Milk: The Deadly Poison. Englewood Cliffs, NJ: Argus Publishing, 1998.

22. National Dairy Council. Guide to Good Eating, 6th ed. Rosemont, IL, 1999.

23. Thompson S. New milk effort promises fame with cap game. Advertising Age April 24, 2000:34.

24. National Fluid Milk Processor Promotion Board and National Dairy Council. Advertisement. New York Times August 3, 1999:F6. The ad quotes medical experts and is signed by a "Calcium Summit Coalition" of about 30 academic and professional societies and institutions. It discloses the dairy industry's sponsorship in small print along the side of the page.

25. Schmitt E. Milk on her lip, a cabinet chief raises eyebrows. New York Times February 3, 1998:A14.

26. Draft U.S. dietary guidelines hit by National Dairy Council. Food Regulation Weekly March 20, 2000:10–11. National Dairy Council commends new dietary guidelines (press release). Rosemont, IL: National Dairy Council, May 30, 2000.

27. Uhlmann M. A sugar debate that's not so sweet. The Inquirer (Philadelphia) April 10, 2000. Online: **http://www.phillynews.com/inquirer/**. Accessed April 10, 2000. The article quoted me: "People should eat less sugar to have a healthy diet . . . the last thing in the world Americans need is more calories."

28. Sacks FM, Svetkey LP, Vollmer WM, et al. Effects on blood pressure of reduced dietary sodium and the Dietary Approaches to Stop Hypertension (DASH) diet. N Engl J Med 2001;344:3–10.

29. MacGregor GA, de Wardener HE. Salt, Diet & Health. Neptune's Poisoned Chalice: the Origins of High Blood Pressure. Cambridge, England: Cambridge University Press, 1998. Godlee F. The food industry fights for salt. British Medical J May 18, 1996:1239–1240. For decidedly different views, see Taubes G. The (political) science of salt. Science 1998;281:898–907, and Dietary sodium and blood pressure (letters). N Engl J Med 2001;344:1716–1719.

30. Press release. Oakville, CA: Robert Mondavi Winery, March 13, 1991.

31. Cates TL. Letter to Patricia Taylor, Director Alcohol Policies Project, Center for Science in the Public Interest. Washington, DC: Department of the Treasury, November 27, 1990. Mr. Cates was chief of the Industry Compliance Division, BATF.

32. Renaud S, De Lorgeril M. Dietary lipids and their relation to ischaemic heart disease: from epidemiology to prevention. J Internal Medicine 1989;225 (suppl 1): 39–46. Renaud S, De Lorgeril M. Wine, alcohol, platelets, and the French paradox for coronary heart disease. Lancet 1992;339:1523–1526.

33. Dodd TH, Morse S. The impact of media stories concerning health issues on food product sales: management planning and responses. J Consumer Marketing 1994;11(2):17–24. Dolan C. Wineries and government clash over ads that

toast health benefits of drinking. Wall Street J October 19, 1992:B1,B8. Bureau of Alcohol, Tobacco and Firearms. Health Claims in the Labeling and Advertising of Alcoholic Beverages. Washington, DC: Department of the Treasury, August 2, 1993.

34. Beringer vineyards drops plan for "health" neckhanger. Food Labeling News November 12, 1992:13,14.

35. CBS "60 Minutes." To your health (transcript). New York: Columbia Broadcasting System, November 5, 1995.

36. Carmichael LA. Comments to the Dietary Guidelines Advisory Committee. San Francisco, January 11, 1995.

37. Burros M. In an about-face, US says alcohol has health benefits. New York Times January 2, 1996:A1,C2.

38. Abramson H. Uncle Sam Never Said Drink for your Health. The Marin Institute for the Prevention of Alcohol and Other Drug Problems, Summer 1996:1–7.

39. Steinhardt L, Hacker G. Vintage Deception: The Wine Institute's Manipulation of Scientific Research to Promote Wine Consumption. Washington, DC: Center for Science in the Public Interest, 1997.

40. Skrzycki C. To your health: vintners poised for more positive labeling. Washington Post July 11, 1997:G1.

41. De Luca JA. Letter to George Hacker and Sara Kayson, Co-Chairs, Coalition for the Prevention of Alcohol Problems, Center for Science in the Public Interest. San Francisco, CA: Wine Institute, August 13, 1997.

42. Thurmond S. Letter to Donna E. Shalala, Secretary DHHS. Washington, DC: U.S. Senate, March 23, 1998.

43. O'Connell V. Labels suggesting the benefits of drinking wine look likely. Wall Street J October 26, 1998:B1,B4.

44. Treasury announces actions concerning labeling of alcoholic beverages (press release). Washington, DC: Department of Treasury, February 5, 1999.

45. U.S. government approves Wine Institute's dietary guidelines label statement (press release). San Francisco, CA: Wine Institute, February 5, 1999.

46. Stout D. Government allows labels about wine's benefits. New York Times February 6, 1999:A13. Massing M. Wine's unfortunate new labels (op-ed). New York Times February 9, 1999.

47. Teinowitz I. Clinton offers legislation on alcohol ad warnings. Advertising Age February 15, 1999:6.

48. Stout D. Bill would bar health referral on wine label. New York Times February 23, 1999:A16.

49. Stout D. Senator's efforts threaten wine makers' celebration. New York Times March 1, 1999:A14. This article quotes me as admitting "how incredibly naïve we were" in thinking that our subcommittee could write dietary guidelines based just on science.

50. Anderson N. The Washington Connection: State delegation uncorks wine politics. Los Angeles Times April 27, 1999. Online: http://www.latimes.com/. Accessed April 28, 1999.

51. Thurmond S. Feds may investigate validity of dietary guidelines: senator is concerned public policy compromised (press release). Washington, DC: U.S. Senate, March 1, 1999.

52. International Food Information Council. Are You Listening? What Consumers Tell Us About Dietary Recommendations. Online: http://ificinfo.health.org/. Accessed November 19, 1999.

PART II WORKING THE SYSTEM

Some of the material in Part II draws on work published previously, used here with permission: Nestle M. Food lobbies, the food pyramid, and U.S. nutrition policy. *International J Health Services* 1993;23:483–496 (courtesy Baywood Publishing Co.). Food lobbies and U.S. dietary guidance policy. In: Kiple KF, Ornelas-Kiple CK, eds. *The Cambridge World History of Food and Nutrition*, Vol II. Cambridge, England: Cambridge University Press, 2000:1628–1643. Food company sponsorship of nutrition research and professional activities. *Public Health Nutrition* 2001;4(October).

CHAPTER 4. INFLUENCING GOVERNMENT: FOOD LOBBIES AND LOBBYISTS

1. For the history of lobbying, see Milbrath LW. The Washington Lobbyists. Chicago, IL: Rand McNally, 1963. Berry JM. The Interest Group Society. Boston MA: Little, Brown, 1984. Browne WP. Private Interests, Public Policy, and American Agriculture. Lawrence, KA: University Press of Kansas, 1988.

2. Madison J. The Federalist No. 10. In: Wills G, ed. Hamilton A, Madison J, Jay J. The Federalist Papers (1787), New York: Bantam, 1982:43,45.

3. Lobbying Disclosure Act of 1995 (Public Law 104-65). 109 Stat. 691, December 19, 1995.

4. Center for Responsive Politics. Influence, Inc: Lobbyists Spending in Washington, 1999 edition. Online: **http://www.opensecrets.org/**. Accessed February 20, 2000.

5. Schmitt E. New lobbying rules, from bagels to caviar. New York Times February 11, 1996:32.

6. Stout D. Tab for Washington lobbying: $1.42 billion. New York Times July 29, 1999:A14.

7. Paarlberg D. American Farm Policy: A Case Study of Centralized Decision-Making. New York: John Wiley, 1964. Kramer J. Agriculture's role in government decisions. In: Gardner BL, Richardson JW, eds. Consensus and Conflict in U.S. Agriculture. College Station, TX: Texas A & M Press, 1979:204–241.

8. Morgan D. Trying to lead the USDA through a thicket of politics. Washington Post July 5, 1978: A8. In 1992, after 27 terms in office, Mr. Whitten stepped down from the Agriculture committee chair as a result of a minor stroke; he did not seek reelection in 1994 and died the following year at the age of 85.

9. Morgan D. "Plain, poor sister" is newly alluring. Washington Post July 4. 1978:A1,A8.

10. Guither HD. The Food Lobbyists: Behind the Scenes of Food and Agripolitics. Lexington, MA: Lexington Books, 1980.

11. See: Congressional Quarterly Service. Legislators and the Lobbyists. Washington, DC, 1965 and 1968. Ridgeway J. The agenda setters: Washington's lobbyists set special interests against the public interest. Village Voice June 16, 1998:55. Abramson J. The business of persuasion thrives in the nation's capital. New York Times September 29, 1998:A1,A22.

12. Jacobson M. Nutrition Scoreboard. New York: Avon Books, 1974:197–198.

13. McGraw M. A case of "very vested interest." Kansas City Star December 10, 1991:A6.

14. Sarasohn J. Ex-USDA Chief Glickman joins Akin Gump. Washington Post February 8, 2001:A21.

15. Storm R. FDA scientist moves to herb industry. HerbalGram48, 2000:13.

16. General Accounting Office. Letter from Acting General Counsel Robert P. Murphy to the Honorables George E. Brown, Jr., David Obey, and Bernard Sanders, Washington, DC, October 19, 1994.

17. Common Cause. The influence of PACs, and soft money laundromat: soft money donors from the agribusiness industry for the 1997–1998 election cycle. Online: **http://www.commoncause.org/**. Accessed February 23, 2000.

18. Center for Public Integrity. Safety Last: The Politics of E. coli and Other Food-Borne Killers. Washington, DC, 1998.

19. Califano JA. Throw the rascals out sooner. New York Times Book Review September 27. 1992:7. Also see: Bowers J. Political Action Committees: Selected References, 1989–1991. Congressional Research Service: Washington, DC, 1991.

20. Public Citizen's Congress Watch. An Ocean of Milk, a Mountain of Cheese, and a Ton of Money: Contributions from the Dairy PAC to Members of Congress. Washington, DC, 1982.

21. Brooks JC, Cameron AC, Carter CA. Political action committee contributions and U.S. congressional voting on sugar legislation. American J Agricultural Economics 1998;80:441–454.

22. Cantor JE. Soft and Hard Money in Contemporary Elections: What Federal Law Does and Does Not Regulate. Washington, DC: Congressional Research Service, January 10, 1997. Online: **http://www.opensecrets.org/parties/**. Accessed February 23, 2000.

23. McCauley M, Cohen A. They Love to Fly . . . and it Shows: An Analysis of Privately-Funded Travel by Members of the U.S. House of Representatives 101st Congress (1989–1990). Washington, D.C., 1991.

24. Lewis C, Center for Public Integrity. The Buying of Congress. New York: Avon Books, 1998.

25. See: Silverstein K. Washington on $10 Million a Day. Monroe, ME: Common Courage Press, 1998. Bartlett DL, Steele JB. Big money and politics: who gets hurt? Time February 7, 2000:38–41.

26. See: Dosal PJ. Doing Business with the Dictators: A Political History of United Fruit in Guatamala, 1899–1944. Wilmington, DE: Scholarly Resources, 1993. When Guatamala attempted to nationalize its fruit plantations in 1954, the company induced the Central Intelligence Agency to organize the removal of that country's president.

27. The Mother Jones 400: Mother Jones' third annual survey of the top 400 political donors. Mother Jones November/December 1998:48–67.

28. Bartlett DL, Steele JB. How to become a top banana. Time February 7, 2000:42–56.

29. DePalma A. Citing European banana quotas, Chiquita says bankruptcy looms. New York Times January 17, 2001:A1,C15. Chiquita sues Europeans, citing banana-quota losses. New York Times January 26, 2001:C5. U.S. and Europeans agree on deal to end banana trade war. New York Times April 12, 2001:C1.

30. General Accounting Office. Sugar Program: Supporting Sugar Prices Has Increased Users' Costs While Benefiting Producers (GAO/RCED-00-126). Washington, DC, June 2000.

31. General Accounting Office. Sugar Program: Changing Domestic and International Conditions Require Program Changes (GAO/RCED-93-84). Washington, DC, April 1993.

32. Ingersoll B. Big sugar seeks bailout, gives money to help get way. Wall Street J April 27, 2000:A28.

33. Wilkinson A. Big Sugar: Seasons in the Cane Fields of Florida. New York: Knopf, 1989.

34. Bartlett DL, Steele JB. Sweet deal: why are these men smiling? The reason is in your sugar bowl. Time November 23, 1998:81–82. For an alternative interpretation, see Pogrebin A. Time on big sugar: a not-so-sweet deal. Brill's Content July/August, 1999:44–45.

35. Office of the Independent Counsel. Referral to the United States House of Representatives pursuant to Title 28, United States Code, § 595 (c), September 9, 1998 ("The Starr Report"). Online: **http://www.nytimes.com/specials/starr/**. Accessed February 24, 2000. The quotations appear in the Narrative, Section III. January–March 1996: Continued Sexual Encounters. D. President's Day (February 19) Break-Up.

CHAPTER 5. CO-OPTING NUTRITION PROFESSIONALS

1. Owen BM, Braeutigam R. The Regulation Game: Strategic Use of the Administrative Process. Cambridge, MA: Ballinger, 1978:7.

2. Rosenthal B, Jacobson M, Bohm M. Feeding at the company trough. Congressional Record August 26, 1976:H8974–H8977. Center for Science in the Public Interest. Integrity in Science. **http://www.cspinet.org/integrity**. Accessed May 16, 2001.

3. Cannon G. The Politics of Food. London: Century Hutchinson, 1987.

4. American Dietetic Association. Online: **http://www.eatright.org/**. Accessed April 13, 2000.

5. Shell ER. The Hippocratic wars. New York Times Magazine June 28, 1998: 34–38.

6. Messina M, Erdman JW. Introduction: Third International Symposium on the Role of Soy in Preventing and Treating Chronic Disease. J Nutrition 2000: 130(suppl):653s–711s.

7. Nestle M, ed. Mediteranean Diets: Science and Policy Implications. Am J Clin Nutr 1995;61(suppl):1313s–1427s.

8. Wazana A. Physicians and the pharmaceutical industry: is a gift ever just a gift? JAMA 2000;283:373–380.

9. Wilde P. Media coverage spurs fad for vitamin pills, after year-long industry effort. Nutrition Week May 22, 1992:1–6. This account describes how the vitamin industry used a Hoffman-LaRoche–sponsored conference at the New York Academy of Medicine to generate favorable media reports on vitamin supplements.

10. Avoid financial "correctness": insistence that authors declare business interests in papers is beside the point (editorial). Nature 1997;385:469.

11. Campbell P, Dhand R. Nature insight: obesity ("produced with support from The Roche Group"). Nature 2000;404:631–677. The section is flanked by advertisements for The Roche Group and includes six papers by various authors, the last by Bray GA & Tartaglia LA on "Medicinal strategies in the treatment of obesity."

12. Blumenthal D, Campbell EG, Causino N, Louis KS. Participation of life-science faculty in research relationships with industry. N Engl J Med 1996;335: 1734–1739.

13. Wadman M. Study discloses financial interests behind papers. Nature 1997;385:376.

14. Stelfox HT, Chua G, O'Rourke K, Detsky AS. Conflict of interest in the debate over calcium-channel antagonists. N Engl J Med 1998;338:101–106. Barnes DE, Bero LA. Why review articles on the health effects of passive smoking reach different conclusions. JAMA 1998;279:1566–1570. Bero LA. Accepting commercial sponsorship: disclosure helps—but is not a panacea. British Medical J 1999;319:653–654.

15. Rausser G. Crowding In Public Good Research: The Case of UC Berkeley's Plant and Microbial Biology Department. Enclosure to letter to author, October 21, 1998. Dr. Rausser is Dean of the College of Natural Resources at UC Berkeley.

16. College of Natural Resources, University of California Berkeley. Online: http://www.nature.berkeley.edu/. Accessed April 18, 2000. Among other interesting items on this Web site, articles point out that Dean Rausser earns more than a million dollars a year from a consulting arrangement that "went public."

17. The critic: Berring R. Is Berkeley off course? The dean's rebuttal: Rausser GC. Fueling the research engine. Both in California Monthly February 1999. Online: http://www.alumni.berkeley.edu/monthly/. Accessed April 18, 2000. The Morrill Act of July 2, 1862 established land-grant colleges: the "leading object shall be . . . to teach such branches of learning as are related to agriculture

and the mechanic arts . . . in order to promote the liberal and practical education of the industrial classes in the several pursuits and professions of life." Online: http://www.nasulgc.org/. Accessed April 19, 2000.

18. MacIlwain C. Berkeley teams up with Novartis in $50m plant genomics deal. Nature 1998;396:5.

19. General Accounting Office. Technology Transfer: Administration of the Bayh-Dole Act by Research Universities (GAO/RCED-98-126). Washington, DC, May 1998.

20. Dalton R. Berkeley dispute festers over biotech deal. Nature 1999;399:5. Press E, Washburn J. The kept university. Atlantic Monthly March 2000:39–54.

21. American Council on Science and Health. About ACSH. Online: http://www.acsh.org. Accessed April 15, 2000.

22. Harnik P. Voodoo Science, Twisted Consumerism: The Golden Assurances of the American Council on Science and Health. Washington, DC: Center for Science in the Public Interest, 1982. The ACSH: forefront of science, or just a front? Consumer Reports May 1994:319.

23. Squires S. Food and choice: Heart Association's plan to endorse certain products is a bold gamble in educating a confused public. Washington Post Health July 5, 1988:9.

24. Parachini A. Food fight: Heart Association plan to label "healthy" foods drawing fire from agencies, nutritionists. Washington Post August 2, 1988: E1,E6.

25. Sugarman C. What price approval? Heart Association's plan raises food firms' pressure. Washington Post August 30, 1989:E1,E4.

26. Benson JS, Acting FDA Commissioner. Letter to Myron L. Weisfeldt, M.D., president of the American Heart Association, January 24, 1990.

27. Burros M. Private food labeling plan opens amid criticism. New York Times February 1, 1990:A1,B8. The statement is attributed to Dr. Jeffrey Blumberg of Tufts University.

28. Angier N. Heart Association cancels its program to rate foods. New York Times April 3, 1990:A1,C6.

29. Kellogg Company. Letter addressed to Dear Health Professional (press release). Battle Creek, MI, February 1997.

30. American Heart Association. Food certification program. Online: http://americanheart.org/. Accessed April 15, 2000.

31. National Action Plan to Improve the American Diet: A Public/Private Partnership. Executive Summary. Washington, DC: Association of State and Territorial Health Officials, 1993.

32. USDA. USDA joins with the Dietary Guidelines Alliance to promote common-sense dietary advice (press release). Washington, DC, March 13, 1997.

33. Dietary Guidelines Alliance. Reaching Consumers with Meaningful Health Messages: A Handbook for Nutrition and Food Communicators. Chicago, IL, 1996.

34. Burros M. Additives in advice on food. New York Times November 15, 1995:C1,C5.

35. American Dietetic Association. Position of the American Dietetic Association: nutrition education for the public. J Am Diet Assoc 1996;96:1183–1187.

36. Gallagher A. Taking a stand on emerging issues. J Am Diet Assoc 2000; 100:410.

37. Kellogg claim for heart benefits challenged by CSPI. Food Regulation Weekly July 3, 2000:10. A court decision in 2001 forced the FDA to approve this claim (see Table 31, Chapter 11).

38. American Dietetic Association. Code of ethics for the profession of dietetics. J Am Diet Assoc 1988;88:1592–1593 and 1999;99:109–113.

39. See: Conflict-of-interest articles by McNutt K and by Rock CL. J Am Diet Assoc 1999;99:29–30,31–32.

40. Tufts University School of Nutrition Science and Policy. Nutrition Navigator (Web site). Online: **http://www.navigator.tufts.edu/**. Accessed February 25, 2000.

41. Jacobson MF. Tufts "Navigator" Web site: misleading advice (press release). Washington, DC: Center for Science in the Public Interest, February 11, 1998.

42. O'Brien P. Dietary shifts and implications for US agriculture. Am J Clin Nutr 1995;61(suppl):1390s–1396s. Subar AF, Heimendinger J, Patterson BH, et al. Fruit and vegetable intake in the United States: the baseline survey of the Five A Day for Better Health program. Am J Health Promotion 1995;9:352–360.

43. National Cancer Institute. 5-A-Day. Online: **http://www.5aday.gov/**. Accessed April 22, 2000. Stables G, Heimendinger J, eds. 5 A Day for Better Health: Monograph. Bethesda, MD: National Cancer Institute, 2001.

44. Potter JD, Finnegan JR, Guinard J-X, et al. 5 A Day for Better Health Program Evaluation Report. Bethesda, MD: National Cancer Institute, 2000.

45. Brody JE. Experts assail report declaring curb on cholesterol isn't needed. New York Times June 1, 1980:A1. Wade N. Food Board's fat report hits fire. Science 1980;209:248–249.

46. Krimsky S, Rothenberg LS. Financial interest and its disclosure in scientific publications. JAMA 1998;280:225–226. Martin JB, Kasper DL. The evolving ties between the university and industry. New Engl J Med 2000;343;1647–1649.

47. British Medical J. Declaration of competing interest: guidance for authors. Online: **http://www.bmj.com/**. Accessed July 17, 1999.

48. Krimsky S, Rothenberg LS, Kyle G, Stott P. Financial interests of authors in scientific journals: a pilot study of 14 publications. Science and Engineering Ethics 1996;2:395–410. Krimsky S, Rothenberg LS. Conflict of interest policies in science and medical journals: editorial practices and author disclosures. Science and Engineering Ethics 2001;7:205–218.

49. Rothman KJ. Conflict of interest: the new McCarthyism in science. JAMA 1993;269:2782–2784.

50. Commercial Sponsorship in the Royal College of Paediatrics and Child Health. London: Royal College of Paediatrics and Child Health, 1999.

51. Kassirer JP. Financial indigestion. JAMA 2000;284:2156–2157.

52. Bero LA. Disclosure policies for gifts from industry to academic faculty (editorial). JAMA 1998;279:1031. American Association of University Professors.

Statement on corporate funding of academic research. Academe May–June 2001: 68–70.

CHAPTER 6. WINNING FRIENDS, DISARMING CRITICS

1. Baquet D, Johnston D. U.S. expanding scope in review of gifts to Agriculture secretary. New York Times August 7, 1994:A1,A24. Johnston D. Agriculture chief quits as scrutiny of conduct grows. New York Times October 4, 1994: A1,A16.

2. Greenhouse L. High court voids theory used to press independent counsel's cases over gifts to Espy. New York Times April 28, 1999:A26.

3. Lewis NA. As trial ends, Espy jury is left with 2 views of defendant: ethically lax or dedicated. New York Times December 1, 1998:A22. The Espy verdict (editorial). New York Times December 3, 1998:A30.

4. Labaton S. Agriculture chief in '93–94 cabinet is indicted by U.S. New York Times August 28, 1997:A1,A26.

5. Executive tells of gifts for ex-Agriculture chief. New York Times September 12, 1996:A17. Lardner G. Mondavi to pay $150,000 in penalties. Washington Post July 22, 1998:A8.

6. Aide to Espy is convicted in lying trial. New York Times December 2, 1997: A20.

7. Did the devil make him do it? (Talk of the Town). The New Yorker October 17, 1994:45.

8. Mr. Espy resigns (editorial). New York Times October 4, 1994:A20.

9. Burros M. Agriculture Dept. scraps poultry bacteria plan. New York Times October 27, 1994:A20.

10. Van Natta D, Lacey M. Access proved vital in last-minute race for Clinton pardons. New York Times February 25, 2001:A1,A14.

11. Blisard WN, Blaylock JR. Generic Promotion of Agricultural Products. Washington, DC: USDA/ERS, 1989. General Accounting Office. Agricultural Marketing: Comparative Analysis of U.S. and Foreign Promotion and Research Programs (GAO/RCED-95-171). Washington, DC, April 1995.

12. Cloud DS. When Madison Avenue talks, farm-belt members listen. Congressional Quarterly November 11, 1989: 3047–3051.

13. Blisard N, Blayney D, Chandran R, Allshouse J. Analyses of Generic Dairy Advertising, 1984–1997. Washington, DC: USDA/ERS, 1999.

14. Felsenthal E. Should government market pork and peaches? Wall Street J November 26, 1996:B1,B10.

15. Greenhouse L. Agricultural marketing effort is ruled constitutional. New York Times June 26, 1997:D25.

16. Becker E. Unpopular fee makes activists of hog farmers. New York Times June 11, 2001:A1,A15.

17. Stauber JC, Rampton S. Toxic Sludge Is Good for You: Lies, Damn Lies and the Public Relations Industry. Monroe, ME: Common Courage Press, 1995.

18. Howard C, Howard F, Lawrence R, et al. Office prenatal advertising and its effect on breast-feeding patterns. Obstetrics & Gynecology 2000;95:296–303.

19. Cone TE. History of infant and child feeding: from the earliest years through the development of scientific concepts. In: Bond JT, Filer LJ, Leveille GA, et al., eds. Infant and Child Feeding. New York: Academic Press, 1981:4–34. Apple RD. Mothers and Medicine: A Social History of Infant Feeding, 1890–1950. Madison, WI: University of Wisconsin Press, 1987.

20. Williams CD. Milk and murder. In: Baumslag N, ed. Primary Health Care Pioneer: The Selected Works of Dr. Cicely D. Williams. Geneva: World Federation of Public Health Associations and UNICEF, 1986.

21. Baumslag N, Michels DL. Milk, Money, and Madness: The Culture and Politics of Breastfeeding. Westport, CN: Bergin & Garvey, 1995.

22. Jelliffe DB. Commerciogenic malnutrition? Food Technology February 1971:55–56.

23. Muller M. The Baby Killer: a War on Want Investigation into the Promotion and Sale of Powdered Baby Milks in the Third World. London: War on Want, 1974.

24. Chetley A. The Politics of Baby Foods: Successful Challenges to an International Marketing Strategy. New York: St. Martin's Press, 1986. Sethi SP. Multinational Corporations and the Impact of Public Advocacy on Corporate Strategy: Nestlé and the Infant Formula Controversy. Boston: Kluwer Academic Publishers, 1994. See also: INFACT. Online: http://www.infact.org/ Accessed June 4, 2001.

25. Van Esterik P. Beyond the Breast–Bottle Controversy. New Brunswick, NJ: Rutgers University Press, 1989; and The politics of breastfeeding: an advocacy perspective. In: Stuart-Macadam P, Dettwyler KA, eds. Breastfeeding: Biocultural Perspectives. New York: Aldine de Gruyter, 1995:145–165.

26. Subcommittee on Health and Scientific Research of the Committee on Human Resources, United States Senate. Marketing and Promotion of Infant Formula in the Developing Nations, 1978. 95th Congress, Second Session, May 23, 1978. Washington, DC, 1978:127–128. On pp. 608–619, the producer, Peter Krieg, describes Nestlé's attempt to discredit the film, Bottle Babies, which he filmed in Kenya in 1975.

27. Ciocca HG, Assistant Secretary, Nestlé, Inc. Letter addressed to "Dear Friend," White Plains, NY, December 18, 1978.

28. The Nestlé Company, Inc. The Infant Formula Controversy: A Nestlé View. New York: White Plains, November 1978.

29. World Health Assembly. International Code of Marketing of Breast-Milk Substitutes. Geneva: WHO, 21 May 1981. Shubber S. The International Code of Marketing of Breast-Milk Substitutes: An International Measure to Protect and Promote Breast-Feeding. The Hague: Kluwer Law International, 1998.

30. Richter J. Engineering of Consent: Uncovering Corporate PR (Briefing 6). Sturminster Newton: The Corner House, March 1998.

31. Dobbing J, ed. Infant Feeding: Anatomy of a Controversy 1973–1984. London: Springer-Verlag, 1988.

32. Sethi SP. Multinational Corporations and the Impact of Public Advocacy on Corporate Strategy: Nestlé and the Infant Formula Controversy. Boston: Kluwer Academic Publishers, 1994.

33. Meier B. Battle for baby formula market: Pediatric Academy named in lawsuits. New York Times June 15, 1993:D1,D17. Water R. Nestlé loses infant formula suit. Financial Times (London), June 21, 1995:32.

34. Cracking the Code: Monitoring the International Code of Marketing of Breast-Milk Substitutes. London: Interagency Group on Breastfeeding Monitoring, January 1997.

35. Breaking the Rules, Stretching the Rules. Penang (Malasia): International Baby Food Action Network, 1998.

36. Heinrich J. International Congress of Nutrition: formula for sponsors. The Gazette (Montreal) July 30, 1997:A5.

37. The Network. Feeding Fiasco: Pushing Commercial Infant Foods in Pakistan. Islamabad: Association for Rational Use of Medication in Pakistan, 1998.

38. De Cock KM, Fowler MG, Mercier E, et al. Prevention of mother-to-child HIV transmission in resource-poor countries. JAMA 2000;283:1175–1182.

39. Miotti PG, Taha TET, Kumwenda NI, et al. HIV transmission through breastfeeding: a study in Malawi JAMA 1999;282:744–749. Coutsoudis A, Pillay K, Spooner E, et al. Influence of infant-feeding patterns on early mother-to-child transmission of HIV-1 in Durban, South Africa: a prospective cohort study. Lancet 1999;354:442–443. Nduati R, John G, Mbori-Ngacha D, et al. Effect of breastfeeding and formula feeding on transmission of HIV-1. JAMA 2000;283:1167–1174.

40. WHO Collaborative Study Team. Effect of breastfeeding on infant and child mortality due to infectious diseases in less developed countries: a pooled analysis. Lancet 2000;355:451–455.

41. Chetley A. Infant feeding row. Lancet 1994;343:1030–1031.

42. Meier B. In war against AIDS, battle over baby formula re-ignites. New York Times June 8, 1997:1,16. Gottlieb S. UN amends policy on breast feeding. British Medical J 1998;317:297. Latham MC, Preble EA. Appropriate feeding methods for infants of HIV infected mothers in sub-Saharan Africa. British Medical J 2000;320:1656–1660.

43. Bellamy C. Unicef and baby food manufacturers (letter). British Medical J 2000;321:960.

44. Freedman AM, Stecklow S. As Unicef battles baby-food makers, African infants sicken and die. Wall Street J December 5, 2000:A1,A18. Formula for disaster. Wall Street J Europe, December 6, 2000.

45. Nduati R, Richardson BA, John G, et al. Effect of breastfeeding on mortality among HIV-1 infected women: a randomized trial. Lancet 2001;357:1651–1655. Newell M-L. Does breastfeeding really affect mortality among HIV-1 infected women? Lancet 2001;357:1634–1635.

46. Fawzi WW, Hunter DJ. Vitamins in HIV disease progression and vertical transmission. Epidemiology 1998;9:457–466. Coutsoudis A, Pillay K, Kuhn L, Coovadia HM. Randomized trial testing the effect of vitamin A supplementation

on pregnancy outcomes and early mother-to-child HIV-1 transmission in Durban, South Africa. AIDS 1999;13:1517–1524.

CHAPTER 7. PLAYING HARDBALL: LEGAL AND NOT

1. Greenpeace (London). What's wrong with McDonald's? The out-of-print original factsheet—subject of the libel action, 1986. Online: **http://www.mcspot light.org/**. Accessed March 10, 2000. This Web site provides a chronology of the McLibel trial with clickable links to relevant documents on both sides of the case, trial transcripts, witness lists, news accounts, and photographs.

2. Vidal J. McLibel: Burger Culture on Trial. New York: New Press, 1997. Mr. Vidal covered the trial for the London Guardian.

3. Guttenplan DD. McJustice in Britain. The Nation July 14, 1997:6–7.

4. Lyall S. Golden arches are victorious, but bloodied, in a British Court. New York Times June 20, 1997:A1,A9.

5. Bogus CT. Ronald McDonald is a bully (book review). The Nation November 24, 1997:31–32.

6. Kuczynski A. Winfrey breaks new ground with magazine. New York Times April 3, 2000:C1,C15.

7. Intolerable Risk: Pesticides in Our Children's Food. New York: Natural Resources Defense Council, February 27, 1989. The chemical name for Alar is daminozide. It breaks down to form the carcinogen "unsymmetrical dimethylhydrazine" (UDMH).

8. Sugarman C. The alarm over Alar: what's a consumer to do about apples? Washington Post March 8, 1989:E1,E14.

9. Dowd M. "I'm President," so no more broccoli! New York Times March 23, 1990:A14.

10. Vegetable-rights bill vetoed. New York Times May 1, 1991:A16.

11. Goetz T. After the Oprah crash. Village Voice April 29, 1997:39–41.

12. Guebert A. Who's Paul Engler and why's he still suing Oprah? Illinois Agrinews May 15, 1998:A5.

13. Overdone beef (editorial). Boston Globe January 24, 1998:A14. Oldenburg A. Supporters contend they're Oprah's fans, not followers. USA Today January 20, 1998:1A,2A.

14. Oprah Winfrey makes debut as star witness. New York Times February 24, 1998:A10.

15. Verhovek SH. Turf was cattlemen's, but jury was Winfrey's: TV host calls verdict free-speech victory. New York Times February 27, 1998:A10.

16. Attorney, expert clash in "Oprah" show. Illinois Agrinews February 6, 1998:A1,A11. Also see: Rampton S, Stauber J. Shut up and eat: the lessons of the Oprah trial. The Nation February 16, 1998:10.

17. Stein N. Banana peel. Columbia Journalism Review September/October, 1998:46–51. The article at issue is Gallagher M, McWhirter C. Chiquita secrets revealed: hidden control crucial to overseas empire. Cincinnati Enquirer May 3, 1998:s1–s18.

18. See: An apology to Chiquita. Cincinnati Enquirer June 28, 1998:A1. Associated Press. Judge got contributions from Chiquita execs, special prosecutor. Cincinnati Enquirer July 10, 1998. Online: **http://www.enquirer.com/**. Accessed February 4, 2000.

19. Frantz D. Word of honor: for a reporter and a source, echoes of a broken promise. New York Times April 11, 1999:D3. Cotts C. Bananarama. Village Voice May 4, 1999:32.

20. Pear R. FTC studying infant formula in price inquiry. New York Times December 31, 1990:A1,A30.

21. Burton TM. Legal beat: Abbott agrees to pay $32.5 million to settle infant-formula case. Wall Street J May 28, 1996:A25.

22. Nobel BP. Price fixing and other charges roil a once-placid market. New York Times July 28, 1991:F5. WIC is the Special Supplemental Program for Women, Infants, and Children.

23. Meier B. What prompted investigations into pricing of baby formula. New York Times January 19, 1991:A54.

24. Eichenwald K. Former Archer Daniels executives are found guilty of price fixing. New York Times September 18, 1998:A1,C2. Top Archer Daniels Midland executive steps down (January 26, 1999:C2). Videotapes take star role at Archer Daniels trial (August 4, 1998:C1,C8). Three sentenced in Archer Daniels Midland case (July 10, 1999:C1,C14). The Informant: A True Story. New York: Broadway Books, 2000.

25. Barboza D. Archer Daniels executive said to tell of price fixing talks with Cargill counterpart. New York Times June 17, 1999:C6. Tearing down the facade of "Vitamins Inc." (October 10, 1999:C1,C11).

26. Andrews EL. Roche officers say scandal is a surprise. New York Times May 22, 1999:C1,C5.

27. Barboza D. Six big vitamin makers are said to agree to pay $1.1 billion to settle pricing lawsuit. New York Times September 8, 1999:C2. Fried JP. New York state to get $25 million in vitamin antitrust case. New York Times October 11, 2000:C6.

28. Sproul MF. Vitamin C (for conspiracy) does no harm. Wall Street J September 15, 1999:A32.

29. Mokhiber R. Top 100 criminals of the decade. Online: **http://www. corporatepredators.org/**. Accessed December 26, 2000. Also see: Labaton S. The world gets tough on price fixers. New York Times June 3, 2001:BU1,BU7.

30. Milbrath LW. The Washington Lobbyists. Chicago, IL: Rand McNally, 1963.

31. Lewis C, The Center for Public Integrity. The Buying of Congress. New York: Avon Books, 1998. Kluger R. Ashes to Ashes: America's Hundred-Year Cigarette War, the Public Health, and the Unabashed Triumph of Philip Morris. New York: Alfred A. Knopf, 1996.

32. Jacobson M. Nutrition Scoreboard. New York: Avon Books, 1974: 197–198.

PART III. EXPLOITING KIDS/CORRUPTING SCHOOLS

Portions of Part III appeared previously as Nestle M. Soft drink "pouring rights": marketing empty calories. Public Health Reports 2000;115:308–319 (With permission of Oxford University Press)

1. DHHS. Healthy People 2010: Understanding and Improving Health. Washington, DC, 2000. Online: **http://www.health.gov/healthypeople**. Accessed June 13, 2001.

2. Andrew M, Nord M, Bickel G, Carlson S. Household Food Security in the United States, 1999. Washington, DC: USDA/ERS, 2000. Online: **http://www.ers.usda.gov**. Accessed June 13, 2001.

CHAPTER 8. STARTING EARLY: UNDERAGE CONSUMERS

1. Troiano RP, Flegal KM, Kuczmarski RJ, et al. Overweight prevalence and trends for children and adolescents. Archives of Pediatric and Adolescent Medicine 1995;149:1085–1091.

2. Muñoz KA, Krebs-Smith SM, Ballard-Barbash R, Cleveland LE. Food intakes of US children and adolescents compared with recommendations. Pediatrics 1997;100:323–329.

3. Marquis J. Eating habits put teens at risk, study says. Los Angeles Times September 26, 2000:A1,A16.

4. Cavadini C, Siega-Riz AM, Popkin BM. US adolescent food intake trends from 1965 to 1996. Archives of Disease in Childhood 2000;83:18–24. Lin B-H, Guthrie J, Frazão E. Quality of children's diets at and away from home: 1994–1996. FoodReview January–April 1999:1-10.

5. McNeal JU. The Kids Market: Myths and Realities. Ithaca, NY: Paramount Publishing, 1999.

6. McNeal JU. Kids as Customers: A Handbook of Marketing to Children. New York: Lexington Books, 1992. Stipp H. New ways to reach children. Am Demographics 1993;15:51–56.

7. McNeal JU. Children as Consumers. Austin: University of Texas Bureau of Business Research, 1964.

8. Hays CL. Advertising: Campbell Soup hopes a new campaign aimed at children will help bolster sagging sales. New York Times May 20, 1998:D6. Also see: Hays CL. Bridging a "Generation Next" Gap. New York Times January 31, 1999:C2.

9. Kramer L. McD's tweaks "tween" marketing campaign. Advertising Age February 8, 1999:4,73.

10. Lauro PW. Coaxing the smile that sells. New York Times November 1, 1999:C1,C20.

11. Stanbrook L. The politics of advertising to children. In: Smith G, ed. Children's Food: Marketing and Innovation. London: Blackie Academic & Professional, 1997:94–118.

12. Barwise TP. How much does food and drink advertising influence children's diet? In: Smith G, ed. Children's Food: Marketing and Innovation. London: Blackie Academic & Professional, 1997:126–151.

13. Teinowitz I. Nader's commercial alert fires first at telemarketing. Advertising Age September 21, 1998:44.

14. Hays CL. Advertising: a call for restrictions on psychological research by advertisers into products for children. New York Times October 22, 1999:C6.

15. Fox G. Harvesting Minds: How TV Commercials Control Kids. Westport, CN: Praeger, 1996.

16. Jackson C, Peifer M. The cola wars: does the media influence your choice of cola and can you taste the difference between different brands? Science fair project, St. Ignatius elementary school, Portland, Oregon, May 25, 1999. The project won first prize. Quoted with permission.

17. American Academy of Pediatrics. Children, adolescents, and television. Pediatrics 1990;85:1119–1120.

18. Mifflin L. A growth spurt is transforming TV for children. New York Times April 19, 1999:A1,A21. Diaz A-CP. Kids use media nearly 40 hours a week: study. Advertising Age November 29, 1999:28.

19. Center for Science in the Public Interest. Survey of advertising on children's TV, press release, July 1, 1992.

20. Cotugna N. TV ads on Saturday morning children's programming—what's new? J Nutrition Education 1988;20:125–127. Kotz K, Story M. Food advertisements during children's Saturday morning television programming: are they consistent with dietary recommendations? J Am Diet Assoc 1994;94:1296–1300.

21. Clancy-Hepburn K, Hickey AA, Nevill G. Children's behavior responses to TV food advertisements. J Nutrition Education 1974;6:93–96. Taras HL, Sallis JF, Patterson TL, et al. Television's influence on children's diet and physical activity. J Developmental and Behavioral Pediatrics 1989;10:176–180.

22. Dietz WH, Gortmaker SL. Do we fatten our children at the television set? Obesity and television viewing in children and adolescents. Pediatrics 1985;75:807–812. Dietz WH, Strasburger VC. Children, adolescents, and television. Current Problems in Pediatrics 1991;21:8–31.

23. Goldsmith MF. Youngsters dialing up cholesterol levels? JAMA 1990;263:2976.

24. Grube JW, Wallack L. Television beer advertising and drinking knowledge, beliefs, and intentions among schoolchildren. Am J Public Health 1994;84:254–259.

25. Rajecki DW, McTavish DG, Rasmussen JL, et al. Violence, conflict, trickery, and other story themes in TV ads for food for children. J Applied Social Psychology 1994;24:1685–1700.

26. Fabricant G. The young and restless audience. New York Times April 8, 1996:D1,D8.

27. Thompson S. Cereal makers entice online kids. Advertising Age July 3, 2000:20,22.

28. Kirkpatrick DD. Snack foods become stars of books for children. New York Times September 22, 2000:A1,C17.

29. The Oreo Cookie Counting Book. New York: Little Simon, 2000. The other book is McGrath BB. Kellogg's Froot Loops! Counting Fun Book. New York: HarperFestival, 2000. Both books were priced at $5.99 in early 2001.

30. Oreo. ABCs of marketing to kids. Parsippany, NJ: Nabisco, 1998.

31. General Accounting Office. Public Education: Commercial Activities in Schools (GAO/HEHS-00-156). Washington, DC, September 2000.

32. Stead D. Corporations, classrooms and commercialism: some say business has gone too far. New York Times Education Life January 5, 1997:30–47.

33. Wynns J. Yes: selling students to advertisers sends the wrong message in the classroom. Advertising Age June 7, 1999:26. The author is identified as commissioner of the San Francisco Unified School District Board of Education. A companion piece, by J. Kane, is entitled "No: Ad dollars can provide needed funds to buy computers and train teachers."

34. Hoynes W. News for a captive audience: an analysis of Channel One. Extra! May/June 1997: 11–17.

35. Miller MC. How to be stupid: the lessons of Channel One. Extra! May/June 1997:18–23. Sawicky MB, Molnar A. The hidden costs of Channel One: estimates for the fifty states. Milwaukee, WI: University of Wisconsin, Center for the Analysis of Commercialism in Education, April 1, 1998.

36. Hays CL. Channel One's mixed grades in schools. New York Times December 5, 1999:C1,C14,C15.

37. Jacobson M, Maxwell B. Corporations invade the classroom: have schools become the last great marketing frontier? Rethinking Schools 1994;9(2):3,24. Molnar A. Giving Kids the Business: The Commercialization of America's Schools. Boulder, CO: Westview Press, 1996.

38. Consumers Union. Captive Kids: Commercial Pressures on Kids at School. Yonkers, NY: Consumers Union Educational Services, 1995.

39. Levine J, Gussow JD. Nutrition professionals' knowledge of and attitudes toward the food industry's education and marketing programs in elementary schools. J Am Diet Assoc 1999;99:973–976.

40. Farber PJ. Schools for sale. Advertising Age October 25, 1999:22–26. Manning S. Students for sale: how corporations are buying their way into America's classrooms. The Nation September 27, 1999:11-18. New outcry raised against Channel One. New York Times June 11, 2001:C13.

41. Poppendieck J. Breadlines Knee-Deep in Wheat: Food Assistance in the Great Depression. New Brunswick, NJ: Rutgers University Press, 1986.

42. Oliveira V. Decline in nutrition assistance expenditures continued in 1999. FoodReview 2000;23(2):35–43.

43. Citizens' Commission on School Nutrition. White Paper on School-Lunch Nutrition. Center for Science in the Public Interest, December 1990. Olson CM. Joint position of Society for Nutrition Education (SNE), the American Dietetic Association (ADA), and American School Food Service Association (ASFSA): school-based nutrition programs and services. J Nutrition Education 1995;27: 58–61.

44. USDA. National school lunch program and school breakfast program: nutrition objectives for school meals; proposed rule. Federal Register 59: 30218–30251, June 10, 1994.

45. USDA. School meals initiative for healthy children. Alexandria, VA, June 1994. For recent information, see: http://www.usda.gov/. Accessed June 12, 1999.

46. US General Accounting Office. School Lunch Program: Role and Impacts of Private Food Service Companies (GAO/RCED-96-217). Washington, DC, August 1996.

47. Price C, Kuhn B. Public and private efforts for the National School Lunch Program. FoodReview 1996;19(2):51–57.

48. Morse D. School cafeterias are enrolling fast-food franchisees. Wall Street J July 28, 1998:B2.

49. Lee L. School's back, and so are the marketers. Wall Street J September 15, 1997:B1,B6.

50. Sheraton M. School lunch utopia: no impossible dream. New York Times May 20, 1976:C32. Burros M. A school turns "yucks" into "yums" for new foods. New York Times May 4, 1994:C4.

CHAPTER 9. PUSHING SOFT DRINKS: "POURING RIGHTS"

1. Jacobson MF. Liquid Candy: How Soft Drinks are Harming America's Health. Washington, DC: Center for Science in the Public Interest, 1998.

2. Ellison RC, Singer MR, Moore LL, et al. Current caffeine intake of young children: amount and sources. J Am Diet Assoc 1995;95:802–804. Barboza D. More hip, higher hop: caffeinated drinks catering to excitable boys and girls. New York Times August 22, 1997:D1,D5.

3. Daft L, Arcos A, Hallawell A, et al. School Food Purchase Study: Final Report. Washington, DC: USDA, October 1998.

4. Morton JF, Guthrie JF. Changes in children's total fat intakes and their food group sources of fat, 1989–1991 versus 1994–1995: implications for diet quality. Family Economics Nutrition Review 1998;11(3):44–57.

5. Wilson JWS, Enns CW, Goldman JD, et al. Data tables: combined results from USDA's 1994 and 1995 Continuing Survey of Food Intakes by Individuals and 1994 and 1995 Diet and Health Knowledge Survey, June 1997. Online: http://www.barc.usda.gov/bhnrc/foodsurvey/. Accessed July 12, 2000.

6. Harnack L, Stang J, Story M. Soft drink consumption among U.S. children and adolescents: nutritional consequences. J Am Diet Assoc 1999;99:436–441.

7. Ludwig DS, Peterson KE, Gortmaker SL. Relation between consumption of sugar-sweetened drinks and childhood obesity: a prospective, observational analysis. Lancet 2001;357:505–508.

8. Ismail AI, Burt BA, Eklund SA. The cariogenicity of soft drinks in the United States. J Am Dental Association 1984;109:241–245. Minnesota Dental Association. Sip all day, get decay. Online: http://www.mndental.org. Accessed June 17, 2001. St. Paul, MN: 2000. Wyshak G. Teenaged girls, carbonated

beverage consumption, and bone fractures. Archives of Pediatrics & Adolescent Medicine 2000;154:610–613.

9. Endicott CR. 100 leading national advertisers, 43rd annual report. Advertising Age September 28, 1998 (suppl):s3–s50. The 45th annual report appeared September 25, 2000:s1–s58. Chura H. Pepsi plans biggest-ever urban push. Advertising Age April 9, 2001:1,38.

10. The biggest change in the American diet in the '90s? . . . would you believe soft drinks! Yahoo Finance March 2, 1998. Online: **http://biz.yahoo.com/**. Accessed March 3, 1998. The fastest-growing foods were soft drinks, presweetened cereals, bagels, toaster pastries, and pizza, in that order.

11. Coca-Cola Company. Online: **http://www.cocacola.com/**. Accessed February 3, 1999.

12. Diet Pepsi, 100% uh huh. On the Fridge. Washington Post August 4, 1993:C2. The bottles are manufactured by the Munchkin Bottling Co, Los Angeles, CA.

13. Siener K, Rothman D, Farrar J. Soft drink logos on baby bottles: do they influence what is fed to children? J Dentistry for Children 1997;64:55–60.

14. Hays CL. Bridging a "generation next" gap. New York Times January 31, 1999:C2.

15. General Accounting Office. Public Education: Commercial Activities in Schools (GAO/HEHS-00-156). Washington, DC: September, 2000. Also see: Gross D. Pepsi-State. University Business March/April 1998:35–40.

16. Hays CL. Today's lesson: soda rights: consultant helps schools sell themselves to vendors. New York Times May 21, 1999:C1,C9.

17. Cherkassky I. Getting the exclusive. Beverage World October 1998: 97–101.

18. The Center for Commercial-Free Public Education, 1714 Franklin Street, #100-306, Oakland CA 94612 (Online: **www.commercialfree.org**).

19. Hays CL. Be true to your cola, rah! rah! Battle for soft-drink loyalties moves to public schools. New York Times March 10,1998:D1,D4.

20. North Syracuse Central School District. Agreement with the Coca-Cola Bottling Company of New York, Inc., July 1, 1998.

21. Nolan M. Public to have say on cola deal. Post Standard (Syracuse, NY), December 14, 1998:B1. Cermak M. Coke, school district ink deal. Times Union (Albany, NY), June 3, 1999.

22. Bushey J. District 11's Coke problem. Harper's Magazine February 1999:26–27.

23. Zorn RL. The great cola wars: how one district profits from the competition for vending machines. Am School Board J February, 1999:31–33.

24. Kaufman M. Pop culture: health advocates sound alarm as schools strike deals with Coke and Pepsi. Washington Post Health March 23, 1999:12,15, 16,19.

25. Wiley HW. 1001 Tests of Foods, Beverages and Toilet Accessories Good and Otherwise: Why They Are So. New York: Hearst's International Library, 1914:19.

26. National Soft Drink Association, Appellant, v. J.R. Block, Secretary, Department of Agriculture, et al. 721 F. 2d 1348 (U.S. Court of Appeals, D.C. Circuit. 1983). The judge's opinion contains a pithy summary of the history prior to 1983.

27. Legislative history, Public Law 91-248. School lunch program—expansion. House report No. 91-81, March 17, 1969. U.S. Code Congressional and Administrative News, 1970:3014.

28. School Lunch Program—Expansion. Public Law 91-248, 84 Stat. 214, May 14, 1970. USDA.

29. Legislative history, Public Law 95-166 (National School Lunch Act . . . of 1977). U.S. Code Congressional and Administrative News, 1977:3573.

30. USDA. National School Lunch Program and School Breakfast Program. Proposed rule. Federal Register 44:40004–40014, July 6, 1979. Also see: Final rule. Federal Register 45:6758–6772, January 29, 1980.

31. USDA. National School Lunch Program and School Breakfast Program: Competitive Foods. Final rule. Federal Register 50:20545–20547, May 17, 1985. Also see: Code of Federal Regulations. USDA 7 CFR § 210 et seq., January 1, 1986.

32. Pear R. Senator, promoting student nutrition, battles Coca-Cola. New York Times April 26, 1994:A20.

33. U.S. Senate. Report 103-300. Better Nutrition and Health for Children Act of 1994. 103rd Congress, 2nd Session. July 1, 1994.

34. Pear R. Soda industry tries to avert a school ban. New York Times May 17, 1994:A15.

35. Legislative history, Senate Report 103-300, § 203. Competitive foods of minimal nutritional value. U.S. Code Congressional and Administrative News, 1994:3718. Also see: Healthy Meals for Healthy Americans Act of 1994. Public Law 103-448 § 203, 108 Stat. 4699 and 4738.

36. USDA. National School Lunch Program and School Breakfast Program: School Meals Initiative for Healthy Children: Final Rule. Federal Register 60:31187–31222, June 13, 1995. Quotation: p. 31203.

37. New York State Education Law. Sale of certain sweetened food in schools—prohibition. Chapter 674, § 915. August 6, 1987.

38. Lawmakers are ready to enlist in the Cola wars. Nutrition Week May 14, 1999:6. Senator Leahy introduced the Better Nutrition for School Children Act of 1999 (106th Congress, 1st Session).

39. Story M, Hayes M, Kalina B. Availability of foods in high schools: is there cause for concern? J Am Diet Assoc 1996;96:123–126.

40. General Accounting Office. School lunch program: role and impacts of private food service companies (GAO/RCED-96-217). Washington, DC, August 1996.

41. Fox MK, Crepinsek MK, Connor P, Battaglia M. School Nutrition Dietary Assessment Study-II. Washington, DC: USDA, 2001.

42. Community Food Resource Center. Nonprofit group sues board of education for illegally selling non-nutritious foods (press release). New York, April 22, 1999. The Center is a New York City-based advocacy group for school meal programs; it filed its case, Morales, Jimenez, Silver, et al. v. New York

Board of Education, in the U.S. Eastern District Court, Kings County, April 13, 1999. The press release quoted a letter that I and others signed in support of the suit.

43. Caldwell D, Nestle M, Rogers W. School nutrition services. In: Marx E, Wooley SF, eds. Health Is Academic: A Guide to Coordinated School Health Problems. New York: Teachers College Press, 1998:195–223.

44. USDA. National school lunch program and school breakfast program: nutrition objectives for school meals; proposed rule. Federal Register 59:30218–30251, June 10, 1994.

45. Contento I, Balch GI, Bronner YL, et al. The effectiveness of nutrition education and implications for nutrition education policy, programs, and research: a review of research. IV. Nutrition education for school-aged children. J Nutrition Education 1995;27:298–311. Wildey MB, Pampalone SZ, Pelletier RL, et al. Fat and sugar levels are high in snacks purchased from student stores in middle schools. J Am Diet Assoc 2000;100:319–322.

46. DHHS. Healthy People 2010. Washington, DC, 2000.

47. Flaherty J. With schools the battleground, a new kind of cola war breaks out. New York Times February 3, 1999:B10.

48. It's about money (editorial). The Patent Trader (Northern Westchester, NY), November 25, 1998:A34. Sheehan J. Why I said no to Coca-Cola. Rethinking Schools 1999;14:Winter, 1999. Online: **www.rethinkingschools.org/**. Accessed September 8, 2000.

49. Wood F. Soda deals are too sweet for schools to pass up. Newark Star-Ledger January 3, 1999:3.

50. USDA. Tips for Using the Food Guide Pyramid for Young Children 2 to 6 Years Old (Program Aid 1647). Washington, DC, 1999.

51. Nestle M, Jacobson MF. Halting the obesity epidemic: a public health policy approach. Public Health Reports 2000;115:12–24.

52. USDA. Foods Sold in Competition with USDA School Meal Programs: A Report to Congress. January 12, 2001. Online: **http://www.fns.usda.gov**. Accessed May 11, 2001.

53. Hard line on soft drinks. Nutrition Week April 13, 2001:1-2. Leahy P, et al. The Better Nutrition for School Children Act of 2001, April 6, 2001. Online: **http://thomas.loc.gov** (S. 745, 107th Congress, 1st Session). Accessed June 12, 2001.

54. Lourey B. Minnesota soda pop bill: Where do we go from here? Presentation to the University of Minnesota's Symposium on "Soft Drinks in Schools: Exploring the Issues," June 7, 2001. Representatives of the Minnesota Soft Drink Association attended that meeting (at which I spoke) and distributed a press release notable for its strong defense of pouring rights contracts ("Soft drink companies have had successful local business partnerships with schools for decades," "A sedentary lifestyle is the leading cause of obesity," "Many factors contribute to tooth decay, including the types of foods that are consumed") and its citation of favorable research, much of it funded by the industry.

55. Zernike K. Coke to dilute push in schools for its products. New York Times March 14, 2001:A14. King P. New Coca-Cola marketing pours it on for education. Advertising Age March 26, 2001:20.

56. Wynns J. Yes: selling students to advertisers sends the wrong message in the classroom. Advertising Age June 7, 1999:26.

PART IV. DEREGULATING DIETARY SUPPLEMENTS

Parts of this section are drawn, with permission of the Society for Nutrition Education, from Nestle M. Dietary supplement advertising: a matter of politics, not science. J Nutrition Education 1999;31:278–282.

1. Report of the Commission on Dietary Supplement Labels. Washington, DC: DHHS Office of Disease Prevention and Health Promotion, November 1997.

2. Blendon RJ, DesRoches CM, Benson JM, et al. Americans' views on the use and regulation of dietary supplements. Archives of Internal Medicine 2001; 161:805–810.

CHAPTER 10. SCIENCE VERSUS SUPPLEMENTS: "A GULF OF MUTUAL INCOMPREHENSION"

1. Silverglade B, Jacobson MF, eds. Functional foods—Public Health Boon or 21st Century Quackery? Washington, DC: Center for Science in the Public Interest, 1999. Also see: Schrijver J, Helsing E, Dukes G, Bruce A, eds. Use and Regulation of Vitamin and Mineral Supplements: A Study with Policy Recommendations. Groningen, The Netherlands: Styx Publications, 1993.

2. Balch JF, Balch PA. Prescription for Nutritional Healing, 2nd ed. Garden City Park, NY: Avery Publishing Group, 1997.

3. Physicians' Desk Reference for Herbal Medicines. Montvale, NJ: Medical Economics Company, 1998.

4. Snow CP. Two Cultures and the Scientific Revolution: The Rede Lecture. London, Cambridge University Press, 1959.

5. Dietary Supplement Health and Education Act of 1994 (DSHEA). Public Law 103–417, 103rd Congress, 21 USC 301. Oct 25, 1994.

6. Medical foods are an exception to this rule. They are designed to treat specific medical conditions (such as diabetes) for which health claims can be made.

7. Federal Trade Commission. FTC policy statement regarding advertising substantiation (March 11, 1983). FTC policy on deception (October 14, 1983). FTC guides concerning use of endorsements and testimonials in advertising (May 21, 1975, amended Jan 31, 1980). Online: http://www.ftc.gov/. Accessed March 13, 1999.

8. Federal Trade Commission. Dietary supplements: an advertising guide for industry. Washington, DC, 1998. FDA. Guidance for industry: notification of a health claim or nutrient content claim based on an authoritative statement of a scientific body. Washington, DC, June 11, 1998. Online: www.cfsan.fda.gov. Accessed August 5, 1998. FDA. Regulations on statements made for dietary

supplements concerning the effect of the product on the structure or function of the body; proposed rule. Federal Register 63:23624–23632, April 29, 1998.

9. Nutritional foods industry touts gains stemming from DSHEA. Food Labeling & Nutrition News, September 1995:37.

10. Young JH. American Health Quackery. Princeton, NJ: Princeton University Press, 1992:90–102,165–181.

11. Hutt PB. Government regulation of health claims in food labeling and advertising. Food, Drug and Cosmetic Law J 1986;41:3–73.

12. Apple RD. Vitamania: Vitamins in American Culture. New Brunswick, NJ: Rutgers University Press, 1996.

13. FDA. Foods for special dietary uses. Dietary foods. Federal Register 27:5815–5818, June 20, 1962.

14. FDA. Foods for special dietary uses. Dietary foods. Federal Register 31:8521–8527, June 18, 1966.

15. Boffey PM. Nader's raiders on the FDA: science and scientists "misused." Science 1970;168:349–352. For a compelling account of the FDA's shortcomings in these events, see: Turner JS. The Chemical Feast. Washington, DC: Center for Study of Responsible Law, 1970 (Penguin Books edition, 1976).

16. FDA. Food and food products: definitions, identity, and label statements. Federal Register 38:20702–20750, August 2, 1973. Quotation: p. 20708. For an account of these events, see: Kassel MA. From a history of near misses: the future of dietary supplement regulation. Food and Drug Law J 1994;49:237–269.

17. Public Law 94-278, 94th Congress, April 22, 1976.

18. Gladwell M. Vitamin makers, FDA renewing long battle. Washington Post February 7, 1988:H1,H6.

19. FDA. Vitamin and mineral drug products for over-the-counter human use: establishment of a monograph; notice of proposed rulemaking. Federal Register 44:16126-16201, March 16, 1979.

20. NFPA opens dialogue with FDA on health claims for food labels. Food Chemical News, May 21, 1984:36–37.

21. Brandt supports Kellogg All-Bran cancer education efforts. Food Chemical News November 5, 1984:42.

22. CSPI asks for food industry moratorium on health claims. Food Chemical News November 12, 1984:51–53.

23. Letter to author from Alan Levy, Chief of the Consumer Studies Branch, FDA Center for Food Safety and Applied Nutrition, April 30, 1999.

24. FTC's Crawford lauds Kellogg's All-Bran ad. Food Chemical News December 10, 1984:13–16.

25. Continued FDA–FTC split on food health claims suggested at NFPA meeting. Food Chemical News February 18, 1985:3–7.

26. All-Bran anti-cancer message is not a health claim, Kellogg's Costley says. Food Chemical News May 6, 1985:28–29.

27. Ippolito PM, Mathios AD. Health claims in advertising and labeling. Washington, DC: Federal Trade Commission, August 1989. Levy AS, Stokes RC.

Effects of a health promotion advertising campaign on sales of ready-to-eat cereals. Public Health Reports 1987;102:398–403.

28. Colford SW. Food marketers let health claims simmer. Advertising Age March 19, 1985:12

29. Pear R. Labeling for food to be broadened: F.D.A. to allow industry to put health benefit statements on various products. New York Times August 18, 1985:A29.

30. Hile says FDA is ready to open door a little to health claims. Food Chemical News March 11, 1985:36–40. CRN urges advance warning of health claim problems before FDA action. Food Chemical News April 8, 1985:4–5.

31. CRN asks distinction between nutritional and therapeutic claims. Food Chemical News June 24, 1985:53–56.

32. FDA. Food labeling: public health messages on food labels and labeling. Federal Register 52:28843–28849, August 4, 1987.

33. Sugarman C. Political skirmish over FDA proposal: debate persists on issue of product health claims. Washington Post February 17, 1988:E1,E14.

34. Committee on Public Health. Statement and resolution regarding proposed revision of Food and Drug Administration regulations concerning disease-related health claims on labels. Bulletin of the New York Academy of Medicine 1987;63(3):410–416.

35. Tillotson JE. The controversy over health claims on labels: where will it all end? Food Technology 1988;42(12):106–108.

36. Sugarman C. Update on health-claim labeling. Washington Post December 21, 1988:E14. Also see: Hilts PJ. F.D.A. is preparing new rules to curb food label claims. New York Times October 31, 1989:A1,C18.

37. Hilts PJ. Panel says White House delayed effort to curb food health claims. New York Times November 15, 1990:B14.

38. Hickman BW, Gates GE, Dowdy RP. Nutrition claims in advertising: a study of four women's magazines. J Nutrition Education 1993;25:227–235. The magazines were Better Homes & Gardens, Good Housekeeping, Ladies' Home Journal, and McCall's.

39. Hilts PJ. In reversal, White House backs curbs on health claims for food. New York Times February 9, 1990:A1,A22.

40. Sugarman C. The new chow hounds: states join forces to monitor product claims. Washington Post September 21, 1988:E1,E12. Burros M. Eating well: the "food police" keep busy with health claims. New York Times February 27, 1991:C3. Meier B. Kellogg files slander suit. New York Times April 3, 1991:C4.

CHAPTER 11. MAKING HEALTH CLAIMS LEGAL:
THE SUPPLEMENT INDUSTRY'S WAR WITH THE FDA

1. FDA. Food labeling: health messages and label statements; reproposed rule. Federal Register 55:5176–5192, February 13, 1990. Quotation: p. 5192.

2. Hilts PJ. In reversal, White House backs curbs on health claims for food. New York Times February 9, 1990:A1,A22.

3. FDA failure to develop health claims policy for foods criticized in House report as "kowtowing" to OMB. The Blue Sheet November 21, 1990:10–11. Also see: Hilts PJ. Panel says White House delayed effort to curb food health claims. New York Times November 15, 1990:B14.

4. Kessler DA. The federal regulation of food labeling: promoting foods to prevent disease. New Engl J Med 1989;321:717–722. Noble BP. After years of deregulation, a new push to inform the public. New York Times October 27, 1991:F5.

5. Hilts PJ. U.S. plans to make sweeping changes in labels on food. New York Times March 8, 1990:A1,B8.

6. Sugarman C. In a state over labels: federal proposal raises questions about who will be in charge. Washington Post March 21, 1990:E1,E3.

7. Burros M. U.S. agency seeks uniform labeling: in a reversal, Sullivan says federal standards should pre-empt local laws. New York Times June 28, 1990: A20.

8. FDA racing with Congress on food labeling rules. Nutrition Week June 28, 1990:3.

9. Roufs JB. Review of L-tryptophan and eosinophilia-myalgia syndrome. J Am Diet Assoc 1992;92: 844–850.

10. FDA. Food labeling: general requirements for health claims for food. Federal Register 58:2066–2941, January 6, 1993.

11. Gorman C. The fight over food labels. Time July 15, 1991:53–56.

12. FDA. Food labeling: Reference Daily Intakes and Daily Reference Values; mandatory status of nutrition labeling and nutrient content revision. Federal Register 56:60366–60878, November 27, 1991. Also see: USDA. Nutrition labeling of meat and poultry products. Federal Register 56:60302–60364, November 27, 1991.

13. Sagon C. New labels: more filling, less fluff. The FDA and USDA to issue long-awaited proposals. Washington Post November 6, 1991:E1,E16. Also see: USDA, OMB skirmish over nutrition labeling proposal. Food Chemical News November 4, 1991:27–29.

14. Moratorium on regulations may wreck labeling plans. Nutrition Week January 31, 1992:2–3.

15. Dietary Supplements Task Force: Final Report. Washington, DC: FDA, May 1992.

16. Williams L. F.D.A. steps up effort to control vitamin claims. New York Times August 9, 1992:1,34.

17. Williams L. A correction: no plan to classify high-potency vitamins as drugs. New York Times August 16, 1992:L33. Yes, F.D.A. wants to block sale of vitamins (letters). New York Times September 8, 1992:A18.

18. Yankelovich, Skelly and White/Clancy Shulman. Public attitudes toward the use and regulation of vitamins, minerals, and herbs. Farmingdale, NY: The Nutritional Health Alliance, September 18, 1992.

19. Sinzinger K. Supplements and Sen. Hatch. Washington Post September 22, 1992:E4.

20. Leaflet: "Can we stop the FDA this year? It's now or never." Farmingdale, NY: Nutritional Health Alliance, 1993.

21. Honest food labels? Fat chance. New York Times November 18, 1992: A26. Also see: Burros M. Strict new rules on food labeling are being delayed: a dispute within cabinet. New York Times November 8, 1992:A1,A38. Ingersoll B. Cabinet officials' dispute may allow Clinton to decide food-labeling issue. Wall Street J November 10, 1992:A6.

22. Burros M. U.S., ending dispute, decides what food labels must tell. New York Times December 3, 1992:A1,B13.

23. FDA. Food labeling. General provisions; nutrition labeling; label format; nutrient content claims; health claims . . . final rules. Federal Register 58: 2066–2941, January 6, 1993. Quotation: p. 2503.

24. FDA. Food labeling: nutrient content claims, definition of term: healthy. Final rule. Federal Register 59:24232–24250, May 10, 1994. Proposed rule was at Federal Register 58:2944, January 6, 1993.

25. Burros M. F.D.A. imposing stricter rules on food labels. New York Times May 5, 1994:A20.

26. FDA. Dietary supplements: general requirements for nutrition labeling: proposed rules. Federal Register 58:33690–33751, June 18, 1993.

27. Burros M. F.D.A. is again proposing to regulate vitamins and supplements. New York Times June 15, 1993:A25.

28. FDA proposed rules biased, limit information, CRN charges. Council for Responsible Nutrition News, September 1993:1–2.

29. Weisskopf M. In the vitamin wars, industry marshals an army of citizen protesters. Washington Post September 14, 1993:A7.

30. Nutritional Health Alliance. Campaign '93: health freedom political action guide. Dallas, TX: NHA Action Center, 1993.

31. Nutritional Health Alliance. Fax update: NHA and allies intensify grassroots campaign. Farmingdale, NY, June 17, 1993.

32. Burros M. F.D.A. wins regulation of supplements by default. New York Times December 15, 1993:C4.

33. FDA. Unsubstantiated Claims and Documented Health Hazards in the Dietary Supplement Marketplace. Washington, DC: DHHS, July 1993.

34. Diet supplements attacked by F.D.A. New York Times July 30, 1993:A17. Also see: Nadel MVS. Letter to Senators. FDA regulation of dietary supplements (GAO/HRD-93-28R), July 2, 1993.

35. FDA. Food labeling: health claims and label statements; folate and neural tube defects: proposed rule. Federal Register 58:53254–53297, October 14, 1993.

36. CRN petitions FDA for labeling revisions. Council for Responsible Nutrition News, December 1993:1,10.

37. Hatch OG. Congress versus the Food and Drug Administration: how one government health agency harms the public health. J Public Policy and Marketing, 1994;13(1):151–152.

38. Silverglade B. The vitamin wars—marketing, lobbying, and the consumer. J Public Policy and Marketing 1994;13(1):152–154.

39. Congress passes dietary supplement bill. Council for Responsible Nutrition News, November 1994:1–2, 4–5,9.

40. Gains in the vitamin war (editorial). New York Times October 20, 1994:A26.

41. The Keystone National Policy Dialogue on Food, Nutrition, and Health: Final Report. Keystone, CO, and Washington, DC: The Keystone Center, March 1996.

42. Report of the Commission on Dietary Supplement Labels. Washington, DC: DHHS Office of Disease Prevention and Health Promotion, November 1997.

43. Food and Drug Modernization Act of 1997 (FDAMA), Public Law 105-115 (§303, §304). Online: http://thomas.loc.gov/. Accessed October 8, 1998.

44. General Mills. A whole new way to defend yourself [full-page advertisement]. New York Times July 12, 1999:A7. FDA. Health claim notification for whole grain foods. Washington, DC, July 1999. Online: http://vm.cfsan.fda.gov/. Accessed July 18, 2000.

45. FDA. Guidance for industry: notification of a health claim or nutrient content claim based on an authoritative statement of a scientific body. Washington, DC, June 11, 1998. Online: http://vm.cfsan.fda.gov/. Accessed August 5, 1998.

46. FDA proposes guidelines for nutritional support statements; CRN responds. Council for Responsible Nutrition News, July 1998:9,12. See: FDA. Regulations on statements made for dietary supplements concerning the effect of the product on the structure or function of the body; proposed rule. Federal Register 63:23624–23632, April 29. 1998.

47. FDA. Food labeling: health claims; interim final rules. Federal Register 63:34084–34117, June 22, 1998.

48. Burton D. Dietary supplement health and education act: is the FDA trying to change the intent of Congress? Opening statement. House Committee on Government Reform. March 25, 1999. Online: http://www.house.gov/reform/hearings/. Accessed April 9, 1999.

49. Pearson v. Shalala. DC Circuit Court of Appeals, 164 F 3rd 650. January 15, 1999.

50. Pharmanex Inc. v. Shalala. US District Court, Central Division, Utah. February 16, 1999. An appeals court later overruled this decision and affirmed the FDA's contentions that Cholestin is not tradition red yeast rice, that it contains the drug lovastatin, and that marketing it as a supplement is a ploy to evade laws (U.S. court of Appeals, 10th Circuit, July 21, 2000.) In response, Pharmanex briefly suspended sales but soon reintroduced Cholestin with a new ingredient.

51. FDA. Guidance for industry: significant scientific agreement in the review of health claims for conventional foods and dietary supplements, December 22, 1999. Online: http://vm.cfsan.fda.gov/. Accessed January 20, 2000.

52. FDA health claims' denial is contrary to Pearson: DeFazio. Food Regulation Weekly January 17, 2000:19.

53. Heart researchers voice support for omega-3 fatty acids claim. Food Regulation Weekly January 10, 2000:18–19.

54. Dietary supplements: FDA responds to McIntosh on *Pearson* implementation. Food Regulation Weekly May 22, 2000:7–9.

55. FDA. Regulations on statements made for dietary supplements concerning the effect of the product on the structure or function of the body. Federal Register 65:999–1050, January 6, 2000.

56. FDA cuts new disease definition from structure/function final rule. Food Regulation Weekly January 10:2000:3–4.

57. Stolberg SG. F.D.A. draws fire for a rule on supplements and pregnancy. New York Times February 4, 2000:A16.

58. New supplement rule from FDA eases restrictions on claims. Nutrition Week January 7, 2000:1,2. Later, the FDA corrected an "oversight" and added this statement to the beginning of the claim: "It is known that diets low in saturated fat and cholesterol may reduce the risk of heart disease." See: Food Chemical News March 12, 2001:19–20.

59. FDA. Letter regarding dietary supplement health claim for omega-3 fatty acids and coronary heart disease. Online: **http://vm.cfsan.fda.gov/**. Accessed January 28, 2001.

60. Kessler G. Decision in Pearson v. Thompson. United States District Court for the District of Columbia, May 7, 2001. Tommy Thompson replaced Donna Shalala as DHHS secretary in January 2001 when President George W. Bush took office. Also see: Wallace P. FDA will not appeal Pearson ruling on folic acid health claim. Food Chemical News June 4, 2001:28.

61. Angell M, Kassirer JP. Alternative medicine—the risks of untested and unregulated remedies. N Engl J Med 1998;339:839–841. In an editorial later that year, JAMA said much the same thing: "There is no alternative medicine. There is only scientifically proven, evidence-based medicine supported by solid data or unproven medicine, for which scientific evidence is lacking." See: Fontanarosa PB, Lundberg GD. Alternative medicine meets science. JAMA 1998;280:1618–1619.

62. Unregulated dietary supplements (editorial). New York Times September 19, 1998:A14.

63. Knowles D. Nutritional supplement industry leaders form new alliance for research and education. News release. Sarasota FL: Corporate Alliance for Intergrative Medicine, Inc., September 23, 1998.

64. Wallace P. Industry to counter negative reports on supplements. NNFA members urged to make efforts to protect political gains. Food Chemical News June 11, 2001:23,24.

65. Cordaro J. Cordaro urges industry to seize the future, act today. Council for Responsible Nutrition News, November 1998:2,11.

CHAPTER 12. DEREGULATION AND ITS CONSEQUENCES

1. General Accounting Office. Food Safety: Improvements Needed in Overseeing the Safety of Dietary Supplements and "Functional Foods" (GAO/RCED-00-156). Washington, DC, July 2000. Wallace P. Herbal supplement use up by 269% in three years, study finds. Food Chemical News May 26, 2001:22–23.

2. Dodd TH, Morse S. The impact of media stories concerning health issues on food product sales: management planning and responses. J Consumer Marketing 1994;11(2):17–24. Storlie J, O'Flaherty MJ, Hare K. Food or supplement? Choosing the appropriate regulatory path. Food Technology 1998;52(12):62–69.

3. DHHS. Dietary supplements now labeled with more information. HHS News March 23, 1999. Online: http://vm.cfsan.fda.gov/. Accessed June 3, 1999. Wallace P. GMA threatens FDA with lawsuit unless Pearson is applied to foods. Food Chemical News March 26, 2001:1,24,25.

4. Drug/supplement products have become a top FDA priority. Food Regulation Weekly June 12, 2000:6. Ono Y. Marketers walk thin line, selling food products with medicinal lure. Wall Street J September 23, 1996:B10.

5. Heber D, Yip I, Ashley JM, et al. Cholesterol-lowering effects of a proprietary Chinese red-yeast-rice dietary supplement. Am J Clin Nutr 1999;69: 231–236. The study was funded in part by Pharmanex; the lead investigator was identified as co-chair of the Pharmanex Medical Advisory Board.

6. Stolberg SG. Drug agency moves against an anti-cholesterol product. New York Times May 21, 1998:A17. Also see: Havel RJ. Dietary supplement or drug? The case of Cholestin. Am J Clin Nutr 1999;69:175–176.

7. Report of the Commission on Dietary Supplement Labels. Washington, DC: DHHS Office of Disease Prevention and Health Promotion, 1997.

8. The FDA reports this information on its Web site. Online: http://vm.cfsan. fda.gov/. Accessed April 9, 1999.

9. Wallace P. FDA appears to make headway on dietary supplement resources. Food Chemical News March 26, 2001:16–17. Sharpe R. FDA tries to find right balance on drug approvals. Wall Street J April 29, 1999:A24.

10. Dickinson A. CRN testifies to Congressional committee about DSHEA implementation. Council for Responsible Nutrition News, March/April 1999:6,12 (see note 35).

11. Grady D. Vitamin O products are fraud, agency says. New York Times March 18, 1999:A20. Federal Trade Commission. "Operation Cure.All" wages new battle in ongoing war against Internet health fraud (press release). Washington, DC, June 14, 2001. Online: http://www.ftc.gov/. Accessed June 16, 2001.

12. Hathcock JN. Vitamins and minerals: efficacy and safety. Am J Clin Nutr 1997;66:427–437. Dr. Hathcock is a former FDA scientist who now directs research for the Council for Responsible Nutrition. For different views, see: Kava R. Vitamins and Minerals: Does the Evidence Justify Supplements? New York: American Council on Science and Health, 1995. Mertz W. A balanced approach to nutrition for health: the need for biologically essential minerals and vitamins. J Am Diet Assoc 1994;94:1259–1262.

13. The Alpha-Tocopherol, Beta Carotene Cancer Prevention Study Group. The effect of vitamin E and beta carotene on the incidence of lung cancer and other cancers in male smokers. N Engl J Med 1994;330:1029–1035. Omenn G, Goodman GE, Thornquist MD, et al. Effects of a combination of beta carotene and vitamin A on lung cancer and cardiovascular disease. N Engl J Med

1996;334:1150-1155. For industry comments, see: Council for Responsible Nutrition. Vitamin & Mineral Safety: a Summary Review. Washington, DC: CRN, 1997.

14. Gorman C. Vitamin overload? Your One-A-Day is still OK, but swallowing supplements by the megadose may be dangerous. Time November 10, 1997: 84. Brody JE. In vitamin mania, millions take a gamble on health. New York Times October 26, 1997:1,28,29

15. Dickenson A. Optimal Nutrition for Good Health: the Benefits of Nutritional Supplements. Washington, DC: Council for Responsible Nutrition, 1998.

16. Bendich A, Mallick R, Leader S. Potential health economic benefits of vitamin supplementation. Western J Medicine 1997;166:306–312. Dr. Bendich is a scientist at Roche Vitamins; the other authors work for Pracon. The study was funded by Hoffman-LaRoche, Inc.

17. USDA and DHHS. Dietary Guidelines for Americans, 5th ed. Washington, DC, 2000. The 4th edition appeared in 1995.

18. Liebman B. 3 vitamins and a mineral: what to take. Nutrition Action Healthletter 1998;25(4)1,3–7. CSPI's bottom line: take a one-a-day with folic acid, vitamin D, vitamin B12 (if over age 50), calcium, and, maybe, vitamin E. Also see: Position of the American Dietetic Association: vitamin and mineral supplementation. J Am Diet Assoc 1996;96:73–77.

19. Physicians' Desk Reference for Herbal Medicines. Montvale, NJ: Medical Economics Company, 1998. Ernst E. Harmless herbs? A review of the recent literature. Am J Medicine 1998;104:170–178.

20. Wilt TUJ, Ishani A, Start G, et al. Saw palmetto extracts for treatment of benign prostatic hyperplasia: a systematic review. JAMA 1999;280:1604–1609. Abourjaily P. Feverfew: a practical review. Nutrition in Clinical Care 1999; 2:(2):87–94. The authors of these studies report no commercial interests in these supplements.

21. Le Bars P, Katz MM, Berman N, Itil TM, et al. A placebo-controlled, double-blind, randomized trial of an extract of ginkgo biloba for dementia. JAMA 1997;278:1327-1332. The study was supported by Dr. William Schwabe Pharmaceuticals, a European manufacturer of ginkgo extracts; it reported modest improvements in some—but not all—outcome measures. In contrast, see: van Dongen MCJM, van Rossum E, Kessels AGH, et al. The efficacy of ginkgo for elderly people with dementia and age-associated memory impairment: new results of a randomized clinical trial. J Am Geriatrics Society 2000;48:1183–1194. This independent study concludes that ginkgo is ineffective.

22. Herbal Rx: the promises and pitfalls. Consumer Reports March 1999: 44–48. ConsumerLab. Latest results. Online: **http://www.consumerlab.com/**. Accessed June 16, 2001. Hemphill C. Putting dietary supplements to the test. New York Times June 20, 2000:F7.

23. Kassel MA. From a history of near misses: the future of dietary supplement regulation. Food and Drug Law J 1994;49:237–269. Also see: Camire ME, Kantor MA. Dietary supplements: nutritional and legal considerations. Food Technology 1999;53(7):87–96.

24. FDA. FDA public health advisory: reports of valvular heart disease in patients receiving concomitant fenfluramine and phentermine, July 8, 1997. FDA Medical Bulletin, Summer 1997.

25. Gower T. Weight loss the herbal way: no all-natural silver bullet. New York Times June 13, 1999:WH13. I paid $14.99 for 60 ephedra capsules in January 2001.

26. FDA. Dietary supplements containing ephedrine alkaloids; withdrawal in part. Federal Register 64:17474–17477, April 3, 2000.

27. FDA. Dietary supplements containing ephedrine alkaloids: proposed rule. Federal Register 62:30678–30724, July 4, 1997.

28. House science panel scrutinizes FDA's ephedrine proposal. Food Regulation Weekly March 23, 1998:8.

29. General Accounting Office. Dietary supplements: uncertainties in analyses underlying FDA's proposed rule on ephedrine alkaloids (GAO/HEHS/GGD-99-90). Washington, DC, July 1999. Office of Inspector General. Adverse Event Report System for Dietary Supplements: An Inadequate Safety Valve. Washington, DC: DHHS, April 2001. Online: http://www.hhs.gov/oig/oei. Accessed June 16, 2001.

30. Howe K. FDA stops tracking herbal remedies. San Francisco Chronicle February 14, 2000:A1,A8.

31. FDA. Dietary supplements containing ephedrine alkaloids; availability. Federal Register 64:17510–17512, April 3, 2000.

32. CRN provides expert testimony at ephedra/ephedrine hearings. CRN News, March 2000. Also see: FDA AERs show ephedra is safe when used correctly: CRN. Food Regulation Weekly April 3, 2000:13–14. AERs are adverse events reports.

33. Pearson, Shaw question use of AERs in new ephedra proposals. Food Regulation Weekly June 5, 2000:6–7.

34. Haller CA, Benewitz NL. Adverse cardiovascular and central nervous system events associated with dietary supplements containing ephedra alkaloids. N Engl J Med 2000;343:1833–1838.

35. Burton D. Dietary supplement health and education act: is the FDA trying to change the intent of Congress? Opening statement. House Committee on Government Reform. March 25, 1999. Online: http://www.house.gov/reform/hearings/. Accessed April 9, 1999.

36. Vermeersch JA, Swenerton H. Consumer responses to nutrition claims in food advertisements. J Nutrition Education 1979;11(1):22–26.

37. Hickman BW, Gates GE, Dowdy RP. Nutrition claims in advertising: a study of four women's magazines. J Nutrition Education 1993;25:227–235.

38. Levy AS, Stokes RC. Effects of a health promotion advertising campaign on sales of ready-to-eat cereals. Public Health Reports 1987;102:398–403.

39. Levy AS, Derby BM, Roe BE. Consumer impacts of health claims: an experimental study. Washington, DC: Food and Drug Administration, January 1997. Online: http://vm.cfsan.fda.gov/. Accessed May 29, 1999.

40. Teisl MF, Levy AS, Derby BM. The effects of education and information source on consumer awareness of diet–disease relationships. J Public Policy and Marketing 1999;18:197–207.

41. Ippolito PM, Mathios AD. Health Claims in Advertising and Labeling: A Study of the Cereal Market. Washington, DC: Federal Trade Commission, August 1989.

42. Mathios AD, Ippolito P. Health claims in food advertising and labeling: disseminating nutrition information to consumers. In: Frazão E. America's Eating Habits: Changes & Consequences. Washington, DC, 1999:189–212.

43. Fullmer S, Geiger CJ, Parent CRM. Consumers' knowledge, understanding, and attitudes toward health claims on food labels. J Am Diet Assoc 1991;91:166–171.

44. Murphy D, Hoppock TH, Rusk MK. Generic copy test of food health claims in advertising. Washington, DC: Federal Trade Commission, November 1998. Online: **http://www.ftc.gov/**. Accessed May 29, 1999. Quotations: Appendix A, Figures 2–4.

45. Levy A, Derby B. Report on dietary supplement labeling focus groups. Washington, DC: FDA, September 30, 1999.

46. Geiger CJ. Health claims: history, current regulatory status, and consumer research. J Am Diet Assoc 1998;98:1312–1322.

47. Ernst E. Harmless herbs? A review of the recent literature. Am J Medicine 1998;104:170–178.

48. Gilhooley M. Testimony. Hearing of the House Committee on Government Reform on Dietary Supplements, March 25, 1999. Online: **http://www.house.gov/reform/hearings/**. Accessed April 9, 1999.

49. Profile. A medical crusader for editorial freedom: fired editor George D. Lundberg makes it a religion to serve the interests of patients. Scientific American 1999;280(5):32–33. Dr. Lundberg says he was accused of "elevating" the scientific credibility of alternative therapies by devoting an entire issue of JAMA to alternative medicine on November 11, 1998.

50. Young JH. American Health Quackery. Princeton, NJ: Princeton University Press, 1992.

PART V. INVENTING TECHNO-FOODS

1. Mr. Drescher used the term *techno-foods* in a program announcement for an Oldways Preservation & Exchange Trust conference in Beverly Hills, California, September 25, 1991.

Some of the material in Part V is adapted from Nestle M. Traditional models of healthy eating: alternatives to "techno-food." J Nutrition Education 1994;26:241–245, and Folate fortification and neural tube defects: policy implications. J Nutrition Education 1994;26:287–293 (reprinted with permission of the Society for Nutrition Education); also, The selling of Olestra. Public Health Reports 1998;113:508–520 (with permission of Oxford University Press).

CHAPTER 13. GO FORTH AND FORTIFY

1. McGinnis JM, Nestle M. The Surgeon General's Report on Nutrition and Health: policy implications and implementation strategies. Am J Clin Nutr 1989;49:23–28.

2. Public Health Service. Promoting Health, Preventing Disease: Objectives for the Nation. Washington, DC, 1980.

3. DHHS. The Surgeon General's Report on Nutrition and Health. Washington, DC, 1988. Quotations: pp. 3, 19.

4. DHHS. Healthy People 2000: National Health Promotion and Disease Prevention Objectives. Washington, DC, 1990.

5. DHHS. Healthy People 2000: Midcourse Review and 1995 Revisions. Washington, DC, 1995. Also see: First major drop in food product introductions in over 20 years. FoodReview 1997;20(3):33–35.

6. Frazão E, Allshouse JE. Size and growth of nutritionally improved foods market. Washington, DC: USDA, 1996.

7. Silverglade B, Jacobson MF, eds. Functional Foods—Public Health Boon or 21st Century Quackery? Washington, DC: Center for Science in the Public Interest, 1999.

8. Markel H. "When it rains it pours": endemic goiter, iodized salt, and David Murray Cowie, MD. Am J Public Health 1987;77:219–229.

9. Sebrell WH. A fiftieth anniversary—cereal enrichment. Nutrition Today January/February, 1992:20–21. Leveille GA. Food fortification—opportunities and pitfalls. Food Technology 1984;38(1):58–63.

10. Lachance PA, Bauernfeind JC. Concepts and practices of nutrifying foods. In: Bauernfeind JC, Lachance PA, eds. Nutrient Additions to Food: Nutritional, Technological and Regulatory Aspects. Trumbull, CT: Food & Nutrition Press, Inc., 1991:19–86. Quotation: p. 49.

11. White House Conference on Food, Nutrition and Health. Final Report. Washington, DC, 1970.

12. FDA. General principles governing the addition of nutrients to foods: notice of proposed rulemaking. Federal Register 39:20900–20904, June 14, 1974.

13. Chemical note: Foods and tissues contain the vitamin in the folate (reduced) form, which is metabolically active but unstable. Supplements provide it as folic acid (oxidized), which is stable and inactive but is readily converted to folate in the body. The terms are often used interchangeably.

14. Lindenbaum J, Rosenberg IH, Wilson PWF, et al. Prevalence of cobalamin deficiency in the Framingham elderly population. Am J Clin Nutr 1994;60:2–11. Tucker KL, Mahnken B, Wilson PWF, et al. Folic acid fortification of the food supply: potential benefits and risks for the elderly population. JAMA 1996; 276:1879–1885.

15. Oakley GP. Let's increase folic acid fortification and include vitamin B-12. Am J Clin Nutr 1997;65:1889–1890. But see: Gaull GE, Testa CA, Thomas PR, Weinreich DA. Fortification of the food supply with folic acid to prevent neural tube defects is not yet warranted. J Nutrition 1996;126:773s–780s.

16. Food Department, Roche Chemical Division. Vitamin nutrition and the American consumer: a position paper for industry. Nutley, NJ: Hoffman-La Roche, Inc., 1978.

17. Bontenbal E. Mineral fortification of food products: adding value to existing products. The World of Ingredients, January/February 1995:12–13. Also see:

Elliott JG. Application of antioxidant vitamins in foods and beverages. Food Technology, 1999;53(2):46–48.

18. Food and Nutrition Board. Recommended Dietary Allowances, 10th ed. Washington, DC: National Academy Press, 1989.

19. Food and Nutrition Board. Dietary Reference Intakes. Washington, DC: National Academy Press, 1997, 1998, 2000, 2001.

20. Bente L, Gerrior S. The U.S. food supply series and dietary guidance. Washington, DC, USDA, 1998:1–2.

21. Carr AC, Frei B. Toward a new Recommended Dietary Allowance for vitamin C based on antioxidant and health effects in humans. Am J Clin Nutr 1999;69:1087–1107.

22. Pennington JAT, Hubbard VS. Derivation of Daily Values used for nutrition labeling. J Am Diet Assoc 1997;97:1407–1412.

23. Collins C. Latest round in orange juice wars. New York Times January 26, 1995:D3.

24. Burros M. At last, a vitamin pill wrapped in a tortilla. New York Times July 7, 1999:F5. Dilbertos, named after the Scott Adams business cartoon character, were designed to be eaten in cars or at desks.

25. Sugarman C. Magic bullets: pumped-up foods promise to make us happier and healthier. We'll see. Washington Post October 21, 1998:E1,E3,E6. Pszczola DE. Nutraceuticals that take the form of candy and snacks. Food Technology 1999;53(10):74–80.

26. Hollingsworth P. Retargeting candy as functional food. Food Technology 1999;53(12):30.

27. Breaking: how cereal maker makes life healthier. Advertising Age September 28, 1998:70. Beatty S, Balu R. Kellogg packs vitamins in cereal and sugar-coats a pitch to parents. Wall Street J February 17, 1999:B8. Full-page advertisements ran in major U.S. newspapers from August through October 1998 and featured one to five cereals in each. See, for example, New York Times August 28:A15, September 27:24, October 6:A15, October 21:A9, October 25:32, and USA Today October 13:7D.

28. Advertisement for Kellogg's FoodService ("breakfast is just the beginning"), J Am Diet Assoc 1999;99:157.

29. Candy D. Is the box half-full or half-empty? Top cereal maker fights to retain eroding share. New York Times November 28, 1998:C1,C15. Also see: Cantor S. Cereals dash for growth. The World of Ingredients, May/June 1999:26–30.

30. Candy D. Kellogg to scale back hometown operations. New York Times June 18, 1999:C18.

31. Thompson S. Kellogg cans K-sentials ads for brand work. Advertising Age November 29, 1999:4.

32. I am indebted to Dr. Jeffrey Backstrand for suggesting the comparison between the health effects of folate and those of iron fortification in an early draft of an unpublished paper, "Optimizing growth and development through food fortification: public health implications."

33. Putnam JJ, Allshouse JE. Food Consumption, Prices, and Expenditures, 1970–1997. Washington, DC: USDA, April 1999.

34. Centers for Disease Control and Prevention. Ten great public health achievements—United States. 1900–1999. JAMA 1999;281:1481.

35. Popkin BM, Siega-Riz AM, Haines PS. The nutritional impact of food fortification in the United States during the 1970s. Family Economics and Nutrition Review 1996;9 (4):20–30. Park YK, Sempos CT, Barton CN, et al. Effectiveness of food fortification in the United States: the case of pellagra. Am J Public Health 2000;90:727–738.

36. Crane NT, Wilson DB, Cook A, et al. Evaluating food fortification options: general principles revisited with folic acid. Am J Public Health 1995;85:660–666.

37. Jacques PF, Selhub J, Bostom AG, et al. The effect of folic acid fortification on plasma folate and total homocysteine concentrations. N Engl J Med 1999;340:1449–1454. Honein MA, Paulozzi LJ, Mathews TJ, et al. Impact of folic acid fortification of the US food supply on the occurrence of neural tube defects. JAMA 2001;285:2981–2986.

38. Looker AC, Dallman PAR, Carroll MD, et al. Prevalence of iron deficiency in the United States. JAMA 1997;277:973–976.

39. Rouault TA. Hereditary hemochromatosis. JAMA 1993;269:3152–3154.

40. Yang Q, McDonnell SM, Khoury MJ, et al. Hemochromatosis-associated mortality in the United States from 1979–1992: an analysis of multiple-cause mortality data. Annals of Internal Medicine 1998;129:946–953. For a different view, see: Gable CB. Hemochromatosis and dietary iron supplementation: implications from U.S. mortality, morbidity, and health survey data. J Am Diet Assoc 1992;92:208–212.

41. Health-related claims can boost food sales, business professor says. Food Regulation Weekly May 1, 2000:11–12.

42. Christopher C. Is fortification unnecessary technology? Food Product Development 1978;12(4):24–25.

43. Mertz W. Food fortification in the United States. Nutrition Reviews 1997;55:44–49.

CHAPTER 14. BEYOND FORTIFICATION: MAKING FOODS FUNCTIONAL

1. Grocery Manufacturers insist health claims for all foods are legal. Food Regulation Weekly April 24, 2000:17.

2. Brody JE. Fortified foods could fight off cancer. New York Times February 19, 1991:C1.

3. Hasler CM. Functional foods: their role in disease prevention and health promotion. Food Technology 1998;52(11):63–70. Hathcock JH. Safety and regulatory issues for phytochemical sources: "designer foods." Nutrition Today November/December 1993:23–25.

4. Storlie J, O'Flaherty MJ, Hare K. Food or supplement? Choosing the appropriate regulatory path. Food Technology 1998;52(12):62–69.

5. General Accounting Office. Food Safety: Improvements Needed in Overseeing the Safety of Dietary Supplements and "Functional Foods." (GAO/RCED-00-156). Washington, DC, July 2000. Also see: Nutrition Business J. Online: **http://www.nutritionbusiness.com/**.

6. Stipp D. Engineering the future of food. Fortune September 28, 1998: 128–144.

7. The new foods: functional or dysfunctional: are 'nutraceuticals' foods, supplements, drugs—or baloney? Consumer Reports on Health 1999;11(6):1–5. Heasman M, Mellentin J. Herbs—hope or hype? The World of Ingredients May/June 1999:48–52. DHHS. Dietary supplements now labeled with more information. HHS News March 23, 1999. Online: **http://vm.cfsan.fda.gov**. Accessed June 3, 1999.

8. FDA hits New York company for adding herbal products to snacks. Food Regulation Weekly February 21, 2000:17.

9. Allied Domecq, Seagram power up extreme drinks. Advertising Age April 17, 2000:1,70.

10. FDA. FDA issues letter to industry on foods containing botanical and other novel ingredients. FDA Talk Paper, February 5, 2001. Online: **http://www.fda.gov/foi/warning.htm/**. Accessed June 18, 2001. Lash S. FDA warns food producers that use supplements. Food Chemical News June 11, 2001:1,25–27.

11. Barnes JE. Coke and Procter & Gamble in joint marketing venture. New York Times February 22, 2001: C4. Also see: McAlindon TE, LaValley MP, Gulin JP, Felson DT. Glucosamine and chondroitin for treatment of osteoarthritis: a systematic quality assessment and meta-analysis. JAMA 2000;283: 1469–1475. Towheed TE, Anastassiades TP. Glucosamine and chondroitin for treating symptoms of osteoarthritis: evidence is widely touted but incomplete (editorial). JAMA 2000;283:1483–1484. Barnes JE, Winter G. Stressed out? Bad knee? Relief promised in a juice. New York Times May 27, 2001: A1,A18.

12. Bloomberg News. Oat foods can tout benefits to heart: cereal, bread firms planning ad push after FDA ruling. San Francisco Examiner January 22, 1997:D2.

13. Pollack J. Ordinary people star in new fall Quaker effort. Advertising Age August 17, 1998:42.

14. Liebman B. Oat bran: part II. Nutrition Action Healthletter July/August 1989:9–11.

15. Swain JF, Rouse IL, Curley CB, Sacks FM. Comparison of the effects of oat bran and low-fiber wheat on serum lipoprotein levels and blood pressure. N Engl J Med 1990;322:147–152.

16. Humble CG. Oats and cholesterol: the prospects for prevention of heart disease. Am J Public Health 1991;81:159–160. Ripsin CM, Keenan JM, Jacobs DR, et al. Oat products and lipid lowering: a meta-analysis. JAMA 1992;267: 3317–3325.

17. Pollack J. Kellogg takes light approach for Ensemble, and Kellogg's new ensemble features an old ingredient. Advertising Age April 19, 1999:3,86, and November 9, 1998:90.

18. Lantner RR, Espiritu BR, Zumerchik P, Tobin MC. Anaphylaxis following ingestion of a psyllium-containing cereal. JAMA 1990;264:2534–2536. Also see: Roy A. Doubts over benefits of a hearty breakfast. The Times (London) January 7, 1990:C9.

19. Burros M. The 'food' police keep busy with health claims. New York Times February 27, 1991:C3.

20. Meier B. Kellogg files slander suit. New York Times April 3, 1991:C4.

21. F.D.A. questions use of grain in 3 cereals. New York Times October 1, 1989:28.

22. Thompson S. Kellogg loses appetite for Ensemble products. Advertising Age November 8, 1999:1,125.

23. FDA. Food labeling: health claims; soy protein and coronary heart disease: proposed rule. Federal Register 63:62977–63015, November 19, 1998.

24. Messina M, Erdman JW, eds. The role of soy in preventing and treating chronic disease. Am J Clin Nutr 1998;68(Suppl):1329s–1544s.

25. van Raaij JMA, Katan MB, Hautvast JGA, Hermus RJJ. Effects of casein versus soy protein diets on serum cholesterol and lipoproteins in young healthy volunteeers. Am J Clin Nutr 1981;34:1261–1271. Erdman JW, Fordyce E. Soy products and the human diet. Am J Clin Nutr 1989;49:725–737.

26. Angier N. Health benefits from soy protein: study finds potent weapon in lowering cholesterol. New York Times August 3, 1995:A1,A22. Anderson JW, Johnstone BM, Cook-Newell ME. Meta-analysis of the effects of soy protein intake on serum lipids. N Engl J Med 1995;333:276-282.

27. Leibman B. The soy story. Nutrition Action Healthletter September 1998: 1–7.

28. Nilausen K, Meinertz H. Lipoprotein(a) and dietary proteins: casein lowers lipoprotein(a) concentrations as compared with soy protein. Am J Clin Nutr 1999;69:419–425. McMichael-Phillips DF, Harding C, Morton M, et al. Effects of soy-protein supplementation on epithelial proliferation in the histologically normal human breast. Am J Clin Nutr 1998;68:1431s–1436s.

29. Kilman S. Food firms to tout health benefits of soybeans. Wall Street J October 26, 1999:B10.

30. Thompson S. Bestfoods packs $20 mil behind NutraBlend launch. Advertising Age June 26, 2000:30.

31. Pollack J. J&J readies U.S. intro of Benecol nutraceutical. Advertising Age September 28, 1998:67.

32. Sharpe R. J&J's cholesterol-lowering spread to be sold as food, not supplement. Wall Street J January 27, 1999:B8. F.D.A. may block margarine aimed at lowering cholesterol. New York Times November 8, 1998:27.

33. Hicks KB, Moreau RA. Phytosterols and phytostanols: functional food cholesterol busters. Food Technology 2001;55:63–67.

34. Johnson & Johnson provides more data on Benecol product. Wall Street J November 6, 1998:B6.

35. Hendriks HFJ, Weststrate JA, Meijer GW. Spreads enriched with three different levels of vegetable oil sterols and the degree of cholesterol lowering in normocholesterolaemic and mildly hypercholesterolaemic subjects. European J Clinical Nutrition 1998;53:319–332 (a second paper follows at 334–343). The investigators work for Unilever, parent company of Take Control margarine.

36. Sharpe R. FDA clears Unilever unit's margarine substitute. Wall Street J May 3, 1999:B4.

37. Rumbelow H. Food that cuts cholesterol has a fat price. The Times (London) March 30, 1999:8.

38. Kuczynski A. Media talk: commercial puts reporter in tight spot. New York Times June 14, 1999:C14.

39. O'Connell V. New pitches set for anticholesterol foods. Wall Street J December 11, 1998:B8. The Benecol Web site is http://www.benecol.com/. Take Control site is at www.takecontrol.com. Both were accessed July 9, 1999.

40. Hollingsworth P. Margarine: the over-the-top functional food. Food Technology 2001;55:59–62.

41. Thompson S. Dysfunctional foods: McNeil, Unilever lines thin out. Advertising Age July 24, 2000:1,52. Winslow R. Johnson & Johnson changes sales focus to doctors for anticholesterol spread. Wall Street J December 2, 1999:B20. Taste test: cholesterol cutters. Consumer Reports September 1999:9.

42. Silverglade B, Jacobson MF, eds. Functional Foods—Public Health Boon or 21st Century Quackery? Washington, DC: Center for Science in the Public Interest, 1999.

43. Clinton, SK. Lycopene: chemistry, biology, and implications for health and disease. Nutrition Reviews 1998;56:35–51.

44. Health-related claims can boost food sales, business professor says. Food Regulation Weekly May 1, 2000:11–12.

CHAPTER 15. SELLING THE ULTIMATE TECHNO-FOOD: OLESTRA

1. FDA. Food additives permitted for direct addition to food for human consumption: Olestra; final rule. Federal Register 61:3118–3166, January 30, 1996.

2. Lawson KD, Middleton SJ, Hassall CD. Olestra, a nonabsorbed noncaloric replacement for dietary fat: a review. Drug Metabolism Review 1997;29:651–703.

3. General Accounting Office. FDA Premarket Approval: Process of Approving Olestra as a Food Additive (GAO/HRD-92-86). Washington, DC, 1992.

4. Procter & Gamble. Conference materials. Reshaping the modern diet: the fat reduction challenge. New Orleans, LA: January 18, 1989.

5. Food and Drug Administration. FDA approves fat substitute, olestra (press release). HHS News January 24, 1996.

6. Center for Science in the Public Interest. White Paper on Olestra. Washington, DC: CSPI, December 25, 1995.

7. Suttie JW, Ross AC, eds. Assessment of the nutritional effects of olestra. J Nutrition 1997;127(8s):1539s–1728s. Sandler RS, Zorich NL, Filloon TG, et al. Gastrointestinal symptoms in 3181 volunteers ingesting snack foods containing olestra or triglycerides: a 6-week randomized, placebo-controlled trial. Annals of Internal Medicine 1999;130:253–261. The lead author and one other are identified as consultants to P&G.

8. Blackburn H. Olestra and the FDA. N Engl J Med 1996;334:984–986.

9. De Graaf C, Hulshof T, Weststrate JA, Hautvast JGA. Nonabsorbable fat (sucrose polyester) and the regulation of energy intake and body weight. Am J Physiology 1996;270:R1386–R1393. Weststrate JA, van het Hof KH. Sucrose polyester and plasma carotenoid concentrations in healthy subjects. Am J Clin Nutr 1995;62:591–597. The investigators work for Unilever, which sponsored the research. Members of this team also worked on TakeControl margarine.

10. Krinsky NI, Sies H, eds. Antioxidant vitamins and **beta**-carotene in disease prevention. Am J Clin Nutr 1995;62(6 suppl):1299s–1540s. Kelly SM, Shorthouse M, Cotterell JC, et al. A 3-month, double-blind controlled trial of feeding with sucrose polyester in human volunteers. British J Nutrition 1998;80:41–49. Geusau A, Tschachler E, Meixner M, et al. Olestra increases faecal excretion of 2,3,7,8-tetrachlorodibenzo-p-dioxin. Lancet 1999;354:1266–1277.

11. Lemonick MD. Are we ready for fat-free fat? Time January 8, 1996: 53–61.

12. Lawrence J. How P&G's hopes for food division's future got mired in FDA quicksand. Advertising Age May 2, 1994:16–17.

13. House of Representatives Committee on the Judiciary. Patent term extensions: report together with dissenting views to accompany H.R. 5475. Washington, DC, August 3, 1992:1–18.

14. U.S. Senate Committee on the Judiciary. Patent extension hearing. 102nd Congress, First Session. Senate Hearing 102-824, August 1, 1991. Washington, DC, 1992. Quotations: 277, 458–459.

15. Stern G. Six groups oppose P&G bid to extend patent on olestra. Wall Street J January 3, 1992:B3. The groups were Center for Science in the Public Interest, Consumer Federation of America, Consumers Guild, Government Accountability Project, National Consumers League, and Public Voice for Food and Health Policy.

16. House of Representatives, Committee on the Judiciary. Patent term extensions. Report together with dissenting views (to accompany H.R. 5475), August 3, 1992. U.S. Senate Committee on the Judiciary. Private patent extensions. Report 102-414, September 22, 1992:1–15.

17. House of Representatives Committee on the Judiciary. Hearing before the Subcommittee on Intellectual Property and Judicial Administration on H.R. 3379: interim patent extensions. 103rd Congress, First Session, October 29, 1993. The law was the Patent and Trademark Office Authorization Act of 1993 (Public Law 103-179), December 3, 1993.

18. FDA. Determination of regulatory review period for purposes of patent extension; Olean. Federal Register 62:763–764, January 6, 1997.

19. Pollack J, Sloan P. P&G enlists political savvy to sell Olean. Advertising Age September 30, 1996:4. Narisetti R. Anatomy of a food fight: the olestra debate. Wall Street J July 31, 1996:B1. Collins G. Crunch time for a fake fat: will America take the bait? New York Times August 24, 1997:F1,F12,F13.

20. Candey D. Fat-free fanfare as Procter starts shipping out olestra. New York Times February 11, 1998:D2. Parker-Pope T. P&G dresses up olestra in farm images. Wall Street J February 11, 1998:B6.

21. Narisetti R. P&G is ready to fight back for olestra. Wall Street J September 23, 1996:B8, and November 29, 1996:B4.

22. Deogun N. Fat-free snacks aren't wowing Frito customers. Wall Street J September 14, 1998:B1.

23. Candey D. Low fat's lowered expectations: Procter & Gamble overestimates America's olestra craving. New York Times July 21, 1999:C1,C25.

24. Mandatory olestra warnings should be dropped: Frito-Lay. Food Regulation Weekly January 3, 2000:15–16, and March 6, 2000:22–23.

25. Cracker with disputed additive is tested. New York Times August 26, 2000:B2.

26. McHugh SL. Off target on Olean (letter). Advertising Age October 4, 1999:34. Mr. McHugh is identified as senior manager for public relations at P&G.

27. Edgers G. Fat chance. Boston Phoenix July 12, 1996:20–22. Silverstein K. Procter & Gamble's academic "white hats." Multinational Monitor November, 1997:13.

28. Horowitz B. Fake fat's big test: olestra. USA Today June 19, 1997:1B,2B. Kleiner K. Fake fat leak fuels funding fury. New Scientist 1997;156:15.

29. Middleton SJ. Procter & Gamble responds on olestra (letter). Public Health Reports 1999;114:5–6 (my article was at 1998;113:508–520). Dr. Middleton is senior nutrition scientist at P&G. The company does not include my article or other studies finding problems with olestra among the bibliographies it routinely mails to health professionals.

30. Bachrach J. The President's private eye. Vanity Fair September 1998: 192–216. Silverstein K. Corporate enemies, corporate friends: did food industry "put out the money" for attacks on nutritionists? Extra! May/June 1997:24–25. Levine D. Attack of the food police. Reader's Digest 1997; March:69–73.

31. Patterson RE, Kristal AR, Peters JC, et al. Changes in diet, weight, and serum lipid levels associated with olestra consumption. Archives of Internal Medicine 2000;160:2600–2604.

32. Newmark-Sztainer D, Kristal AR, Thornquist MD, et al. Early adopters of olestra-containing foods: who are they? J Am Diet Assoc 2000;100:198–204, and 2000;100:576–579.

33. Putnam JJ, Allshouse JE. Food consumption, prices, and expenditures, 1970–1997. Washington, DC: USDA, 1999. The USDA depends on industry to supply data on production of food commodities, but the artificial-sweetener industry refuses to provide this information. Until 1991, the USDA estimated production from use in diet soft drinks, but it could no longer do so after the use of artificial sweeteners extended to many other products.

34. Hampl JS, Sheeley AE, Schnepf MI. Sounding the alarm for misuse of olestra-containing foods in binge-eating disorders (letter). J Am Diet Assoc 1998;98:971.

35. Silverglade B, Jacobson MF, eds. Functional Foods—Public Health Boon or 21st Century Quackery? Washington, DC: Center for Science in the Public Interest, 1999.

36. Brophy B, Schardt D. Functional foods. Nutrition Action Healthletter, 1999;26 (April):1,3-7.

37. Gussow J. A chicken little in our future? (interview). Nutrition Action Healthletter 1991;18(1):5-7.

CONCLUSION: THE POLITICS OF FOOD CHOICE

1. Parts of this chapter draw on material previously published as: Nestle M. Ethical dilemmas in choosing a healthful diet: Vote with your fork! Proceedings of the Nutrition Society (UK) 2000;59:619-629 (with permission), and Nestle M. Jacobson MF. Halting the Obesity Epidemic: A Public Health Policy Approach. Public Health Reports 2000;115:12-24 (courtesy of Michael Jacobson and Oxford University Press).

2. Applebaum RS. Commentary. Food Policy 1999;24:265-267.

3. Anderson D. Americans get fatter, but refuse to die. How naughty. Wall Street J June 8, 2000:A24.

4. Bernstein MF. A big fat target. Wall Street J August 28, 1997:A14.

5. Kluger R. Ashes to Ashes: America's Hundred-Year Cigarette War, the Public Health, and the Unabashed Triumph of Philip Morris. New York: Alfred A. Knopf, 1996. Advocacy Institute. Smoke & Mirrors: How the Tobacco Industry Buys & Lies Its Way to Power & Profits. Washington, DC: Advocacy Institute, 1998. Glantz SA Balbach ED. Tobacco War: Inside the California Battles. Berkeley: University of California Press, 2000.

6. A manipulated dichotomy in global health policy (editorial). Lancet 2000;355:1023.

7. McGinnis JM, Foege WH. Actual causes of death in the United States. JAMA 1993;270:2207-2212. Gallo AE. Fewer food products introduced in last 3 years. FoodReview 1999;22(3):27-29.

8. Malm HM. Ethical considerations in dietary recommendations. American Society of Preventive Oncology, 14th annual meeting, Washington, DC, March 6, 2000.

9. Clancy KL. Ethical issues in food processing and marketing, or a nutritionist talks about "moral fiber." Agriculture, Change and Human Values, Proceedings of a Multidisciplinary Conference. Gainesville, FL: University of Florida, October 18-21, 1982. Gussow JD & Clancy K. Dietary guidelines for sustainability. J Nutrition Education 1986;18:1-5.

10. Gussow JD. Can industry afford a healthy America? CNI Weekly Report June 7, 1979:4-7.

11. O'Brien P. Dietary shifts and implications for US agriculture. Am J Clin Nutr 1995;61(suppl):1390s–1396s. Young CE, Kantor LS. Moving Toward the Food Guide Pyramid: Implications for U.S. Agriculture. Washington, DC: USDA, 1999.

12. Kennedy E, Offutt S. Commentary: alternative nutrition outcomes using a fiscal food policy. British Medical J 2000;320:304–305.

13. Ralston K. How government policies and regulations can affect dietary choices. In: Frazão E, ed., America's Eating Habits: Changes & Consequences. Washington, DC: USDA, 1999:331–370.

14. Reger B, Wootan MG, Booth-Butterfield S, Smith H. Using mass media to promote healthy eating: a community-based demonstration project. Preventive Medicine 1999;29:414–421.

15. Blaylock J, Smallwood D, Kassel K, et al. Economics, food choices, and nutrition. Food Policy 1999;24:269–286.

16. Jacobson MF, Brownell KD. Small taxes on soft drinks and snack foods to promote health. Am J Public Health 2000;90:854–857.

17. French SA, Story M, Jeffery RW. Environmental influences on eating and physical activity. Annual Review of Public Health 2001;22:309–335. Huang KS. Prices and incomes affect nutrients consumed. FoodReview May–August 1998: 11–15. Marshall T. Exploring a fiscal food policy: the case of diet and ischaemic heart disease. British Medical J 2000;320:301–304.

18. Piller C. No surprise: new economy faces old problem of poverty. Los Angeles Times May 31, 1999:C3.

19. Gould SJ. The lying stones of Würzburg and Marrakech. Natural History 1998;107(3):90.

20. Rotblat J. A Hippocratic oath for scientists (editorial). Science 1999; 286:1475.

21. McEachern L. The Angelica Home Kitchen. New York: Roundtable Inc., 2000:19.

22. Norwich W. Salad days. New York Times Magazine August 13, 2000: 52–56.

23. Ritzer G. The McDonaldization of Society: An Investigation Into the Changing Character of Contemporary Social Life, rev. ed. Thousand Oaks, CA: Pine Forge Press, 1996.

24. Jacobson MF, Mazur LA. Marketing Madness: A Survival Guide for a Consumer Society. Boulder CO: Westview Press, 1995.

25. Slow Food U.S.A. Taste and culture (leaflet). New York, 2000 (online: **http://www.slowfood.com**).

APPENDIX: ISSUES IN NUTRITION AND NUTRITION RESEARCH

1. This Appendix was adapted in part from Nestle M. Nutrition in public health and preventive medicine. In: Wallace RB, ed. Maxcy-Rosenau-Last Public Health & Preventive Medicine, 14th ed. Norwalk, CN: Appleton & Lange, 1998:1081–1089 (with permission of The McGraw-Hill Companies).

2. Any nutrition textbook is a good source of basic information, but the "Bible" is Shils ME, Olson JA, Shike M, Ross AC, eds. Modern Nutrition in Heath and Disease, 9th ed. Philadelphia, PA: Lippincott Williams & Wilkins, 1999.

3. Food and Nutrition Board. Dietary Reference Intakes. Washington, DC: National Academy Press, 1997, 1998, 2000, 2001. Online: **http://www.iom.edu.**

4. Maxwell S, Frankenberger TR. Household Food Security: Concepts, Indicators, Measurements: A Technical Review. New York and Rome: United Nations Children's Fund and International Fund for Agricultural Development, 1992.

5. Popkin BM. The nutrition transition and its health implications in lower-income countries. Public Health Nutrition 1998;1(1):5–21.

6. DHHS. Healthy People 2010, Vol 1. Washington, DC, 2000.

7. Willett W. Nutritional Epidemiology, 2nd ed. New York: Oxford University Press, 1998.

8. Pauling L. Vitamin C and the Common Cold. San Francisco: WH Freeman, 1970.

9. Karlowski TR, Chalmers TC, Frenkel LD, et al. Ascorbic acid for the common cold: a prophylactic and therapeutic trial. JAMA 1975;231:1038–1042.

10. Hrobjartsson A, Gotzsche PC. Is the placebo powerless?—An analysis of clinical tri als comparing placebo with no treatment. N Engl J Med 2001; 344:1594–1602.

11. Lee RD, Nieman DC. Nutritional Assessment, 2nd ed. St. Louis, MO: Mosby, 1996. Also see: Basiotis PP, Lino M, Dinkins JM. Consumption of food group servings: people's perceptions vs. reality. Nutrition Insights 20, October 2000. Online: **http://www.usda.gov/cnpp.**

12. Putman JJ, Allshouse JE. Food Consumption, Prices, and Expenditures, 1970–1997. Washington, DC: USDA, 1999.

13. Harnack LJ, Jeffrey RW, Boutelle KN. Temporal trends in energy intake in the United States: an ecologic perspective. Am J Clin Nutr 2000;71:1478–1484.

14. General Accounting Office. Food nutrition: better guidance needed to improve reliability of USDA's food composition data (GAO/RCED-94-30). Washington, DC, October 1993.

LIST OF TABLES

439

LIST OF FIGURES

INDEX

Note: Page numbers with the letter *t* indicate pages with tables and page numbers with the letter *f* indicate pages with figures.

Abbott Laboratories, 167
Added value, 17–19, 18f
Additives, feed additives, 168
Advertising, 21–23
  and check-off programs, 142–145, 144f
  to children, 22–23, 161, 174, 176,
    178–188, 370
    criticism of, 179–180
    Internet, 183
    McDonald's, 178, 181, 184f, 185
    methods of, 178, 183, 184f, 185,
      186f, 187–188, 187t
    in schools, 188–191
    soft drinks, 185, 186f, 200–202
    television advertising, 180–183
  and dietary change, 369
  expenditures, 12t, 21–22, 23f, 179
  health claims in, 315–316
    for dietary supplements, 236
    for functional foods, 322–323, 327,
      328, 329, 331, 332–333, 334,
      335f, 336
    impact on consumers, 287–291
    for infant formula, 147–148, 148f,
      154 166–167
    milk campaign, 80–81, 82f
  of philanthropic programs, 22, 24
  regulatory authority over, 227, 228t,
    229
  See also Kellogg; Marketing
Advertising Age, 333
Advertising Guide for Industry, 229
Agricultural committees, congressional
  as agricultural establishment, 97
  expanded functions of, 98
  farm state members on, 97–98

  and lobbyist-sponsored trips, 106
  and PAC contributions, 103–104
Agricultural subsidies, 19
Agriculture Department. *See* U.S.
    Department of Agriculture (USDA)
AIDS crisis, and infant formula marketing,
  156–158
Alar scare, 162
Alcoholic beverages
  diseases associated with, 380
  guidelines on, 71, 84–85, 90–91, 364t
  herbal supplemented, 321
  industry health claims for, 85–91
Allergies, 326
Alliances, corporate-professional, 125–126
Alzheimer's disease, 306
American Academy of Pediatrics (AAP),
  154, 166, 183
American Cancer Society, 113t
American College of Nutrition, 113t
American Council on Science and Health,
  113t, 122–123, 129
American Dietetic Association, 46, 57
  ethics code of, 129
  food industry ties, 12t, 113, 113t, 115,
    116, 126–129, 127f, 128t, 310
  and olestra, 352
  nutrition fact sheets, 127, 128t, 129
  PAC contributions of, 103, 105t
  Web site of, 129–130
American Egg Board, 132
American Heart Association (AHA), 39,
  43, 48, 100, 113t
  HeartCheck program of, 123–125, 125f,
    317t
American Herbal Products Association,
  101
American Journal of Clinical Nutrition,
  113, 114–115, 351
American Journal of Public Health, 308

Journal of the American Dietetic Association, 133, 144, 310, 323, 332
Journal of the American Medical Association, 114, 293
Journal of Nutrition, 112, 114, 133, 351
Journal of Nutrition Education, 112
Jungle, The (Sinclair), 163, 233

Kava kava, 320
Kellogg, 12*t*
  All-Bran campaign, 239–245, 241*f*, 286
  health claims of, 128–129, 240–242, 245, 247, 257*t*, 286–289, 309, 310, 316*t*, 341
  functional food products, 322, 325–328, 326*f*
  HeartCheck program, 124–125
  K-sentials campaign, 308–310
  marketing to children, 189*t*, 190
  Psyllium cereals, 325, 326*f*, 327
  ties to NCI, 240
  vitamin lawsuit, 169
Kennedy, Edward M., 149–152
Kessler, David, 249, 258, 345
Ketchup, as functional food, 334, 335*f*, 336
Keys, Ancel and Margaret, 39
Kohlberg Kravis Roberts, 14*t*
Koop, C. Everett, 122
Kraft Foods, 14*t*, 64, 102, 105*t*, 113*t*, 129, 169, 189*t*, 329

Labeling
  for dietary supplements, 223, 229–230, 239, 275
  for foods, 123–124, 129, 239–242, 240–242, 249–252, 255–258, 257*t*, 264, 341
    techno-foods, 315, 317, 319–320, 325
  nutrient standards, of FDA, 307
  and Nutrition Labeling and Education Act of 1990, 235*t*, 245, 250, 255, 256, 306
  regulatory authority over, 129, 227, 228*t*, 229, 235*t*, 251
  for wine, 89–90.
  See also Health claims
Lactose intolerance, 73, 79, 81
Lancet, The, 133
Lawsuits, 159–160
  Chiquita Brands-*Cincinnati Enquirer* case, 165–166
  dietary supplement regulation cases, 257*t*, 265–267, 275–276
  food disparagement cases, 162–165
  and food label health claims, 257*t*
  McDonald's libel case, 160–162
  price fixing cases, 166–170
  school meal program cases, 212–213
  and veggie-libel laws, 162–163
Leahy, Patrick, 210–211
Lee, Philip, 88
"Lesser-evil" foods, 296, 333
Leveille, Gilbert, 305
Levenstein, Harvey, 27
Lewinsky, Monica, 109–110
Lewis, Stephen, 155
Lindner, Carl H., 107, 108
Lipton, 257, 331
Liver cirrhosis, 380, 381*t*
Lobbying
  campaign contributions
    hard money, 102–105, 105*t*
    soft money, 105–106, 107
  and check-off programs, 142–145
  defined, 95, 96
  and dietary guidelines, 3–4
    for alcohol consumption, 85–92
    Dietary Goals, 40–42, 77
    for fat intake, 77–81
    Food Guide Pyramid, 51–53, 57–58, 60*f*
    for salt intake, 83–84
    for sugar intake, 81, 83
  by dietary supplement industry, 242–244, 258–262, 260*f*, 291–292
  and food-labeling rules, 251
  gift-giving, 106, 138–142
  influence on government decisions, 107–110
  number of lobbyists/groups, 99
  for olestra patent extension, 345–347
  pros and cons of, 95–96, 170–171
  regulation of, 96–97, 102, 106, 107, 138–139
  and regulatory agencies, 48, 138–142
  and revolving door job exchanges, 99–102
  social transaction expenditures in, 102
  travel sponsorship in, 106–107
London Greenpeace, 160–161
Low-fat foods, 333–334, 355
Low-sodium foods, 299
Lovastatin, 266
Lugar, Richard, PAC contributions to, 103, 104, 105*t*
Lycopene, 334, 335*f*
Lyman, Howard, 163–164
Lysine, 168

M & M candy, 183. *See* Mars
McDonaldization of Society, The (Ritzer), 374

Designer:	Nola Burger
Compositor:	Michael Bass & Associates
Text:	10/13 Sabon
Display:	Deepdene No. 315 and Futura
Printer:	Edwards Brothers, Inc.
Binder:	Edwards Brothers, Inc.